Williams-Beuren Syndrome

Williams-Beuren Syndrome
Research, Evaluation, and Treatment

EDITED BY

Colleen A. Morris, M.D.

Professor, Department of Pediatrics,
University of Nevada School of Medicine, Las Vegas, Nevada

Howard M. Lenhoff, Ph.D.

Professor Emeritus, Department of Developmental and Cell Biology,
University of California, Irvine, California
and Adjunct Professor, Department of Biology,
University of Mississippi, Oxford, Mississippi

Paul P. Wang, M.D.

Director, Pfizer Global Research and Development,
New London, Connecticut

The
Johns Hopkins University Press
BALTIMORE

The Johns Hopkins University Press
2715 North Charles Street
Baltimore, Maryland 21218-4363
www.press.jhu.edu

Library of Congress Cataloging-in-Publication Data

Williams-Beuren syndrome : research, evaluation,
and treatment / edited by Colleen A. Morris,
Howard M. Lenhoff, and Paul P. Wang.
p. ; cm.
Includes bibliographical references and index.
ISBN 0-8018-8212-5 (hardcover : alk. paper)
1. Williams syndrome.
[DNLM: 1. Williams Syndrome—physiopathology.
2. Cognition.   3. Williams Syndrome—genetics.
4. Williams Syndrome—therapy. QS 677 W689 2006]
I. Morris, Colleen A.   II. Lenhoff, Howard M.
III. Wang, Paul P.
RJ506.W44W554 2006
618.92′0042—dc22   200506473

A catalog record for this book
is available from the British Library.

Contents

Foreword

In the past two decades, we have witnessed remarkable advances in our understanding of the molecular and genetic basis of a multitude of human diseases, common and rare. This notable expansion of knowledge is, in fact, not a revolution in the Kuhnian sense of the word but rather a proof of principle of the molecular genetics paradigm that arose in the second half of the twentieth century. The public and the media are well attuned to these advances in genetic analysis and recognize, often through the public announcements of investigators, that the ultimate promise of genomic knowledge includes improved therapeutics of the diseases at hand. Rarely, though, does the media attention—or even the pages of high-impact scientific publications—focus on simultaneous advances in *phenotype analysis*. Sure, the term *phenomics* is tossed around on occasion and, periodically, even the most prestigious of molecular genetics journals publish commentaries (or letters) giving some copy (some lip service) to the importance of documenting phenotype analysis. But the M.D./Ph.D. student and the junior professor in the academic setting hear that the "future of the field" seems to be in the discovery of genes and how they work in the cell. Ironically, without comprehensive knowledge of phenotype, how will we know "how they work"? Without detailed phenotypic information, how will genotype-phenotype correlations and the translation of knowledge from the laboratory bench to the clinic room occur?

Well, Colleen Morris and her colleagues have risen to the challenge of providing meticulous documentation of phenotype in this monograph, wisely published by the Johns Hopkins University Press. On first glance, one may say that Williams-Beuren syndrome is a "rare" disease and of little significance. This disorder occurs in about 1 in 10,000 to 20,000 children. Yet, all of us in medicine, especially in pediatrics and genetics, know that the challenges in the care of individuals with rare conditions are daunting and no less important than the common problems of the clinic. The work published here represents an important contribution to the molecular genetics paradigm: the establishment of the definition and delineation of a syndrome that is needed in genotype-phenotype investigations. The *definition* of a condition is the cause or molecular basis of the condition, and *delineation* is the pathogenesis, natural history, and variable expressivity of clinical presentation of the syndrome. The authors have addressed all these themes in this book.

Not only have Morris and colleagues illustrated phenotype with the needed precision, but they have particularly focused on the behavioral aspects of phenotype—that is, the *behavioral phenotype*. This now widely used term refers to the cognitive, behavioral, personality, and affective components of a human syndrome. All of those who are interested in delineating and analyzing phenotype, especially behavioral phenotypes, should take heed of this work. It lays out a template for future investigation on related and similar conditions. It dissects and analyzes the components and manifestations of the clinical aspects of Williams-Beuren syndrome. We see discussions of the abnormalities of organ systems, such as the heart; we can review the guidelines for routine health supervision in the care of patients, and here, for a condition most widely known in pediatrics, we learn of the adult side of Williams-Beuren syndrome. But it is the illustration, in needed detail, of behavioral phenotype that is the centerpiece of this book. The authors have provided a model with which we can approach the analysis and documentation of the various components of behavioral phenotype in other syndromes.

I am excited about the availability of this book to the medical, psychology, and genetics communities, as well as to teachers, individuals, and families. Notably, Morris and her colleagues developed a partnership with the Williams Syndrome Association and Williams Syndrome Foundation, which embraced much of the research that led to published work and to this book. Other investigators interested in phenomics in genotype-phenotype analysis can use this book as a framework and guideline for phenotypic analysis. It will be the standard for future excellence in this arena. I look forward to future editions of this monograph and to seeing the model presented here applied with the same precision to other syndromes.

John C. Carey, M.D.

Preface

A quick perusal of the history of research on Williams-Beuren syndrome (WBS) shows that, although the syndrome was first described in the early 1960s (Williams et al. 1961; Beuren et al. 1962), the condition was not widely recognized by physicians and received little attention from research scientists until about twenty years later. During the past two decades, however, interest in WBS has grown at an exponential rate. Of primary importance in generating this attention during the earlier of those years was parental activism. More and more parents found that their children with WBS had similar physical features and atypical behaviors that seemed surprising when contrasted with some of their abilities in language and their generally warm and empathetic personalities.

Parental support organizations began to spring up in several countries. The Infantile Hypercalcaemia Association (IHA) in England was the first, and it was instrumental in bringing WBS to the attention of the medical and research communities. In the 1980s in the United States, the Williams Syndrome Association (WSA) and the Williams Syndrome Foundation (WSF) were established. Like the IHA in England, the WSA and WSF helped researchers find WBS participants and at times provided seed moneys toward research on this syndrome. As a consequence, increasing numbers of researchers, primarily psychologists and physicians, began to define the behavioral, mental, physiologic, and physical characteristics of individuals with WBS. Other parental organizations were set up in Germany, New Zealand, and Australia. Today there are parental support groups in more than twenty countries spread over five continents (see www.wsf.org).

From the 1960s through the 1980s, WBS went by names or nicknames that reflected the amorphous nature of the study and understanding of the syndrome. It was variably called idiopathic infantile hypercalcemia, Williams syndrome, Beuren syndrome, elfin face syndrome, and supravalvular aortic stenosis syndrome. Because the syndrome was described independently by Williams and Beuren and their coworkers within a one-year period, for this book we have chosen to follow the European custom of calling the condition Williams-Beuren syndrome.

By 1990, WBS was beginning to be more narrowly defined by its recognizable characteristics (diagnostic code: "Syndrome NEC 759.89"), and psychological research on the syndrome was mushrooming. Then, in 1993, genetic discoveries led to an explosion of research on WBS. Scientists were able to associate WBS with a specific chromosomal condition, a microdeletion of about twenty genes in one chromosome 7. The first gene identified in the deleted chromosomal segment was the gene for elastin (Ewart et al. 1993), a structural protein associated with arteries, lungs, intestines, skin, and other tissues and organs that have elastic properties. From this discovery came a diagnostic test based on the absence of the gene for elastin from one chromosome 7 (diagnostic code: "Autosomal deletion 758.3").

Most of the ensuing publications on WBS appeared in specialized peer-reviewed academic journals or in compendia/symposia volumes dealing with such subjects as language, behavior, and genetic abnormalities. A few years ago the editors of this book met and decided to produce a volume dedicated broadly to WBS so that researchers, physicians, other health and educational professionals, and parents would have available, in a single publication, information on many aspects of research on WBS and the clinical implications of that research.

The senior editor, Colleen Morris, was selected because of her pioneering research on the "natural history" of people with WBS and because of her role in the breakthrough discovery of the missing elastin gene; she has been able to provide comprehensive coverage of research on WBS. The "elder" editor, Howard Lenhoff, in addition to his research expertise dealing with WBS and musical pitch and his rare experience of being a scientist parent of a WBS musical savant, also brings a background in editing compendia. Tying together the medical, behavioral, and neuroscientific aspects is editor Paul Wang, who has worked with the WBS community as both a pediatrician and a researcher in the cognitive sciences. Together, the editors sought to find outstanding researchers to write chapters that cover the main areas of research in WBS. The resulting compendium provides a model for the detailed study of a genetic syndrome that can be applied to other conditions.

As editors, we had two other goals. First, to put together a concise book that would present current findings from the fundamental research on WBS useful to clinicians and would also provide insights into future research possibilities, we asked all authors to include in their chapters a section dealing with clinical implications and a section, "Future Directions," detailing how they see research in their fields of WBS developing during the next five to ten years. Second, to prevent redundant referrals to the pioneering basic discoveries, Morris has written an overview of research on the medical complications, clinical management, and genetics of WBS. Wang has prepared a similar overview for research on the behavior and neuroscience of WBS. Finally, because research on music cognition in WBS is just starting to take off, Lenhoff (chapter 15) and Levitin and Bellugi (chapter 16) have included similar though more limited overviews.

In addition to the research described in the present volume, we refer readers to two other books. One is a concise summary of some of the pioneering research carried out at the Salk Institute (Bellugi et al. 2001). The other deals with strategies for the behavioral and educational management of WBS (Semel and Rosner 2003). Further information about WBS can also be found at www.wsf.org, www.williams-syndrome.org, www.wsf.uk, and www.berkshirehills.org.

Is this the appropriate time to publish a compendium dealing with research on WBS, or is the field still not sufficiently developed? A rationale for publishing the book now might well be drawn from an analogy offered by our "elder" editor in the preface of his first book, which also dealt with a new field (Lenhoff and Loomis 1961) and which was followed by six additional books as the field became more refined: "Much of the work presented [in this book] is in an early stage. At times we had thought that perhaps [some of] these results are too preliminary and should be compiled [only] after more data have been accumulated. The situation is analogous to the construction of a new building. At times we might feel that all such work should proceed behind walls marked 'Work in Progress. No Admittance.' At other times we are intrigued with the very smell of sawdust and of wet paint. It is in this latter spirit that the volume was compiled" (vi). We believe that aura of "sawdust and wet paint" may bring additional researchers to conclude that the study of WBS is particularly favorable for investigating the relation of genes and behavior, of music and language, and indeed the development and functioning of the human brain.

We thank Wendy Harris and Sarah Shepke of the Johns Hopkins University Press for their help and encouragement and the Williams Syndrome Association and the Williams Syndrome Foundation for their good work.

BIBLIOGRAPHY

Bellugi, U., and St. George, M., eds. 2001. *Journey from cognition to brain to gene: Perspectives from Williams syndrome.* Cambridge: MIT Press, 189 pp.
Beuren, A. J., Apitz, J., and Harmanz, D. 1962. Supravalvular aortic stenosis in association with and without mental retardation and a certain facial appearance. *Circulation* 26:1235–1240.
Ewart, A. K., Morris, C. A., Atkinson, D., Wishan, J., Stermes, K., Spallone, P., Stock, A., Leppert, M., and Keating, M. 1993. Hemizygosity of the elastin locus in a developmental disorder, Williams syndrome. *Nature Genetics* 5:11–16.

Lenhoff, H. M., and Loomis, W. F. 1961. *The biology of hydra and of some other coelenterates: 1961.* Coral Gables: University of Miami Press.

Semel, E., and Rosner, S. R. 2003. *Understanding Williams syndrome: Behavioral patterns and interventions.* Mahwah, NJ: Erlbaum, 456 pp.

Williams, J. C. P., Barrett-Boyes, B. G., and Lowe, J. B. 1961. Supravalvular aortic stenosis. *Circulation* 24:1311–1318.

Contributors

DANIEL ANSARI, Ph.D., Assistant Professor, Department of Education, Dartmouth College, Hanover, New Hampshire

RAANAN ARENS, M.D., Associate Professor of Pediatrics, University of Pennsylvania; Attending Pulmonologist and Medical Director, Sleep Disorders Center, Children's Hospital of Philadelphia, Philadelphia, Pennsylvania

URSULA BELLUGI, Ed.D., Professor, Laboratory for Cognitive Neuroscience, Salk Institute for Biological Studies, La Jolla, California

LINDA CAMPBELL, B.Sc., Doctoral Student, Institute of Psychiatry, King's College London, London, United Kingdom

GITANA CHUNYO, B.A., Language and Cognition Lab Coordinator, Department of Cognitive Science, Johns Hopkins University, Baltimore, Maryland

DANIEL D. DILKS, M.A., Graduate Student, Department of Cognitive Science, Johns Hopkins University, Baltimore, Maryland

ELISABETH M. DYKENS, Ph.D., Professor, Psychology and Human Development, Peabody College, John F. Kennedy Center, Vanderbilt University, Nashville, Tennessee

CARL FEINSTEIN, M.D., Professor, Department of Psychiatry and Behavioral Sciences, Stanford University School of Medicine, Stanford, California

JAMES E. HOFFMAN, Ph.D., Professor, Department of Psychology, University of Delaware, Newark, Delaware

PAIGE KAPLAN, M.B.B.Ch., Professor, Department of Pediatrics, University of Pennsylvania School of Medicine, Philadelphia, Pennsylvania

ANNETTE KARMILOFF-SMITH, Ph.D., Professor and Head, Neurocognitive Development Unit, Institute of Child Health, London, United Kingdom

RONALD V. LACRO, M.D., Assistant Professor, Department of Pediatrics, Harvard Medical School, Boston, Massachusetts

LAURA LAKUSTA, M.A., Graduate Student, Department of Psychological and Brain Sciences, Johns Hopkins University, Baltimore, Maryland

BARBARA LANDAU, Ph.D., Dick and Lydia Todd Professor, Department of Cognitive Science, Johns Hopkins University, Baltimore, Maryland

DANIEL J. LEVITIN, ph.D., Assistant Professor, Department of Psychology, McGill University, Montreal, Quebec, Canada

THORNTON B. A. MASON II, M.D., Ph.D., Assistant Professor, Departments of Neurology and Pediatrics, University of Pennsylvania School of Medicine, Philadelphia, Pennsylvania

CAROLYN B. MERVIS, Ph.D., Professor and Distinguished University Scholar, Department of Psychological and Brain Sciences, University of Louisville, Louisville, Kentucky

LUCY R. OSBORNE, Ph.D., Assistant Professor, Departments of Medicine and Molecular and Medical Genetics, University of Toronto, Toronto, Ontario, Canada

DANIELA PLESA-SKWERER, Ph.D., Research Associate, Department of Anatomy and Neurobiology, Boston University School of Medicine, Boston, Massachusetts

BARBARA R. POBER, M.D., Associate Professor, Harvard Medical School, Boston, Massachusetts

ALLAN L. REISS, M.D., Robbins Professor, Department of Psychiatry and Behavioral Sciences, Stanford University School of Medicine, Stanford, California

JASON E. REISS, M.A., Graduate Student, Department of Psychology, University of Delaware, Newark, Delaware

BETH A. ROSNER, Ph.D., Assistant Research Psychologist, UCLA Neuropsychiatric Institute, Los Angeles, California

GAIA SCERIF, Ph.D., Lecturer, School of Psychology, University of Nottingham, Nottingham, United Kingdom

LESLIE B. SMOOT, M.D., Instructor, Department of Cardiology, Harvard Medical School, Boston, Massachusetts

HELEN TAGER-FLUSBERG, Ph.D., Professor, Department of Anatomy and Neurobiology, Boston University School of Medicine, Boston, Massachusetts

MICHAEL THOMAS, Ph.D., Senior Lecturer, School of Psychology, Birkbeck College, London, United Kingdom

I. Biomedical and Genetic Research

The Dysmorphology, Genetics, and Natural History of Williams-Beuren Syndrome

1

Colleen A. Morris, M.D.

The study of a syndrome typically proceeds in a stepwise fashion reflecting distinct knowledge increments:

1. Discovery: Clinicians recognize a unique pattern of malformations and abnormalities of function in an individual or members of a family. The same pattern is later identified in unrelated individuals.
2. Definition: (a) As more people with the condition are clinically identified, clinicians and researchers elucidate the most pertinent features and develop clinical diagnostic criteria. (b) The differential diagnosis is determined in a larger diagnostic category, such as "syndromes that include both mental retardation and congenital heart disease."
3. Natural history: Researchers catalogue the characteristics of the syndrome over the life span, noting variations of the clinical phenotype with respect to age, gender, and environmental influences, such as treatment.
4. Etiology/delineation: Investigators discover the cause of the syndrome. Etiologic categories include teratogens, mutant genes, and chromosome abnormalities. Elucidation of the etiology often leads to a diagnostic test and provides an opportunity to study the pathogenesis of the syndrome.
5. Genotype-phenotype correlation: The population of clinically affected individuals is examined. With an objective test for diagnosis, researchers can detect both extremes (mild and severe) of the distribution, resulting in a redefinition of the syndrome. The range of the phenotype is better evaluated. Researchers investigate the variability of the phenotype relative to the particular genetic mutation, the genetic background, varying environmental conditions, and the actions of modifying genes. Genetic heterogeneity may be demonstrated for the phenotype, if a mutation in a different gene is found to result in the same clinical syndrome.

In this chapter I provide an overview of the history of medical and genetic research on Williams-Beuren syndrome (WBS).

Discovery

Williams-Beuren syndrome is a multisystem disorder. The first descriptions of the syndrome were incomplete in that they reflected the chief complaint (presentation) of the individuals studied and/or the medical specialty of the observer. Thus, cardiologists emphasized the congenital heart defects, while nephrologists and endocrinologists reported the idiopathic hypercalcemia. Fanconi and colleagues (1952) described infantile hypercalcemia with short stature and congenital malformations. Other early reports of children with the syndrome appeared in the wake of an epidemic of infantile hypercalcemia due to overfortification of foods with vitamin D as part of a public health effort to prevent rickets in Britain. Once the population intake of calcium and vitamin D was adjusted appropriately, Stapleton and colleagues (1957) reported a remaining subset of infants with persistent idiopathic hypercalcemia, failure to thrive, and developmental delay. The early case studies of infantile hypercalcemia noted systolic cardiac murmurs, which were initially thought to be related to the infants' hypermetabolic states. The condition was named *idiopathic infantile hypercalcemia* (IHC). In the early 1960s, cardiologists reported unrelated children who had supravalvular aortic stenosis (SVAS) and mental retardation. SVAS was known as a relatively rare familial cause of left-sided outflow tract obstruction, first described in 1842 (Chevers 1842), with autosomal dominant inheritance documented by Eisenberg et al. (1964). Williams and colleagues (1961) reported on four unrelated children from New Zealand, noting that in addition to all having SVAS and mental retardation, their facial features were similar. In Germany, Beuren and colleagues (1962) also documented the syndrome and in subsequent studies pointed out that peripheral pulmonic stenosis was part of the phenotype and that other systemic arteries could be narrowed. Beuren et al. (1964) described the children as "charming characters" and noted that dental anomalies were common. Geneticists observed that the cardiovascular disease SVAS could occur sporadically (presumed new mutation), could occur in a family (autosomal dominant inheritance), or could occur in association with mental retardation. The latter instances occurred sporadically and were termed *supravalvular aortic stenosis syndrome* (SASS) (Merritt et al. 1963). Black and Carter (1963) pointed out the similarities between the facial features of IHC and SASS. Finally, the various signs and symptoms were recognized as a single entity following the 1964 paper of Garcia and colleagues that described SVAS in a child who had a documented history of infantile hypercalcemia. During this period it was postulated that the cause of the syndrome was hypersensitivity to vitamin D, based on the finding that rabbits exposed to high doses of vitamin D prenatally developed aortic lesions and abnormal craniofacies (Friedman and Roberts 1966).

Besides the names "idiopathic infantile hypercalcemia" and "supravalvular aortic stenosis syndrome," reflecting the symptoms emphasized by early authors, other names in the literature included "Williams elfin facies syndrome," "Williams syndrome" (primarily used in the United States), and

"Williams-Beuren syndrome" (primarily used in Europe). To be as inclusive as possible, we have chosen to use the *Williams-Beuren syndrome* appellation for this volume; fortunately, terms such as "elfin facies" and "cocktail party personality" are no longer in use as syndrome descriptions.

Definition

The clinical diagnosis of WBS depends on recognition of the characteristic dysmorphic facial features, the medical problems resulting from the organ system manifestations such as SVAS, the specific cognitive profile, and the unique personality. The expanded medical phenotype was defined in the 1970s as more individuals with this syndrome were identified (Beuren 1972). The early series reflected biases of ascertainment. The prevalence of SVAS was ~100% in cardiology reports, and the prevalence of hypercalcemia was 100% in endocrine series. However, the landmark paper by Jones and Smith (1975) emphasized the true variability of the phenotype. In a series of nineteen children and young adults evaluated in a genetics clinic, none had a history of hypercalcemia and, although 79% had a heart murmur, SVAS was identified in only 37% and an intracardiac defect in 53% (Jones and Smith 1975). Continued study of WBS has resulted in a more complete picture of the phenotype, as summarized below. Management of the medical complications of WBS is discussed in detail in chapters 4 to 6.

The facial gestalt of WBS is easily recognizable to the experienced observer due to the distinctiveness of the facial features. In the young child, the forehead is broad, the cranium is dolichocephalic, and there is narrowing at the temples. The eyes are striking, with periorbital fullness, medial eyebrow flare, epicanthal folds, a lacy or stellate iris pattern, and strabismus. The tendency of infants with WBS to stare intently at faces (Mervis et al. 2003) draws attention to their eyes. They also have a low nasal root, broad nasal tip, malar flattening, long philtrum, full lips, wide mouth, full cheeks, prominent earlobes, small jaw, and dental malocclusion with small, widely spaced teeth (figs. 1.1 and 1.2). The short stature and infantile facial features such as full cheeks combine to make children with WBS appear younger than their chronological age. With growth, the facial appearance changes. The face of the adult with WBS is typically thin, with a prominent supraorbital ridge, narrow nasal root of normal height, flat mala, wide mouth with full lips, and long philtrum (figs. 1.3 and 1.4). Adults with WBS may appear older than their chronological age because they have early graying of the hair and lax facial skin. As the child gets older, the neck appears long and the shoulders sloping. Kyphosis and lordosis often develop, and there is limitation of the joints, especially fingers, knees, and ankles (Kaplan et al. 1989). These features typically lead to a crouched posture and a stiff, awkward gait.

Growth deficiency in WBS is common and may be prenatal or postnatal.

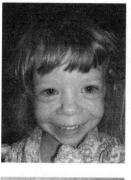

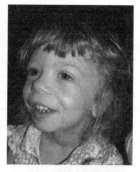

Fig. 1.1.
A three-year-old girl with WBS demonstrates the typical facial appearance, including a broad forehead, bitemporal narrowing, periorbital fullness, stellate iris pattern, full nasal tip, flat mala, full cheeks, wide mouth, full lips, widely spaced teeth, and prominent earlobes.

Fig. 1.2.
An eleven-year-old boy with WBS.

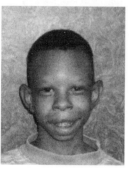

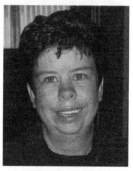

Fig. 1.3.
A thirty-two-year-old woman with WBS.

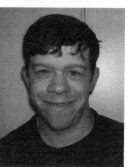

Fig. 1.4.
A twenty-five-year-old man with WBS.

Final adult height is typically less than the third centile but is influenced by the genetic background (parental heights) (Pankau et al. 1992). Puberty may occur early (Partsch et al. 1999, 2002). Endocrine problems may include infantile hypercalcemia, hypothyroidism, and diabetes (Pober et al. 2001). The hypercalcemia typically occurs in the first two years of life and is due to increased absorption of calcium from the gut. The mechanism for the increased absorption is still unknown. Studies of vitamin D metabolism and calcitonin have yielded conflicting results (Kruse et al. 1992).

Microcephaly is common, and neurologic manifestations of WBS include hypotonia, hyperreflexia (especially in the lower extremities), and evidence of cerebellar impairment (Morris et al. 1990; Pober and Szekely 1999). Reduced cerebral volume has been demonstrated by neuroimaging studies, whereas volumes of the cerebellum and superior temporal gyrus are normal (Reiss et al. 2000). Arnold-Chiari malformation has been reported in a few individuals with WBS (Kaplan et al. 1989; Wang et al. 1992), and stroke has also been reported (Ardinger et al. 1994; Wollack et al. 1996).

Ophthalmologic problems include hyperopia, strabismus, and reduced stereo acuity (Sadler et al. 1996; Winter et al. 1996). Chronic otitis media and hypersensitivity to sound are common traits. Malformed or missing teeth and malocclusion have been frequently reported (Hertzberg et al. 1994). The voice is typically hoarse, which is related to elastin deficiency in the vocal cords (Vaux et al. 2003).

The cardiovascular complications of WBS result in the most significant morbidity and mortality, as described in detail in chapter 5. Any artery may be narrowed, but SVAS is most common, detected in 75% of individuals with WBS (Morris et al. 1988). Surgical correction of the aortic lesion is required in 30% (Kececioglu et al. 1993). Common connective tissue abnormalities include soft, loose skin, umbilical hernia, inguinal hernia, bowel and/or bladder diverticula, and joint laxity or contractures.

Developmental delay and/or mental retardation were recognized as key components of the WBS phenotype in the earliest reports. In a landmark paper, Bennett and colleagues (1978) suggested that the psychological profile could aid in diagnosis of WBS. Subsequent studies showed a wide range of full-scale IQ scores in the WBS population (Udwin et al. 1987; Morris et al. 1988), from severe mental retardation to low average intelligence. Most series report a mean IQ of 59 (Mervis et al. 1999a). WBS is characterized by a highly specific cognitive profile, however. There are strengths in verbal short-term memory (Udwin and Yule 1991; Wang and Bellugi 1994) but extreme weakness in visuospatial construction (Mervis et al. 1999b). The WBS cognitive profile has been shown to be independent of IQ and has been quantified by Mervis and colleagues (2000). The functional consequence of the difficulty with visual motor integration includes difficulty with fine motor tasks such as handwriting. Reading is a relative academic strength in people with WBS. For a detailed discussion of these topics, see chapters 8, 9, and 11.

The WBS behavioral phenotype was recognized early in the history of the condition. In 1964, von Arnim and Engel noted "outstanding loquacity . . . ability to establish interpersonal contacts . . . against a background of insecurity and anxiety" (376). Individuals with WBS have impulsivity, attention deficit disorder, overfriendliness, and generalized anxiety (Tomc et al. 1990; Gosch and Pankau 1997; Dykens and Rosner 1999; Klein-Tasman and Mervis 2003; Doyle et al. 2004). Behavior in WBS is further discussed in chapters 10 and 12.

Based on the clinical characteristics, diagnostic scoring systems have been published (Preus 1984; American Academy of Pediatrics Committee on Genetics 2001) to help distinguish WBS from other syndromes that include developmental delay, congenital heart defects, and dysmorphic facial features. Because no feature is found in every individual with WBS, the scoring systems emphasize those traits that are most unique to WBS, such as SVAS. The diagnosis of WBS should be considered for any individual with sporadic SVAS, but those with WBS will have additional findings, such as cognitive impairment. The differential diagnosis of WBS includes Noonan syndrome, Smith-Magenis syndrome, velocardiofacial syndrome, Kabuki syndrome, FG syndrome, Coffin-Lowry syndrome, fragile X syndrome, and fetal alcohol syndrome (Morris 2001) (table 1.1). All of these conditions have some overlap with WBS, but the facial features are different. Most individuals incorrectly diagnosed with WBS have the most nonspecific features of the condition, such as developmental delay or attention deficit disorder.

Natural History

Beginning in the 1980s, parent support organizations, particularly the Infantile Hypercalcaemia Foundation in Britain and the Williams Syndrome Association in the United States, encouraged researchers to study WBS. These groups have provided participants, asked important questions that have guided research, and helped educate communities. Their efforts made natural history studies possible (Martin et al. 1984; Morris et al. 1988, 1990). These studies documented the evolving phenotype of WBS over time, including the change in facial features from the child to the adult, the medical complications with aging, and the prenatal and postnatal growth deficiency. Growth curves specific for WBS were published (Morris et al. 1988; Saul et al. 1988). Children with WBS were often born post-term and were small for gestational age. Infants were found to have a high frequency of feeding problems, failure to thrive, prolonged colic, and multiple episodes of otitis media, necessitating frequent doctor's visits (Morris et al. 1988). Some infants (~40%) required surgery for inguinal hernia, and 15% were documented to have hypercalcemia. Children had delayed developmental milestones (walking and talking at twenty-one months, toileting at thirty-nine months). Esotropia required surgery in ~20%, and hyperopia was treated with corrective lenses. Hypersensitivity to sound was common at all ages. Regarding the cardiovascular disease, peripheral pulmonic stenosis was most commonly detected in infancy and tended to improve with age. In contrast, SVAS could worsen over time. Hypertension had onset in childhood or adolescence; mitral valve prolapse was commonly found in adults. Genitourinary problems included bladder diverticula, which became more frequent with aging. Renal ultrasound demonstrated structural urinary anomalies in 35% (Sforzini

Table 1.1.
Differential Diagnosis of Williams-Beuren Syndrome: Clinical Features

	WBS	NS	SMS	VCFS	KS	FGS	CLS	FRAXA	FAS
Etiology	7q11.23 deletion	PTPN11 mutation	17p11 deletion	22q11 deletion	Unknown	X-linked	X-linked RSK2	X-linked FMR1	Alcohol
OFC	D	I	D	D	D	I	D	I	D
Eye									
Acuity	Hyperopia	Myopia	Myopia			Myopia			
Stabismus	+	+	+	+	+	+			+
Ptosis		+		+	+				+
Other	Stellate iris, periorbital fullness	Downslanting palpebral fissures	Brushfield spots, synophrys	Narrow palpebral fissures	Long palpebral fissures		Hypertelorism		Short palpebral fissures
Ears	OM, Large lobes, hypersensitive	OM, HL; Lowset, posteriorly rotated	OM, HL; Lowset	OM, HL; Small	OM, HL; Large	HL; Small	HL	OM; Large	OM; Small
Cleft palate	+	+	++	+++	+++			+	+
Voice	Hoarse		Hoarse	Hypernasal	Hypernasal		Hoarse		
Face	Long philtrum; prominent lips; wide mouth	Prominent grooved philtrum; webbed neck	Flat face; prominent philtrum	Long face; prominent nose	Short nasal septum; arched eyebrows	Broad forehead; many hair whorls	Broad short nose; lower lip everted		Smooth philtrum; thin upper lip
Jaw	Small	Small	Prominent	Small		Small		Prominent	Small
Heart	SVAS, SVPS, HTN	PS, HCM	ASD	Conotruncal	ASD, coarct Aorta			HTN	ASD, VSD
Inguinal hernia	+	+		+	+	+	+		+
Pectus	+	++					+		+
Lax joints	+				+		+	+	
Elbow	RUS	Cubitus vulgas	RUS						
Fingers	Short		Short	Long	Short		Large		Short
Other	Bowel, bladder diverticula; low calcium	Edema	Scoliosis; pes cavus	Low calcium	Vertebral anomalies	Anal anomalies	Scoliosis	Pes planus; macro-orchidism	

Note: All syndromes in the table are characterized by delayed development, learning disability and/or mental retardation, feeding difficulty in infancy, and an increased incidence of behavioral problems, especially attention deficit hyperactivity disorder. All but one (fetal alcohol syndrome) are associated with hypotonia. Short stature is characteristic of all the syndromes except fragile X syndrome. This table lists many, but not all, distinguishing clinical signs of the syndromes. For a more complete description of the syndromes, the reader is referred to K. L. Jones, *Smith's Recognizable Patterns of Human Malformation*, 5th ed. (Philadelphia: Saunders, 1996).

Abbreviations: WBS, Williams-Beuren syndrome; NS, Noonan syndrome; SMS, Smith-Magenis syndrome; VCFS, velocardiofacial syndrome; KS, Kabuki syndrome; FGS, FG syndrome; CLS, Coffin-Lowry syndrome; FRAXA, fragile X syndrome; FAS, fetal alcohol syndrome; OFC, occipital-frontal (head) circumference; D, decreased; I, increased; OM, otitis media; HL, hearing loss; SVAS, supravalvular aortic stenosis; SVPS, supravalvular pulmonic stenosis; HTN, hypertension; PS, pulmonic stenosis; HCM, hypertrophic cardiomyopathy; ASD, atrial septal defect; VSD, ventricular septal defect; RUS, radioulnar synostosis.

et al. 2002). Urinary frequency was a common symptom at all ages. Gastrointestinal complaints included gastroesophageal reflux, abdominal pain, chronic constipation, rectal prolapse, and colon diverticula. Obesity was reported in 30% to 50% (Morris et al. 1988; Martin et al. 1984; Cherniske et al. 2004). Endocrine problems in adults could include hypothyroidism, diabetes, and, rarely, recurrence of hypercalcemia (Martin et al. 1984; Morris et al. 1990; Pober et al. 2001).

Infants with WBS were noted to be hypotonic and have lax joints. Hypertonicity of the lower extremities and joint limitations, especially tightening of heel cords and hamstrings, occurred with increasing frequency with aging. Kyphosis, lordosis, and a stiff gait were seen in many adults. Cerebellar signs in adults included ataxia and tremor. Behaviorally, infants with WBS tended to be irritable. Attention deficit disorder was typically noted in childhood, and anxiety was common. Adults with WBS usually lived with their parents or in a supervised setting; most had part-time employment (Morris et al. 1990). Typically, both children and adults have had greater strengths in socialization skills than in daily living skills (Morris and Mervis 2000; Mervis et al. 2001).

Etiology/Delineation

Various possible etiologies for WBS were explored as investigators learned more about the syndrome. Early investigations suggested a possible role for vitamin D or calcium teratogenesis (Friedman and Roberts 1966). Later, different chromosome anomalies were reported in individuals with some features of WBS (Burn 1986). There was speculation on the relationship between autosomal dominant SVAS and WBS. Perhaps WBS was an "iceberg dominant"—that is, WBS was the most obvious and severe manifestation of a more variable condition. Grimm and Wesselhoeft (1980) studied 120 families with SVAS; they found some affected family members with hernias, hoarse voice, and some dysmorphic facial features as seen in WBS. To explore this possibility, Ewart and colleagues (1993b) evaluated SVAS families and carefully classified the family members by echocardiography with Doppler to designate individuals as affected, unaffected, or uncertain. Advances in cardiac ultrasound and recombinant DNA technology resulted in the successful linkage study that identified the elastin gene (*ELN*) as the causative gene for SVAS (Ewart et al. 1993b). Subsequently, Morris and colleagues (1993) identified a family with a 6;7 translocation that disrupted the *ELN* gene. The SVAS phenotype cosegregated with the translocation (Morris et al. 1993; Curran et al. 1993). Several mutations in *ELN* have now been identified in SVAS families (Metcalfe et al. 2000). Studies of individuals with WBS revealed haploinsufficiency for *ELN* (Ewart et al. 1993a). Lowery and colleagues (1995) tested the diagnostic assay for WBS that uses fluorescent in

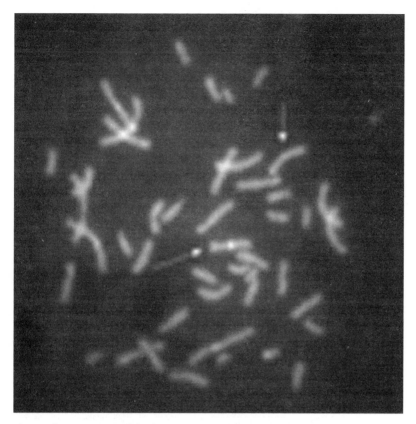

Fig. 1.5. Fluorescent in situ hybridization (FISH) results in WBS. The short arrows point to probes for the end of chromosome 7. The long arrow points to the probe for Cos 1186 from the WBS region, which is present in one chromosome 7 but not the other. *Source:* Morris, CA et al. 2003. GTF21 Hemizygosity Implicated in Mental Retardation in Williams Syndrome: Genotype-phenotype Analysis of Five Families with Deletions in the Williams Syndrome Region, *American Journal of Medical Genetics* 123(1):45–59. Reprinted with permission from Wiley.

situ hybridization (FISH). The test uses a fluorescent marker that hybridizes to a gene or genes in the WBS critical region; a normal result shows a WBS probe on each chromosome 7, whereas only one probe is seen in individuals who have a deletion on one of the chromosomes (fig. 1.5). The deletion has been shown to encompass approximately 1.6 Mb of chromosome 7q11.23. This area contains more than twenty genes (see chapter 2). Because more than one gene contributes to the WBS phenotype, WBS is termed a "contiguous gene syndrome."

Recent studies of the genomic structure of chromosome 7 have provided insight into the mechanism of deletion that causes WBS. The ~1.6 Mb segment of chromosome 7 deleted in WBS is flanked by low-copy repeats (LCRs) made up of gene clusters and pseudogenes. The LCRs predispose to nonallelic homologous recombination in meiosis. The possible outcomes of this unequal crossing over are as follows: (1) deletion of the WSCR, resulting in WBS; (2) duplication of the WSCR; and (3) inversion, which would not cause a phenotypic change in the individual but could predispose to deletion or duplication in offspring. Osborne et al. (2001) found that 4 of 12 parents who transmitted the deleted chromosome had an inversion, and Bayés et al. (2003) reported 21 of 71 individuals with WBS with molecular evidence of a parental inversion. Hobart et al. (2004) reported a prevalence of 7% for this genomic inversion in the general population. By determining the parent of origin of the deleted chromosome in more than two hundred couples, Hobart and colleagues found that 25% of transmitting parents had the inversion. Even though these data show a fivefold increased chance of an affected child for individuals who have this common inversion, the absolute risk is still quite low: the chance for individuals with the inversion is 1 in 2,000, compared with the 1 in 9,500 chance for individuals without the inversion (C. A. Morris, unpublished observations).

Genotype-Phenotype Correlation

With the discovery that WBS was caused by a submicroscopic deletion of 7q11.23, it became possible to investigate the genetic contribution of each aspect of the phenotype. In chapter 2, Osborne details the extensive body of work related to discovery of genes in the WBS region and the research on their function and expression. The contribution of *ELN* haploinsufficiency to the phenotype was the first described. The results of subsequent genotype-phenotype correlation studies are detailed in chapter 3.

Clinical Implications

In the forty years since the early descriptions of Williams-Beuren syndrome, advances in molecular genetics and diagnostic technologies have greatly increased our understanding of the disorder. We now know that WBS is more common than previously estimated; a recent population study has reported a prevalence of 1 in 7,500 (Strømme et al. 2002). A diagnostic laboratory test has made it possible to reliably and quickly distinguish WBS from other conditions associated with developmental delay, and the technique has been used for prenatal diagnosis. People with WBS have a 50% chance with each pregnancy of having a child with WBS; these individuals should receive genetic counseling. Recurrences of WBS in siblings are rare (Kara-Mostefa et al. 1999). Even though the risk of having a second affected child is low, prenatal diagnosis may be offered. Earlier identification of affected individuals and the willingness of those affected and their families to participate in research have resulted in improved recommendations for anticipatory guidance and medical care (American Academy of Pediatrics 2001; Morris 2005). Concomitantly, advances in our understanding of the WBS cognitive and behavioral phenotypes have resulted in improved recommendations for education and therapy (Morris and Mervis 2000; Semel and Rosner 2003). With continued research efforts, improved treatment in many areas should result in improved quality of life for individuals with WBS.

Future Directions

Research on Williams-Beuren syndrome will continue in many areas of clinical medicine. Improved therapeutic strategies will be tested, and as individuals with WBS are diagnosed at younger ages and prospectively evaluated, early treatment will prevent some complications. For some WBS problems, the responses of this select population to therapeutic agents (e.g., drugs for hypertension, medications for attention deficit disorder) can be formally tested in controlled clinical trials. The emerging field of pharmacogenetics, which deals with genetic differences in drug efficacy and reactions, will provide useful information.

Cognition

The study of brain structure and function in people with WBS has been greatly enhanced by improved functional neuroimaging and improved psychological characterization of neurologic development. As the fields continue to progress, WBS will remain a prime subject for study because it has a characteristic cognitive profile. Advances in our understanding of cognition in WBS not only will help with designing educational strategies for people with WBS but will also advance our overall understanding of central nervous system function. It will likely lend insight into problems that affect large segments of the general population, such as those with learning disability and attention deficit disorder.

Behavior

One of the most challenging and fascinating subjects of study is complex human behavior. WBS has generated a great deal of interest in this area because there are many positively viewed aspects of the behavior, such as empathy, affinity for music, and sociability. However, other behavioral traits interfere with adaptive function, such as attention deficit disorder, anxiety, and over-friendliness. Individuals with WBS will benefit from advances in neuropharmacology and improvement in psychotropic medications. Genotype-phenotype correlation studies will be especially important in advancing this field. Study of individuals with WBS will improve our understanding of the genetic underpinnings of anxiety. Therapeutic agents may be tailored to specific genetic antecedents of anxiety, attention deficit disorder, and so forth. Particular behavioral therapies will also be studied. Interactions of biofeedback, behavioral responses, music therapy, and neurophysiologic effects of meditation techniques are only a few of the potential areas of research. In summary, individuals with WBS have much to teach us, and we treasure their contribution to our society.

REFERENCES

American Academy of Pediatrics Committee on Genetics. 2001. Healthcare supervision for children with Williams syndrome. *Pediatrics* 107:1192–1204.

Ardinger, R. H., Jr., Goertz, K. K., and Mattioli, L. F. 1994. Cerebrovascular stenosis with cerebral infarction in a child with Williams syndrome. *American Journal of Medical Genetics* 51:200–202.

Bayés, M., Magano L. F., Rivera N., Flores R., and Pérez Jurado L. A. 2003. Mutational mechanisms of Williams-Beuren syndrome deletions. *American Journal of Human Genetics* 73:131–151.

Bennett, C., La Veck, B., and Sells, C. J. 1978. The Williams elfin facies syndrome: The psychological profile as an aid in syndrome identification. *Pediatrics* 61:303–306.

Beuren, A. J. 1972. Supravalvular aortic stenosis: A complex syndrome with and without mental retardation. *Birth Defects* 8:45–56.

Beuren, A. J., Apitz, J., and Harmjanz, D. 1962. Supravalvular aortic stenosis in association with mental retardation and a certain facial appearance. *Circulation* 27:1235–1240.

Beuren, A. J., Schulze, C., Eberle, P., Harmjanz, D., and Apitz, J. 1964. The syndrome of supravalvular aortic stenosis, peripheral pulmonary stenosis, mental retardation and similar facial appearance. *American Journal of Cardiology* 13:471–482.

Black, J. A., and Carter, R. E. B. 1963. Association between aortic stenosis and facies of severe infantile hypercalcemia. *Lancet* 91:745–748.

Burn, J. 1986. Williams syndrome. *Journal of Medical Genetics* 23:389–395.

Cherniske, E. M., Carpenter, T. O., Klaiman, C., Young, E., Bregman, J., Insogna, K., Schultz, R. T., and Pober, B. R. 2004. Multisystem study of 20 older adults with Williams syndrome. *American Journal of Medical Genetics* 131A:255–264.

Chevers, N. 1842. Observations on the diseases of the orifice and valves of the aorta. *Guys Hospital Reports* 7:387–442.

Curran, M. E., Atkinson, D. L., Ewart, A. K., Morris, C. A, Leppert, M. F., and Keating, M. T. 1993. The elastin gene is disrupted by a translocation associated with supravalvular aortic stenosis. *Cell* 73:159–168.

Doyle, T. F., Bellugi, U., Korenberg, J. R., and Graham, J. 2004. "Everybody in the world is my friend": Hypersociability in young children with Williams syndrome. *American Journal of Medical Genetics* 124A:263–273.

Dykens, E. M., and Rosner, B. A. 1999. Refining behavioral phenotypes: Personality-motivation in Williams and Prader-Willi syndromes. *American Journal of Mental Retardation* 104:158–169.

Eisenberg, R., Young, D., Jacobson, B., and Boito, A. 1964. Familial supravalvular aortic stenosis. *American Journal of Diseases of Children* 108:341–347.

Ewart, A. K., Morris, C. A., Atkinson, D., Jin, W., Sternes, K., Spallone, P., Stock, A. D., Leppert, M., and Keating, M. T. 1993a. Hemizygosity at the elastin locus in a developmental disorder, Williams syndrome. *Nature Genetics* 5:11–16.

Ewart, A. K., Morris, C. A., Ensing, G. K., Loker, J., Moore, C. A., Leppert, M., and Keating, M. 1993b. A human vascular disease, supravalvular aortic stenosis, maps to chromosome 7. *Proceedings of the National Academy of Sciences USA* 90:3226–3230.

Fanconi, G., Giradet, P., Schlesinger, B., Butler, N., and Blade, J. S. 1952. Chronische Hypercalcaemie kombiniert mit Osteosklerose, Hyperazotaemie, Minderwuchs, und kongenitalen Missbildungen. *Helvetica Paediatrica Acta* 7:314–334.

Friedman, W., and Roberts, W. 1966. Vitamin D and the supravalvular aortic stenosis syndrome. *Circulation* 34:77–86.

Garcia, R. E., Friedman, W. F., Kaback, M. M., and Rowe, R.D. 1964. Idiopathic hypercalcemia and supravalvular aortic stenosis. *New England Journal of Medicine* 271:117–120.

Gosch, A., and Pankau, R. 1997. Personality characteristics and behaviour problems in individuals of different ages with Williams syndrome. *Developmental Medicine and Child Neurology* 39:327–533.

Grimm, T., and Wesselhoeft, H. 1980. Zur Genetik Des Williams-Beuren-Syndroms Und Der Isolierten Form Der Supravalvularen Aortenstenose Untersuchungen Von 128 Familien. *Zeitschrift für Kardiologie* 69:168–172.

Hertzberg, J., Nakisbendi, L., Neddleman, H. L., and Pober, B. 1994. Williams syndrome—oral presentation of 45 cases. *Pediatric Dentistry* 16:262–267.

Hobart, H. H., Gregg, R. G., Mervis, C. B., Robinson, B. F., Kimberley, K. W., Rios, C. M., Pani, A. M., and Morris, C. A. 2004. Heterozygotes for the microinversion of the Williams-Beuren region have an increased risk for affected offspring (abstract 891). American Society for Human Genetics, Toronto. www.ashg.org.

Jones, K. L., and Smith, D. W. 1975. The Williams elfin facies syndrome. *Journal of Pediatrics* 86:718–723.

Kaplan, P., Kirschner, M., Watters, G., and Costa, M. T. 1989. Contractures in patients with Williams syndrome. *Pediatrics* 84:895–899.

Kara-Mostefa, A., Raoul, O., Lyonnet, S., Amiel, J., Munnich, A., Vekemans, M., Magnier, S., Ossareh, B., and Bonnefont, J. P. 1999. Recurrent Williams-Beuren syndrome in a sibship suggestive of maternal germ-line mosaicism. *American Journal of Human Genetics* 64:1475–1478.

Kececioglu, D., Kotthoff, S., and Vogt, J. 1993. Williams-Beuren syndrome: A 30-year follow-up of natural and postoperative course. *European Heart Journal* 14:1458–1464.

Klein-Tasman, B. P., and Mervis, C. B. 2003 Distinctive personality characteristics of 8-, 9-, and 10-year-olds with Williams syndrome. *Developmental Neuropsychology* 23:269–290.

Kruse, K., Pankau, R., Gosch, A., and Wohlfahrt, K.1992. Calcium metabolism in Williams-Beuren syndrome. *Journal of Pediatrics* 121:902–907.

Lowery, M. C., Morris, C. A., Ewart, A., Brothman, L., Zhu, X. L., Leonard, C. O., Carey, J. C., Keating, M., and Brothman, A. R. 1995. Strong correlations of elastin deletions, detected by FISH, with Williams syndrome: Evaluation of 235 patients. *American Journal of Human Genetics* 57:49–53.

Martin, N. D. T., Snodgrass, G. J. A. I., and Cohen, R. D. 1984. Idiopathic infantile hypercalcemia: A continuing enigma. *Archives of Disease in Childhood* 59:605–613.

Merritt, D. A., Palmar, C. G., Lurie, P. R., and Petry, E. L. 1963. Supravalvular aortic stenosis: Genetic and clinical studies (abstract). *Journal of Laboratory and Clinical Medicine* 62:995.

Mervis, C. B., Morris, C. A., Bertrand, J., and Robinson, B. F. 1999a. Williams syndrome: Findings from an integrated program of research. In *Neurodevelopmental disorders: Contributions to a new framework from the cognitive neurosciences,* ed. H. Tager-Flusberg, 65–110. Cambridge: MIT Press.

Mervis, C. B., Robinson, B. F., and Pani, J. R. 1999b. Visuospatial construction. *American Journal of Medical Genetics* 65:1222–1229.

Mervis, C. B., Robinson, B. F., Bertrand, J., Morris, C. A., Klein-Tasman, B. P., and Armstrong, S. C. 2000. The Williams syndrome cognitive profile. *Brain and Cognition* 44:604–628.

Mervis, C. B., Klein-Tasman, B. P., and Mastin, M. E. 2001. Adaptive behavior of 4-through 8-year-old children with Williams syndrome. *American Journal on Mental Retardation* 106:82–93.

Mervis, C. B., Morris, C. A., Klein-Tasman, B. P., Bertrand, J., Kwitny, S., Appelbaum, L. G., and Rice, C. E. 2003. Attentional characteristics of infants and toddlers with Williams syndrome during triadic interactions. *Developmental Neuropsychology* 23:243–268.

Metcalfe, K., Rucka, A. K., Smoot, L., Hofstadler, G., Tuzler, G., McKeown, P., Siu, V., Rauch, A., Dean, J., Dennis, N., Ellis, I., Reardon, W., Cytrynbaum, C., Osborne, L., Yates, J. R., Read, A. P., Donnai, D., and Tassabehji, M. 2000. Elastin mutational spectrum in supravalvular aortic stenosis. *European Journal of Human Genetics* 8:955–963.

Morris, C. A. 2005. Williams syndrome. In *Management of genetic syndromes,* 2nd ed., ed. S. B. Cassidy and J. E. Allanson, 655–665. Hoboken, NJ: John Wiley.

Morris, C. A., and Mervis, C. B. 2000. Williams syndrome and related disorders. *Annual Review of Genomics and Human Genetics* 1:461–484.

Morris, C. A., Dilts, C., Demsey, S. A., Leonard, C. O., and Blackburn, B. 1988. The natural history of Williams syndrome: Physical characteristics. *Journal of Pediatrics* 113:318–326.

Morris, C. A., Leonard, C. O., Dilts, C., and Demsey, S. A. 1990. Adults with Williams syndrome. *American Journal of Medical Genetics Supplement* 6:102–107.

Morris, C. A., Loker, J., Ensing, G., and Stock, A. D. 1993. Supravalvular aortic stenosis cosegregates with a familial 6:7 translocation which disrupts the elastin gene. *American Journal of Medical Genetics* 46:737–744.

Osborne, L. R., Li, M., Pober, B., Chitayat, D., Bodurtha, J., Mandel, A., Costa, T., Grebe, T., Cox, S., Tsui, L. C., and Scherer, S. W. 2001. A 1.5 million-base pair inversion polymorphism in families with Williams-Beuren syndrome. *Nature Genetics* 29:321–325.

Pankau, R., Partsch, C.-J., Gosch, A., Oppermann, H. C., and Wessel, A. 1992. Statural growth in Williams-Beuren syndrome. *European Journal of Pediatrics* 151:751–755.

Partsch, C. J., Dreyer, G., Gosch, A., Winter, M., Schneppenheim, R., Wessel, A., and Pankau, R. 1999. Longitudinal evaluation of growth, puberty, and bone maturation in children with Williams syndrome. *Journal of Pediatrics* 134:82–89.

Partsch, C. J., Japig, I., Siebert, R., Gosch, A., Wessel, A., Sippell, W. G., and Pankau, R. 2002. Central precocious puberty in girls with Williams syndrome. *Journal of Pediatrics* 141:441–444.

Pober, B. R., and Szekely, A. M. 1999. Distinct neurological profile in Williams syndrome. *American Journal of Human Genetics Supplement* 65(4):A70.

Pober, B. R., Wang, E., Petersen, K., Osborne, L., and Caprio, S. 2001. Impaired glucose tolerance in Williams syndrome. *American Journal of Medical Genetics* 69:302A.

Preus, M. 1984. The Williams syndrome: Objective definition and diagnosis. *Clinical Genetics* 25:422–428.

Reiss, A. L., Eliez, S., Schmitt, J. E., Straus, E., Lai, Z., Jones, W., and Bellugi, U. 2000. IV. Neuroanatomy of Williams syndrome: A high-resolution MRI study. *Journal of Cognitive Neuroscience* 12 (suppl. 1): 65–73.

Sadler, L. S., Olitsky, S. E., and Reynolds, J. D. 1996. Reduced stereoacuity in Williams syndrome. *American Journal of Medical Genetics* 66:287–288.

Saul, R. A., Stevenson, R. E., Rogers, R. C., Skinner, S. A., Prouty, L. A., and Flannery, D. B. 1988. Growth references from conception to adulthood. *Proceedings of the Greenwood Genetic Center* 7 (suppl. 1): 204–209.

Semel, E., and Rosner, S. R. 2003. *Understanding Williams syndrome: Behavioral patterns and interventions.* Mahwah, NJ: Erlbaum.

Sforzini, C., Milani, D., Fossali, E., Barbato, A., Grumieri, G., Bianchetti, M. G., and Selicorni, A. 2002. Renal tract ultrasonography and calcium homeostasis in Williams-Beuren syndrome. *Pediatric Nephrology* 17:899–902.

Stapleton, T., MacDonald, W. B., and Lightwood, R. 1957. The pathogenesis of idiopathic hypercalcemia in infancy. *American Journal of Clinical Nutrition* 5:533–542.

Strømme, P., Bjornstad, P. G., and Ramstad, K. 2002. Prevalence estimation of Williams syndrome. *Journal of Child Neurology* 17:269–271.

Tomc, S. A., Williamson, N. K., and Pauli, R. M. 1990. Temperament in Williams syndrome. *American Journal of Medical Genetics* 36:345–352.

Udwin, O., and Yule, W. 1991. A cognitive and behavioral phenotype in Williams syndrome. *Journal of Clinical and Experimental Neuropsychology* 13:232–244.

Udwin, O., Yule, W., and Martin, N. 1987. Cognitive abilities and behavioral characteristics of children with idiopathic infantile hypercalcemia. *Journal of Child Psychiatry* 28:297–309.

Vaux, K. K., Wojtczak, H., Benirschke, K., and Jones, K. L. 2003. Vocal cord abnormalities in Williams syndrome: A further manifestation of elastin deficiency. *American Journal of Medical Genetics* 119A:302–304.

Von Arnim, G., and Engel, P. 1964. Mental retardation related to hypercalcemia. *Developmental Medicine and Child Neurology* 6:366–377.

Wang, P. P., and Bellugi, U. 1994. Evidence from two genetic syndromes for a dissociation between verbal and visual-spatial short-term memory. *Journal of Clinical and Experimental Neuropsychology* 16:317–322.

Wang, P. P., Hesselink, J. R., Jernigan, T. L., Doherty, S., and Bellugi, U. 1992. Specific neurobehavioral profile of Williams syndrome is associated with neocerebellar hemispheric preservation. *Neurology* 42:1999–2002.

Williams, J. C. P., Barratt-Boyes, B. G., and Lowe, J. B. 1961. Supravalvular aortic stenosis. *Circulation* 24:1311–1318.

Winter, M., Pankau, R., Amm, M., Gosch, A., and Wessel, A. 1996. The spectrum of ocular features in the Williams-Beuren syndrome. *Clinical Genetics* 49:28–31.

Wollack, J. B., Kaifer, M., LaMonte, M. P., and Rothman, M. 1996. Stroke in Williams syndrome. *Stroke* 27:143–146.

The Molecular Basis of a Multisystem Disorder

2

Lucy R. Osborne, Ph.D.

More than a decade has passed since Williams-Beuren syndrome (WBS) was shown to result from a chromosomal deletion (Ewart et al. 1993), but the underlying genetic basis of most of the symptoms remains a mystery. This is not to suggest that researchers have been idle: at least twenty-six genes have been identified in the commonly deleted region, and progress is being made toward elucidating the role, if any, of each of these genes in the etiology of WBS. For many of the genes, animal models are being generated to better assess the possible contribution of each gene to the complex WBS phenotype, and some of these models have already yielded fascinating insight into the function of specific proteins. In addition, the WBS chromosome segment itself has been the focus of research, with recent data suggesting that the region can undergo other genomic rearrangements that predispose the chromosome to subsequent deletion or may even be associated with clinical symptoms.

The WBS Chromosome Region at 7q11.23
Mechanism of Deletion

Williams-Beuren syndrome is characterized by a common, submicroscopic deletion of 7q11.23, found in more than 95% of individuals with a clinical diagnosis of WBS (Mari et al. 1995; Nickerson et al. 1995; Kotzot et al. 1995; Lowery et al. 1995). Since the WBS deletion was first identified (Ewart et al. 1993), a framework of genomic clones spanning the commonly deleted region has been assembled and used as the basis for gene discovery and characterization of the deleted region (Osborne et al. 1996; Pérez Jurado et al. 1996; X. Meng et al. 1998a; Peoples et al. 2000). The common deletion spans about 1.3 Mb of "unique" DNA comprising at least twenty-three genes—including those thought to contribute to the disorder—flanked by several hundred kilobases of repetitive DNA (Peoples et al. 2000). These flanking regions are chromosome-specific, low-copy repeats (LCRs) that are thought to be directly responsible for the occurrence of the deletion.

Studies have shown that the WBS deletion occurs with approximately equal frequency on the maternally or paternally inherited chromosome, although there have been several reports of a nonsignificant predominance of maternal deletions (Pérez Jurado et al. 1996; Y. Q. Wu et al. 1998; M. S. Wang et al. 1999; L. R. Osborne, unpublished observations). Analyses of markers around the WBS deletion region have shown that the deletion results from unequal recombination between grandparental chromosomes during meiosis in the parent from whom the deleted chromosome stemmed (Urban et al. 1996; Dutly and Schinzel 1996; Baumer et al. 1998). Two-thirds of the deletions were found to have resulted from interchromosomal rearrangements (between the chromosome 7 homologues) and the remainder from intrachromosomal rearrangements (between sister chromatids of the same chromosome 7) (Dutly and Schinzel 1996). It is postulated that the deletion event is precipitated by the presence of the flanking repeats, made up of genes, pseudogenes, and gene clusters that form blocks of sequence known as duplicons (Peoples et al. 2000; Valero et al. 2000).

As has recently become clear, the genome is peppered with LCRs (Bailey et al. 2001; Eichler 2001), some of which directly contribute to genomic disorders such as the microdeletion syndromes (for a review, see Stankiewicz and Lupski 2002). LCRs have been identified flanking the regions commonly deleted in Smith-Magenis syndrome, at 17p11.2 (Chen et al. 1997); hereditary neuropathy with liability to pressure palsies, at 17p12 (Chance et al. 1994); DiGeorge/velocardiofacial syndrome, at 22q11.2 (Edelmann et al. 1999a); Angelman and Prader-Willi syndromes, at 15q12–14 (Amos-Landgraf et al. 1999); and neurofibromatosis type 1, at 17q11.2 (López-Correa et al. 2000)—to name but a few. LCRs promise to prove increasingly important as we learn more about the evolution and rearrangement of the genome.

Although not directly proven in WBS, nonallelic homologous recombination between LCRs has been demonstrated in Smith-Magenis syndrome (Potocki et al. 2000). Investigators have also proposed that recombination between LCRs on homologous chromosomes can result in two reciprocal products—one with a deletion and one with a tandem duplication of the region (Pentao et al. 1992)—and such duplications have indeed been identified. Duplication of 17p12 results in Charcot-Marie-Tooth disease type 1A, with a frequency similar to that of the deletion that causes hereditary neuropathy with liability to pressure palsies (Chance et al. 1994). Less frequent duplications have also been reported for the 17p11.2 Smith-Magenis region (Potocki et al. 2000) and the 22q11.2 velocardiofacial syndrome region (Edelmann et al. 1999b; Ensenauer et al. 2003). Duplications of the WBS region have not been identified to date, for several possible reasons. First, both the 17p11.2 and 22q11.2 deletion/duplication regions are considerably larger than the WBS deletion region, at a ~4,000 kb and between 3,000 and 6,000 kb, respectively, enabling detection of deletion or duplication by conventional cytogenetic analysis. A dup(7q11.23) cannot be identified by standard cytogenetic analysis or by metaphase FISH (fluorescent in situ hybridization), which is commonly used for the molecular diagnosis of the WBS deletion, because the region is too small and duplicated signals would overlap on metaphase chromosomes. Second, the phenotype seen in individuals with dup(17p11.2) or dup(22q11.2) was often less severe than that seen in individuals with the corresponding deletion (Edelmann et al. 1999b; Potocki et al. 2000) and was variable (Potocki et al. 2000; Ensenauer et al. 2003). This suggests that if the hallmark characteristics of WBS are not present in individuals with a 7q11.23 duplication, that population may be very heterogeneous and hard to identify. It is also conceivable that duplication of 7q11.23 does not result in any clinical symptoms or may even produce a more severe phenotype that is incompatible with life. In the small number of individuals in whom dup(7q11.23) could have been identified, given the experimental technique used, none were found to have this duplication (Osborne et al. 2001).

Chromosome 7 Low-Copy Repeats

The LCRs that flank the WBS deletion region and predispose to nonallelic homologous recombination consist of large (~400 kb), actively transcribed stretches of DNA, often referred to as duplicons. There is a single duplicon at the centromeric deletion boundary and two duplicons at the telomeric boundary separated by a stretch of nonrepetitive DNA. To simplify descriptions of the complex structure of the LCRs, each duplicon has been subdivided into blocks of sequence (A, B, and C) that contain the same sets of DNA elements, such as genes, pseudogenes, and genetic markers, with subtle sequence differences (Peoples et al. 2000; Valero et al. 2000; Bayés et al. 2003). These single base differences allow the blocks to be distinguished from one another despite their being ~98% identical at the nucleotide level. The duplicons consist of several genes and pseudogenes and clusters of related genes, many of which are also present in other regions on chromosome 7 (fig. 2.1).

The gene components of the duplicons include *GTF2I, NCF1, GTF2IRD2, STAG3, POM121, FKBP6, NSUN5, TRIM50,* and clusters of *PMS2*-like (*PMS2L*) genes. Of these, functional copies of *FKBP6, TRIM50,* and *GTF2I* are disrupted or deleted at the centromeric and telomeric breakpoints. *NCF1* is not usually included in the deletion but may be included when the telomeric breakpoint lies at a more distal location, as sometimes happens (Robinson et al. 1996; Baumer et al. 1998; M. S. Wang et al. 1999). The inclusion of *NCF1* in a WBS-associated deletion was further supported by the identification of

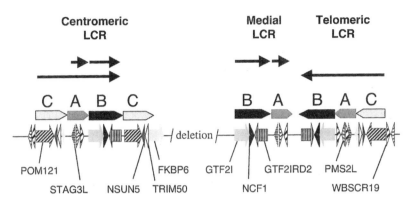

Fig. 2.1. Schematic diagram of the structure of the WBS duplicons. The WBS duplicons have been divided into blocks of nearly identical sequence (A, B, and C, according to Valero et al. 2000), which are shown in their correct orientation in relation to the centromere and telomere. The gene content of these individual blocks is shown at the bottom of the figure, with different shaded boxes representing different gene sequences (as labeled) and arrowheads indicating the direction of transcription where known. The large repeats, in direct and inverted orientation—which contribute to deletion and inversion of the region, respectively—are indicated by arrows at the top of the figure.

two individuals with both WBS and chronic granulomatous disease, which is an autosomal recessive disorder usually caused by mutations in *NCF1* (Görlach et al. 1997). In both cases, one copy of *NCF1* was indeed mutated, and in one case the second copy was in the WBS deletion, as revealed by analysis of somatic cell hybrids generated from the patient (Kabuki et al. 2003; J. M. Gastier, unpublished results).

No functional copy of *STAG3* is predicted at 7q11.23. *STAG3* itself lies distal to the WBS region, at 7q22, although at least five pseudogenes are known, three of them in the WBS duplicons (Pezzi et al. 2000). *POM121* sequences are present in the distal telomeric duplicon and flanking the centromeric duplicon, but we do not yet know whether any of the copies correspond to the actual POM121 gene. The *POM121* story is further complicated by the presence of fusion transcripts between *POM121* and *ZP3* (Kipersztok et al. 1995), which seem to map distal to the WBS deletion region (DeSilva et al. 2002; L. R. Osborne, unpublished observations), and the identification of numerous *POM121*-like sequences located throughout the genome (GenBank, www.ncbi .nlm.nih.gov/Genbank/GenbankSearch.html). Further analysis is needed to determine the exact number, location, and orientation of POM121 genes and to establish whether any of the copies in the WBS duplicons are functional. Intriguingly, *POM121*-like sequences are also found in the LCRs that flank the velocardiofacial syndrome deletion region on chromosome 22q11.2 (Edelmann et al. 1999a).

NSUN5 has three copies—designated *NSUN5A, NSUN5B,* and *NSUN5C*

—one in each C block, flanked by *FKBP6* and *POM121* sequences (Doll and Grzeschik 2001; Merla et al. 2002). Each copy is transcribed, with the largest predicted protein translation coming from *NSUN5A*, but whether any protein products are actually generated from these genes is still unknown. In the case of *GTF2I*, it has been shown that although the pseudogenes are transcribed, protein is translated only from the functional telomeric copy, which also has a unique N-terminus that is not present in the pseudogenes (Pérez Jurado et al. 1998).

The gene clusters consist of numerous, highly similar genes that have homology to the mismatch repair gene *PMS2* (Nicolaides et al. 1995). They are named *PMS2*-like genes (*PMS2L*), and clusters are also present in at least two other regions of chromosome 7: 7q11.22 and 7q22 (Osborne et al. 1997a). The high similarity of these genes makes it difficult to determine the exact number of copies at a given location, and it is unclear whether they are all transcribed—although many are known to be (Horii et al. 1994; Nicolaides et al. 1995).

Given the repetitive nature of the DNA surrounding the common deletion, the precise mapping of deletion breakpoints, which lie in the duplicons, in individual WBS patients is difficult, but the common breakpoints most often lie in the B blocks of sequence that span approximately 120 kb of DNA (Valero et al. 2000; Peoples et al. 2000; Bayés et al. 2003). The breakpoints almost always lie in the centromeric and medial B-block copies but are occasionally seen in the corresponding A blocks (Bayés et al. 2003) (fig. 2.2). Studies of deletion size in patients with WBS have shown that a polymorphic marker D7S489A, located distal to *GTF2I*, usually lies outside the deleted region (Pérez Jurado et al. 1996, 1998; Y. Q. Wu et al. 1998) but was deleted in a small subset of patients (Robinson et al. 1996; Baumer et al. 1998; M. S. Wang et al. 1999).

The B block itself is comprised of exons 13 to 35 of the GTF2I gene, a complete copy of *NCF1*, plus *GTF2IRD2* (*GTF2I* repeat domain containing protein 2), a third member of the *GTF2I* gene family (the second member, *GTF2IRD1*, lies in the common deletion and is present in a single copy only). *GTF2I* has twelve exons at its proximal end that are unique to the functional copy, whereas the pseudogenes have a different 5' end, as if during duplication the repeat unit was juxtaposed onto a transcribed element (also present at 7q22) that forms the first exon of *GTF2IP1* and *GTF2IP2*. The blocks represent 120 kb of continuous homology that is more than 98% identical at the nucleotide level and contains actively transcribed genes. Both the high homology and the high level of transcription from the duplicons may contribute to the frequency of rearrangement in this region. It has been suggested that meiotic homologous recombination requires at least 300 to 500 bp of sequence identity (Reiter et al. 1998) and that the open chromatin formation of actively transcribed regions may facilitate the process (T. C. Wu

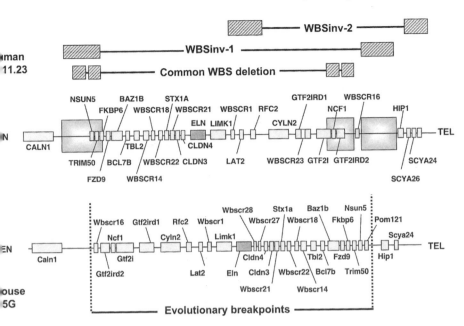

Fig. 2.2. The WBS deletion region at chromosome 7q11.23 in human and 5G in mouse. The WBS deletion region is shown, with known genes represented by boxes and the repetitive duplicons by large shaded boxes flanking the region in human, but not in mouse. The only gene definitely linked to the WBS phenotype, elastin (*ELN*), is shown with darker shading. In human, the common deletion and inversion breakpoints are shown above the 7q11.23 region, with hatched boxes representing the areas to which the breakpoints have been narrowed. In mouse, the region is in the opposite orientation, although flanking regions are in the same orientation; the evolutionary inversion breakpoints are indicated.

and Lichten 1994). Because the similarity of the DNA sequence, not the nature of the sequence itself, is thought to mediate unequal recombination, the breakpoints are unlikely to occur at exactly the same nucleotides in the B block, but there could be a recombination hotspot. A 557 bp hotspot has been associated with the Charcot-Marie-Tooth disease type 1A / hereditary neuropathy with liability to pressure palsies rearrangements (Reiter et al. 1998) and a 2 kb hotspot with the deletions sometimes seen in patients with neurofibromatosis type 1 (López-Correa et al. 2001). In WBS, through analysis of site-specific nucleotide differences between the different copies, a cluster of breakpoints has been narrowed to a 12 kb region in the B block, but further delineation might be impossible because of extremely high sequence homology between the B blocks (Bayés et al. 2003). In approximately 5% of WBS deletions, the breakpoints lie in the centromeric and medial A blocks rather than in the B blocks. These deletions also include *NCF1*, as mentioned earlier, and *GTF2IRD2*, but there is no apparent difference in the presentation of the phenotype in these individuals (Tipney et al. 2004).

The WBS Region in Other Species

The WBS region at 7q11.23 has a region of conserved synteny at the distal end of mouse chromosome 5, which has become the focus of intense study. Initially, several of the genes identified from human 7q11.23 were mapped to mouse chromosome 5G by genetic mapping approaches, but their order along the chromosome was not known (Wydner et al. 1994; Y. K. Wang et al. 1998; Paperna et al. 1998; Pérez Jurado et al. 1999; de Luis et al. 2000). More recently, the Human Genome Project and accompanying sequencing of the mouse genome have allowed the assembly of clone contigs across both regions and a direct comparison of the DNA sequences between species (De-Silva et al. 1999, 2002; Doyle et al. 2000; Martindale et al. 2000; Valero et al. 2000; Bayarsaihan et al. 2002). The region of synteny on mouse chromosome 5 is highly conserved, with each of the genes present in human also present in mouse, except one, WBSCR23. Evidence of this particular gene was found in sequences generated from apes but not those from Old World monkeys or other evolutionarily more distant species (Merla et al. 2002). The presence of a primate-specific gene is intriguing, and it is tempting to speculate that such a gene might play a major role in a disorder that affects such essentially human characteristics as personality and language. The predicted WBSCR23 gene product, however, bears no resemblance to known proteins, and its expression seems to be limited to the skin and some internal organs, making its candidacy for involvement in any neurologic aspects of WBS rather unappealing.

Although highly conserved, the human and mouse chromosome regions have striking differences. First, the LCRs on human 7q11.23 are not found on mouse 5G. The functional genes, along with pseudogene copies, found in the human duplicons are present only as single-copy genes in the mouse (Gtf2i, Gtf2ird1, Ncf1, Pom121, Trim50, Nsun5, and Fkbp6). The genes that are present at 7q11.23 only as pseudogenes are found not at 5G1 but at the region of synteny with the location of their functional human copy (Pms2, Stag3). Second, the duplicons coincide with the evolutionary breakpoints of an inversion, given that the region between Pom121 and Wbscr16 is in the opposite orientation in the mouse, although the flanking genes, Hip1 and Caln1, are in the same position in relation to the centromere and telomere as on human chromosome 7q11.23 (Valero et al. 2000). This coincidence of LCRs and evolutionary breakpoints has also been reported for the Angelman/Prader-Willi syndromes region of 15q11–q13 (Gimelli et al. 2003).

The high similarity of the human duplicons implies that genomic duplication events occurred around the WBS region, and comparative analysis suggests that these events took place in the primate lineage, some time after the divergence of hominoids and Old World monkeys about twenty-three million years ago. These results are in concordance with those found for other regions of the genome associated with human LCRs, such as those involved in Angelman and Prader-Willi syndromes, velocardiofacial syndrome, and Smith-Magenis syndrome. DNA sequence data from a variety of species, including many primates, are currently being deposited in the public databases, making cross-species comparisons possible at the nucleotide level. Analysis of available sequences, in addition to experimental data, suggests that duplication of parts of the WBS region happened both early and very late in the hominoid lineage (L. Pérez Jurado, unpublished results). Macaques (Old World monkeys), like mice, do not harbor WBS LCRs. In orangutan, block C has already duplicated and is present in three copies; in gorilla, block A has duplicated, but only two copies of block C are present. It is estimated that the original generation of LCRs occurred approximately twelve to sixteen million years ago, just before the beginning of the hominoid speciation.

In our closest ancestor, the chimpanzee, block C is present in three copies and block A in two copies, but block B is still unique, suggesting a duplication of these B block sequences after the divergence of the apes and humans about five million years ago. The rapid change in sequence around the WBS region demonstrates a method for genome variation and evolution that has only recently been appreciated. Such bursts of chromosome rearrangement can move genes into different transcriptional environments or generate new genes by combining sequences that were previously at disparate parts of the chromosome (for a review, see Samonte and Eichler 2002).

Genes in the WBS Critical Region

More than twenty genes have now been shown to lie in the common deletion, but only *ELN* has been definitively shown to contribute to any of the symptoms of WBS. The genes code for proteins that span a large range of cellular functions, including many that are not yet known. Many of those identified have simply been named WBSCR, for *W*illiams-*B*euren *s*yndrome *c*hromosome *r*egion, because of the lack of knowledge about their function. Some of the genes had been previously cloned and were merely mapped to this region (e.g., *STX1A*), whereas others originally carried a WBSCR designation but have since had their official nomenclature changed as more has been discovered about their physiologic or biochemical role (e.g., *WBSCR4* has since become *CYLN2*, for *cy*toplasmic *li*nker 2). Several genes were identified and named by different research groups, which led to some confusion in the WBS research community (e.g., *GTF2IRD1* was also named *MusTRD1, CREAM, WBSCR11, GTF3*, and *BEN*). Because of this confusion, efforts are being made to use the approved nomenclature (as determined by the HUGO Gene Nomenclature Committee, www.gene.ucl.ac.uk/nomenclature) when referring to the genes.

Twenty-two genes lie in the common deletion and have been shown to produce a transcript detectable by Northern blot analysis. In addition, at least four other genes have been predicted from sequence analysis and the identification of expressed sequence tags, but as yet we have no experimental evidence to substantiate their designation as genes (*TRIM50, WBSCR24, WBSCR27, WBSCR28*). Further analysis is needed to determine whether these sequences do represent transcribed genes. Given the availability of both human and mouse sequences, plus the publication of genome sequences from numerous other species including apes, it is unlikely that many other coding genes from the WBS region remain to be found—although there may be noncoding RNAs that have not yet been identified.

The genes of the WBS region are listed in table 2.1, in order from centromere to telomere, with their alternative names, GenBank accession numbers, and associated references. The genes that flank the WBS chromosome region but are not usually deleted are also of interest, because a few individuals have larger than usual deletions and often exhibit a more severe phenotype (see chapter 3). The next gene on the centromeric side, immediately outside the duplicon, is calneuron 1 (*CALN1*), a large gene spanning ~400 kb of genomic DNA sequence, which codes for a brain-specific member of the calmodulin superfamily of calcium binding proteins (Y. Q. Wu et al. 2001). The telomeric side of the common deletion is potentially more interesting because several larger deletions extend in this direction (Mizugishi et al. 1998; Y. Q. Wu et al. 1999; Stock et al. 2003; L. R. Osborne, unpublished results). Immediately adjacent to the most telomeric duplicon is the *H*untingtin *i*nteracting *p*rotein *1* gene (*HIP1*), a cofactor in clathrin-mediated vesicle trafficking (Rao et al. 2002). Targeted mutation of *Hip1* in the mouse revealed that homozygous disruption resulted in defects of the spine, abnormal hematopoiesis, and cataracts (Metzler et al. 2003; Oravecz-Wilson et al. 2004). The heterozygous mice, however, were completely normal, suggesting that *HIP1* is unlikely to be relevant to the additional phenotypes associated with larger WBS deletions, such as seizures or more severe mental retardation.

Here the discussion focuses on genes in the deletion region for which we have little information about the function of their protein product or that are unlikely candidates for involvement in WBS. The likely candidates and their functional analysis are discussed in the next section.

NOL/NOP2/Sun Domain Family Member 5 (NSUN5). This gene has three expressed copies in the WBS region, one in each of the C blocks. *NSUN5A*, which lies in the centromeric LCR, has a predicted protein of 466 amino acids; *NSUN5B* and *NSUN5C* have predicted proteins that are truncated before 200 amino acids (Doll and Grzeschik 2001; Merla et al. 2002).

ble 2.1.
nes Identified in the WBS Chromosome Region at 7q11.23

ne	Aliases	GenBank Accession Number Human	Mouse	References
LN1		NM_031468	NM_021371	Y. Q. Yu et al.
BSCR 17	GALNT9	NM_022479	NM_145218	Merla et al. 2002
M121		NM_172020	NM_148392	Valero et al. 2002
UN5	NOL1R; WBSCR20	NM_018044; NM_148956	NM_145414	Doll and Grzeschik 2001; Merla et al. 2002
IM50	Hs.121647; LOC135892; BF522554	NM_178125	NM_178240	De Silva et al. 2002; Ota et al. 2004
BP6		NM_003602	NM_033571	X. Meng et al. 1998b
D9	FZD3	NM_003508	XM_284144	Y. K. Wang et al. 1997
Z1B	WBSCR9; WSTF	NM_023005; NM_032408	NM_011714	Lu et al. 1998; Peoples et al. 1998
L7B		NM_001707; NM_138707	NM_009745	Jadayel et al. 1998; Meng et al. 1998a
L2	WS-betaTRP	NM_012453; NM_032988	NM_013763	Meng et al. 1998a; Perez-Jurado et al. 1998
BSCR14	WS-bHLH	NM_032951–4; NM_032944	NM_021455	Meng et al. 1998; de Luis et al. 2000
BSCR24		NM_177574	NM_177254	De Silva et al. 2002
BSCR18		NM_032317	NM_025362	Merla et al. 2002
BSCR22		NM_017528	NM_025375	Doll and Grzeschik 2001; Merla et al. 2002
X1A	HPC-1	NM_004603	NM_016801	Osborne et al. 1997
BSCR21		NM_031295	NM_145215	Merla et al. 2002
DN3	RVP1; CPETR2; C7orf1	NM_001306	NM_009902	Paperna et al. 1998
DN4	CPETR1	NM_001305	NM_009903	Paperna et al. 1998
BSCR27		NM_152559	NM_024479	Strausberg et al. 2002
BSCR28		NM_182504	NM_029681	Strausberg et al. 2002
V		NM_000501	NM_007925	Ewart et al. 1993
MK1		NM_002314; NM_016735	NM_010717	Frangiskaskis et al. 1996; Osborne et al. 1996; Tassabehji et al. 1996
BSCR1	EIF4H	NM_022170; NM_031992	NM_033561	Osborne et al. 1996
T2	WBSCR5; WBSCR15; NTAL	NM_022040; NM_032463-4; NM_014146	NM_022964	Martindale et al. 2000; Dolye et al. 2000; Brdicka et al. 2002
C2		NM_002914	NM_020022	Osborne et al. 1996; Peoples et al. 1996
LN2	CLIP-115; WBSCR3/4	NM_003388; NM_032421	NM_009990	Osborne et al. 1996; Hoogneraad et al. 1998
F2IRD1	MusTRD1; WBSCR11; BEN; GTF3; CREAM1	NM_016328; NM_005685	NM_020331	Franke et al. 2000; Osborne et al. 1999; Tassabehji et al. 1999
BSCR23		NM_025042	Not present	Merla et al. 2002
F2I	TFII-I; BAP-135; SPIN	NM_032999–3003; NM_001518	NM_010365	Perez-Juardo et al. 1998
F1	p47phox	NM_000265	NM_010876	Görlach et al. 2002
F2IRD2	GTF2IL	NM_173537; NM_001003795	NM_053266	Tipney et al. 2004; Makeyev et al. 2004
BSCR16	R52511	NM_030798	NM_033572	Merla et al. 2002
1		NM_005338	NM_146001	Kalchman et al. 1997; Wanker et al. 1997

NSUN5A has a mouse orthologue, suggesting it is probably the ancestral gene. The other two genes, which do not have mouse orthologues, seem to have arisen through later duplication events and may not be translated. The NSUN5 protein products show some similarity to NOL1, a proliferation-associated antigen that is thought to play a role in regulation of the cell cycle (Fonagy et al. 1993).

Tripartite Motif-Containing 50 (TRIM50). TRIM50 genes are present in each of the three C blocks of the WBS LCRs. TRIM50A, which lies in the centromeric block, is a predicted protein that belongs to the large tripartite motif protein family, members of which typically are composed of three zinc binding domains, a RING, unique B-box type 1 and B-box type 2 domains, followed by a coiled-coil region. TRIM proteins use homomultimerization to identify specific cell compartments (Reymond et al. 2001).

B-Cell CLL/Lymphoma 7B (BCL7B). This is a member of the BCL7 family of proteins, which share an N-terminal motif (Jadayel et al. 1998). The first member (*BCL7A*) was cloned as part of a three-way translocation in a Burkitt's lymphoma cell line and shows homology to the actin binding protein caldesmon. No function has been shown for any of the three family members.

Transducin-Beta Like 2 (TBL2). This gene is predominantly expressed in testis, skeletal muscle, heart, and some endocrine tissues. It codes for a protein of unknown function, containing four putative β-transducin (WD40) repeats (X. Meng et al. 1998a; Pérez Jurado et al. 1999). Other proteins that contain these highly conserved domains are involved in the regulation of a variety of processes, and haploinsufficiency for some is known to cause developmental disorders (e.g., *LIS1* in lissencephaly) (Reiner et al. 1993).

Williams-Beuren Syndrome Chromosome Region 18 (WBSCR18). This intronless gene codes for a member of the DNAJ molecular chaperone family (Merla et al. 2002). These chaperones are protein cofactors shown to minimize the aggregation of newly synthesized proteins (Fink 1999).

Williams-Beuren Syndrome Chromosome Region 22 (WBSCR22). This gene codes for a protein with a predicted S-adenosyl-L-methionine binding motif, usually found in the DNA methylation enzymes, the methyl transferases (Doll and Grzeschik 2001; Merla et al. 2002).

Williams-Beuren Syndrome Chromosome Region 21 (WBSCR21). The WBSCR21 gene codes for a protein predicted to contain an alpha/beta hydrolase fold. This gene seems to generate several ubiquitously expressed, alternatively spliced transcripts, but it is not known whether these are translated into proteins (Merla et al. 2002).

The Claudins (*CLDN3* and *CLDN4*). The claudins are members of a large family of proteins that constitute tight junction strands (Morita et al. 1999). They are necessary for cell-to-cell contacts and are also responsible for the barrier function of epithelial and endothelial tissues. CLDN3 and CLDN4 are unique in this family in that they can also bind *Clostridium perfringens* enterotoxin, with subsequent triggering of toxin-mediated cytolysis (Sonoda et al. 1999). These genes are highly expressed in liver and kidney, and *CLDN3* has also been identified in skin (Tebbe et al. 2002) and possibly in retinal pigment epithelial cilia (Nishiyama et al. 2002).

Williams-Beuren Syndrome Chromosome Region 1 (*WBSCR1*). This ubiquitously expressed gene (Osborne et al. 1996) encodes eukaryotic initiation factor 4H (eIF4H). The factor eIF4H interacts with eIF4A, a helicase that unwinds secondary structure in the 5'-untranslated region of mRNAs, facilitating the binding of the translational machinery. It is postulated that eIF4H stabilizes conformational changes in eIF4A that occur during RNA binding, ATP hydrolysis, and RNA duplex unwinding (Richter et al. 1999; Rogers et al. 2001). As has recently been shown, eIF4H also can form a complex with a herpes simplex virus protein (virion host shutoff, Vhs) (Feng et al. 2001). Vhs accelerates mRNA decay and so helps determine the levels and kinetics of viral and cellular gene expression. It has a preference for the 5' ends of mRNA, and its interaction with eIF4H most likely helps target the RNase to regions of translation initiation (Feng et al. 2001; Everly et al. 2002).

Linker of Activation of T Cells Family Member 2 (*LAT2*). The LAT2 gene was identified from the WBS deletion region as *WBSCR5*, a gene expressed at low levels in many tissues, although more abundant in mast cells (Doyle et al. 2000; Martindale et al. 2000). LAT2 was also independently identified as non-T cell activation linker (NTAL), a structural and possibly also functional homologue of LAT (Brdicka et al. 2002). LAT is an essential molecule for activation of T lymphocytes through their antigen-specific T-cell receptor. LAT2 is expressed in B lymphocytes, natural killer cells, monocytes, and mast cells but not in resting T lymphocytes. Mice lacking *LAT2* do not show overt changes in B-cell development, but their mast cells were found to be hyperresponsive to stimulation via the FcepsilonRI, suggesting the LAT2 negatively regulates mast cell function (Zhu et al. 2004; Y. Wang et al. 2005).

Replication Factor C Subunit 2 (*RFC2*). The RFC2 gene (Osborne et al. 1996; Peoples et al. 1996) corresponds to the 40 kDa ATP binding subunit of replication factor C, also called activator 1, which is an auxiliary factor for the DNA polymerases delta and epsilon (Pan et al. 1993). The RFC complex plays an essential role in both DNA replication and cell checkpoint function (Schmidt et al. 2001), and it has been postulated that a reduction in the availability of RFC2 could lead to a decrease in the amount of RFC complex and subsequently affect DNA replication efficiency, possibly contributing to symptoms such as growth deficiency (Osborne et al. 1996; Peoples et al. 1996).

Williams-Beuren Syndrome Chromosome Region 23 (WBSCR23). This intronless transcript is located in intron 9 of *GTF2IRD1* and on the same strand. Interestingly, this gene is present in the genomic sequence from chimpanzee but not in the sequence from Old World monkey (baboon) or from even more evolutionarily distant species such as mouse, cat, pig, or cow (Merla et al. 2002).

Neutrophil Cytosolic Factor 1 (NCF1). The NCF1 gene product is a component of the phagocyte NADPH oxidase system, mutations of which cause chronic granulomatous disease, an autosomal, recessively inherited disorder of impaired superoxide production (OMIM [Online Mendelian Inheritance in Man catalogue number] 233700). *NCF1* mutation carriers show no phenotype, and, consequently, hemizygosity of this gene does not contribute to the WBS phenotype. The presence of at least two *NCF1* pseudogenes at 7q11.23, however, is thought to be a factor in the high frequency of a GT deletion in exon 2, through either gene conversion or, more likely, partial crossing over between gene and pseudogene (Roesler et al. 2000; Vazquez et al. 2001).

General Transcription Factor 2 I Repeat Domain Containing 2 (GTF2IRD2). This was identified as a gene with similarity to *GTF2I* and *GTF2IRD1* (discussed below) (Tipney et al. 2004; Makeyev et al. 2004). The protein product shares most similarity in structure with GTF2I, from which it seems to have been generated through a duplication event. As mentioned previously, *GTF2IRD2* is sometimes included in the WBS deletion but with no obvious phenotypic effect (Tipney et al. 2004).

Williams-Beuren Syndrome Chromosome Region 16 (WBSCR16). The WBSCR16 gene lies in a unique stretch of sequence sandwiched between the medial and telomeric duplicons (Valero et al. 2000). It encodes a protein with similarity to the RCC1 (regulator of chromosome condensation) G-exchanging factor (Merla et al. 2002).

Functional Analysis of Candidate Genes

Efforts to link individual genes with specific parts of the clinical picture of Williams-Beuren syndrome have followed two paths: first, the study of individuals with atypical deletions of the WBS region, as discussed in chapter 3, and second, the study of the protein products themselves, sometimes through the generation of animal models with deficiencies in specific genes.

Not all genes from the region have been studied, but those that have are discussed here.

Elastin (*ELN*)

The elastin gene lies approximately at the center of the deletion and is the only gene that has been unequivocally linked to any aspect of the WBS phenotype, causing supravalvular aortic stenosis (SVAS) and other vascular stenoses (Curran et al. 1993; Tassabehji et al. 1997; D. Y. Li et al. 1997). Elastin is synthesized as a soluble precursor polypeptide (tropoelastin), which is secreted and then self-assembles into a highly insoluble network of elastic fibers on a scaffold of microfibrils, imparting flexibility and elasticity to the tissues where it is expressed (Uitto et al. 1991). It comprises the bulk of the elastic fibers found in many tissues, including skin, lungs, ligaments, and large blood vessels. Although a reduction in elastin expression is known to cause pathology, the mechanism by which this leads to obstructive vascular disease is only now being understood.

Elastin has traditionally been regarded as a structural protein, but recent experiments in both mice and humans have revealed that it also plays a role in the regulation of smooth muscle cell proliferation. Mouse mutants were generated through targeting of the *Eln* locus by homologous recombination (D. Y. Li et al. 1998a), and the homozygous null mice ($-/-$) died at about postnatal day 4 as a result of obstructive arterial disease. The arterial lumens were obliterated during the third trimester of fetal development, when elastin starts to be highly expressed because of the increased proliferation and reorganization of smooth muscle cells. The heterozygous animals were also found to have an increase in smooth muscle in their arteries, consistent with the finding in humans affected by either WBS or isolated SVAS (D. Y. Li et al. 1998b).

More recent data suggest that this increase in smooth muscle cell proliferation is due to the decrease in elastin synthesis associated with disruption of the elastin gene (Urban et al. 2002). An increase in smooth muscle cell proliferation was seen on co-culturing with fibroblasts from individuals with SVAS or WBS but could be normalized by the addition of exogenous insoluble elastin, suggesting that elastin is an important regulator of cellular proliferation. In a comparison of ELN mRNA and protein levels among individuals with WBS, individuals with SVAS, and controls, elastin expression and deposition in SVAS fibroblasts was roughly half that of controls, whereas in WBS fibroblasts it was only 15% of control levels, despite equal mRNA stability. This finding suggests a possible gene interaction between *ELN* and another gene(s) in the common WBS deletion that exerts transcriptional control over *ELN*. Despite the large discrepancy in levels of elastin synthesis, there does not seem to be a significant difference in the cardiovascular manifestations between SVAS and WBS, although further detailed clinical evaluation is warranted.

FK506 Binding Protein 6 (*FKBP6*)

FK506 binding proteins (FKBP), also known as immunophilins, were originally identified as binding partners for the immunosuppressive drug FK506. They comprise an FK506 binding domain and three protein-protein interaction domains and are thought to act as chaperones to stabilize protein complexes (Nair et al. 1997). *FKBP6*, which was cloned from the WBS deletion region in 1998, was originally reported to have a wide expression profile (X. Meng et al. 1998b), but in the mouse it is restricted to the testis and ovary (Crackower et al. 2003). The only human expressed sequence tags that have been identified are from the testis, suggesting that *FKBP6* may also be gonad-specific in humans.

A mouse deficient in *Fkbp6* was recently generated through homologous recombination (Crackower et al. 2003); the resultant males were aspermic, with hypogonadism and absence of normal pachytene chromosomes. The FKBP6 protein was shown to specifically localize to the synaptonemal complex during meiosis, and the *Fkbp6$^{-/-}$* males had a major disruption in chromosomal stability in meiotic cells, as evidenced by the accumulation of DNA repair proteins (RAD51/DMC1), leading to crisis and meiotic failure. A natural rat mutant (TT) with a histologic phenotype similar to that of the *Fkbp6$^{-/-}$* mouse also exists (Ikadai et al. 1992), and the responsible recessive allele (*as*) was mapped to rat chromosome 12, the region syntenic with the WBS deletion (Noguchi et al. 1999; Bayés et al. 2001). Analysis of *Fkbp6* in this mutant revealed an absence of protein and a deletion of the last coding exon of the gene, thereby implicating *Fkbp6* in this infertile rat mutant (Crackower et al. 2003).

Reduced fertility is not a phenotype known to be associated with WBS (Pober and Dykens 1996), and indeed a father with WBS with deleted *FKBP6* was recently reported (Metcalfe et al. 2005). Also, the absence of any abnormality in mice and rats heterozygous for a mutation in *Fkbp6* suggests there is no haploinsufficiency for *FKBP6*. Given that no other phenotypic abnormalities are present in the animals deficient for *Fkbp6*, this gene is unlikely to play a causative role in WBS.

Frizzled 9 (*FZD9*)

The frizzled 9 gene is one of several mammalian homologues of a gene (*frizzled*) originally cloned from *Drosophila* (Y. K. Wang et al. 1997). The frizzled proteins are Wnt receptors that share a cysteine-rich extracellular domain and seven transmembrane domains. On binding to Wnt proteins, frizzleds function in beta-catenin/T-cell factor (TCF) signaling, a pathway involved in neural development, cell polarity generation, cell fate specification, tumorigenesis, and the self-renewal ability of stem cells. Analysis of *Fzd9* in the developing mouse showed expression in the neural tube, skeletal muscle precursors, craniofacial regions, and nephric ducts, and Fzd9 transcript was also seen in adult heart, brain, testis, and skeletal muscle (Y. K. Wang et al. 1999).

Replacement gene targeting has been used to generate mice without a functional *Fzd9* gene (E. A. Ranheim et al. 2005). These mice show early mortality (40% die before they are six months old), enlarged lymph nodes, and an increase in both spleen and thymus weight compared with littermates. Analysis of the bone marrow showed a severe depletion in the number of pro-B cells, particularly two subtypes named the B and C Hardy subsets, in which the heavy chain is expressed and the cells are undergoing clonal expansion before light chain rearrangement. These results suggest a role for frizzled 9 signaling in lymphoid development, possibly at a stage when B cells undergo self-renewal before further differentiation. Mice heterozygous for *Fzd9* were completely normal, so a major role in the WBS phenotype seems unlikely.

LIM Kinase 1 (*LIMK1*)

LIM kinase 1 (Mizuno et al. 1994) is a LIM domain–containing protein expressed at high levels in the early mouse embryo, the developing nervous system, and the adult brain (Cheng and Robertson 1995; Pröschel et al. 1995). LIMK1 is part of the Rho GTPase signaling pathway that induces reorganization of the actin cytoskeleton during cell morphogenesis and motility and, in the case of neurons, during neurite and axonal growth. LIMK1 has the ability to phosphorylate and thus inactivate cofilin, a protein that mediates the depolymerization of actin in the cytoskeleton (Arber et al. 1998; N. Yang et al. 1998). Several components of the Rho GTPase signaling pathway have already been implicated in X-linked mental retardation, including oligophrenin (Billuart et al. 1998), p21-associated kinase 3 (Allen et al. 1998), GDP dissociation inhibitor 1 (D'Adamo et al. 1998), Rac/Cdc42 guanine nucleotide exchange factor 6 (Kutsche et al. 2000), and the fragile X mental retardation protein (Schenck et al. 2003).

These findings make *LIMK1* an attractive candidate in the neurologic phenotype of WBS. Indeed, *LIMK1* has been implicated as necessary for proper visuospatial constructive cognition (see chapter 3) (Frangiskakis et al. 1996). Unfortunately, genotype-phenotype correlations for *LIMK1* are not consistent with the finding that some individuals who have a *LIMK1* deletion have visuospatial deficits and others do not.

Limk1 knockout mice have been generated, and although they show grossly normal development of the nervous system, they have abnormalities in the dendritic spine structure of neurons in the hippocampus and accompanying changes in both pre- and postsynaptic function (Y. Meng et al. 2002). Dendritic spines make up the majority of the synaptic connections in the hippocampus, and their formation has been shown to be highly dependent on actin filament reorganization. Indeed, it is surprising that neuronal development in the $Limk1^{-/-}$ mice is relatively normal, given that actin dynamics play such an important role in neuronal growth and guidance. Investigators have hypothesized that another LIMK, $Limk2$, may be compensating for loss of $Limk1$, because the two genes are coexpressed in some regions of the brain (Mori et al. 1997).

The $Limk1^{-/-}$ mice also showed altered behavioral responses, including increased locomotor activity and impaired spatial learning (Y. Meng et al. 2002). The mice were tested on the Morris water maze. In this test, the mice swim to a visible platform and subsequently learn to locate the platform when it is submerged at the same position, using visual and spatial cues. When the platform is then moved, still submerged, the mice automatically swim to the learned, original position of the platform and have to locate the new platform position by trial and error. Although the $Limk1^{-/-}$ mice performed well in the initial stages of the test, they took longer to find the repositioned platform and did not show much improvement on subsequent tests. The basis of this spatial learning deficit is not clear, and further studies are required to determine whether the underlying problem is related to the difficulty of the task or other factors such as "overlearning" the initial platform position.

The results from these mice are exciting, but many questions remain. Perhaps the most tantalizing is whether the heterozygous mice exhibit similar morphologic, electrophysiologic, or behavioral abnormalities—something that was not addressed by Y. Meng and colleagues (2002). It would also be interesting to see whether WBS patients have altered dendritic spine morphology, as has been reported for other neurologic disorders including Down syndrome, Rett syndrome, and fragile X syndrome (Kaufmann and Moser 2000). Y. Meng et al.'s study does add weight to the argument that $LIMK1$ hemizygosity plays a role in some aspects of WBS, but, as always, translating behavioral abnormalities from mice to humans must be done with caution.

Cytoplasmic Linker 2 (*CYLN2*)

The CYLN2 gene codes for the cytoplasmic linker protein of 115 kDa, CLIP-115 (De Zeeuw et al. 1997). This is a member of a family of nonmotor microtubule binding proteins called cytoplasmic linkers, which contain homologous microtubule binding motifs. Other members include the mammalian CLIPS, CLIP-170, which associates with the mitotic spindle (Dujardin et al. 1998), and CLIPR-59, which localizes to the Golgi complex (Perez et al. 2002); and the *Drosophila* CLIPs, p150[Glued] (Holzbaur et al. 1991) and CLIP-

190 (Lantz and Miller 1998). These microtubule binding proteins function alongside the kinesin and dynein-related motor proteins to organize the microtubule network in the cell and allow the coordinated movement and localization of organelles. CLIP-115 was initially identified as a protein that bound to a brain-specific organelle of unknown function, the dendritic lamellar body (De Zeeuw et al. 1995); however, analysis of mice lacking CLIP-115 revealed unaffected distribution of these organelles, suggesting that CLIP-115 is not involved in their transport in the cell (Hoogenraad et al. 2002).

Although its role is still unclear, strong expression of *CYLN2* in specific regions of the brain, such as the hippocampus, amygdala, and cerebellum, suggests that hemizygosity for *CYLN2* may contribute to the neurologic features of WBS. In an attempt to clarify the role of CLIP-115 in WBS, Hoogenraad and colleagues (2002) generated mice that were either heterozygous or null for the *Cyln2* gene, and these animals exhibited several features that are hallmarks of WBS. Both $Cyln2^{-/-}$ and $Cyln2^{+/-}$ mice showed mild growth retardation during the first weeks of postnatal development, and this retardation was sustained into adulthood in females but not in males. Neither $Cyln2^{-/-}$ nor $Cyln2^{+/-}$ mice showed gross brain abnormalities, but there were subtle differences in volume of the corpus callosum in the null mice. To test the specific functions of different regions of the brain where CLIP-115 is expressed, the investigators used a variety of behavioral tests. Both $Cyln2^{-/-}$ and $Cyln2^{+/-}$ mice showed impaired motor coordination as measured by running on a wheel and a rotating rod but not by other tests designed to look at different aspects of motor behavior, indicating abnormalities of the cerebellar hemispheres and the paravermis. Furthermore, contextual and cued fear-conditioning experiments revealed that amygdala function was unaffected but hippocampal function was impaired, as was further supported by measurement of synaptic plasticity in hippocampal slices.

The precise impact of reduced levels of CLIP-115 at the cellular level needs further investigation. In cultured fibroblasts from the null mice, microtubule dynamics were not perturbed, but an accumulation of CLIP-170 and dynactin proteins was noted at the plus ends of growing microtubules, where CLIP-115 usually binds. CLIP-170 has previously been shown to interact with LIS1, the lissencephaly gene product (Tai et al. 2002; Coquelle et al. 2002), so a reduction in CLIP-115 could cause brain abnormalities indirectly, through the alteration of CLIP-170 or other components of the dynein motor.

Thus, hemizygosity for CLIP-115 may indeed contribute to some of the symptoms of WBS, notably growth retardation and problems in motor coordination, although whether the same deficits seen in the mouse will manifest in humans remains to be established. Detailed study of individuals who have smaller than usual deletions of the WBS region and are missing *CYLN2* may help confirm that this gene is indeed dosage sensitive. It is also possible that the combined hemizygous deletion of genes involved in the regulation of both the actin (*LIMK1*) and microtubule (*CYLN2*) cytoskeletons may have a greater effect on the growth and differentiation of neurons. The generation of mice that are heterozygous for both genes will help clarify whether a combinatorial effect exists.

Williams-Beuren Syndrome Chromosome Region 14 (*WBSCR14*)

Williams-Beuren syndrome chromosome region 14 contains a basic helix-loop-helix-leucine-zipper motif (bHLHZip) and a bipartite nuclear localization signal, suggesting that it functions as a transcription factor (X. Meng et al. 1998a; de Luis et al. 2000). The helix-loop-helix (HLH) and leucine zipper (Zip) motifs enable protein dimerization before DNA binding (via the basic region) to the E-box upstream sequence of genes (Ferre-D'Amare et al. 1993). WBSCR14 has been identified as a member of a specific subclass of bHLHZip transcription factors, the Myc/Max/Mad superfamily (Cairo et al. 2001) and was shown to bind another member of this family, TCFL4 (MLX) (Billin et al. 1999). Five alternatively spliced human WBSCR14 transcripts have been identified, some of which encode proteins lacking the bHLHZip domains necessary for dimerization and subsequent DNA binding, thus expanding the potential functions for this gene (Cairo et al. 2001).

WBSCR14 has been linked to the regulation of lipogenic enzymes (Uyeda et al. 2002). A high-carbohydrate diet induces transcription of more than fifteen genes involved in the metabolic conversion of glucose to fat, including enzymes of glycolysis and lipogenesis, promoting long-term storage of carbohydrates as triglycerides. The rat orthologue of WBSCR14 (ChREBP) is expressed under a high-glucose diet and inhibited under a high-fat diet and up-regulates these genes, whereas a high-fat diet inhibits ChREBP and slows down glucose utilization (Uyeda et al. 2002; Stoeckman et al. 2004). Thus, WBSCR14 is able to control transcription of lipogenic enzyme genes in response to nutritional and hormonal inputs and may play an important role in disease states such as diabetes, obesity, and hypertension. This suggests that there may be a correlation between deletion of *WBSCR14* and the endocrine abnormalities reported in many individuals with WBS. Investigators have also shown that the action of the WBSCR14:Mlx complex is regulated in part by its association with several 14-3-3 protein isoforms that can actively export it from the nucleus and prevent its participating in transcriptional activation (Merla et al. 2004).

Bromodomain Adjacent to a Leucine Zipper 1 B (*BAZ1B*)

Bromodomain adjacent to a leucine zipper 1B (Lu et al. 1998; Peoples et al. 1998) encodes a novel protein that contains a PHD zinc finger and a bromodomain: two domains commonly found in transcriptional regulators. Expressed throughout the developing and adult human, this protein has recently been shown to be a constituent of two distinct types of chromatin remodeling complex.

BAZ1B was initially identified as part of the WICH (*WSTF-ISWI chromatin remodeling*) complex (Bozhenok et al. 2002). In mouse cells, the WICH complex was shown to specifically associate with pericentromeric heterochromatin, a region of the chromosome thought to be important for maintaining chromosome stability (Bozhenok et al. 2002). Heterochromatin is extremely condensed and consists of hypermethylated DNA and hypoacetylated histones, forming a transcriptionally repressive environment. It is postulated that such condensed chromatin requires special mechanisms and remodeling complexes to allow its replication and assembly, and WICH seems to be such a complex. Whether WICH participates in the establishment of an active origin of replication or plays a role in the postreplication organization of the chromatin is unclear, but its ability to arrange irregular chromatin into a nucleosome array in vitro points to the latter (Bozhenok et al. 2002) The WICH complex is unique in that it binds stably to metaphase chromosomes during mitosis, whereas other chromatin remodeling complexes have been shown to associate with replicating chromosomes during meiosis.

As deduced from its role in heterochromatin remodeling, the hemizygous deletion of *BAZ1B* may affect chromosome stability. Haploinsufficiency of other chromatin remodeling factors has been shown to cause at least two other mental retardation syndromes—X-linked alpha thalassemia with mental retardation (mutations in *ATRX*) (Gibbons et al. 1995) and Rett syndrome (mutations in *MECP2*) (Amir et al. 1999)—but the role of BAZ1B in the cognitive aspects of WBS has still to be determined.

More recently, BAZ1B was found to be a constituent of a large ATP-dependent chromatin remodeling complex named WINAC (*WSTF including nucleosome assembly complex*), which has at least thirteen components (Kitagawa et al. 2003). WINAC was postulated to function during DNA replication, because DNA synthesis was found to be lowered after perturbation of expression of different components of the complex by RNA interference. BAZ1B binds the vitamin D receptor (VDR), where it seems to act as a platform on which the other complex components can then assemble. The VDR is required for the activation of vitamin D–responsive genes. WINAC is thought to bind the vitamin D–responsive elements (VDREs) of promoters via VDR and to rearrange the nucleosome array, so facilitating the binding of additional regulatory complexes.

Studies in WBS fibroblasts showed that VDR and WINAC targeting to VDREs was lower than in normal fibroblasts and that the transactivating function of VDR was impaired (Kitagawa et al. 2003). These deficits could be rescued by overexpression of *BAZ1B*. Impaired VDR function could account for the defects in vitamin D metabolism and the transient hypercalcemia seen in WBS.

Syntaxin 1A (*STX1A*)

Syntaxin 1A is part of the vesicle docking and fusion machinery involved in neurotransmitter release at the presynaptic membrane in neurons (Bennett et al. 1992). It forms a trimeric protein complex, with SNAP-25 and VAMP (Sollner et al. 1993), which has been shown to be essential for neurotransmitter release in *Drosophila* (Schulze et al. 1995). The components of this complex are collectively called SNARE proteins, and the current view of SNARE-mediated exocytosis is that the SNARE proteins on the donor vesicle (v-SNARE: VAMP) and the target membrane (t-SNAREs: SNAP-25 and STX1A) interact to form a stable complex that provides the energy to drive membrane fusion (Weber et al. 1998).

To date, no mouse models with reduced levels of STX1A have been generated, which may reflect a particular dosage sensitivity in the developing mouse. A naturally occurring mouse mutant with one copy of the SNAP-25 gene deleted is hyperactive (Hess et al. 1996), suggesting that hemizygosity for *STX1A* may contribute to the attention deficit–hyperactivity seen in ~70% of individuals with WBS. In addition, an association between *SNAP-25* polymorphisms and attention deficit hyperactivity disorder has been shown in humans (Barr et al. 2000; Mill et al. 2002), but no evidence for such an association has been reported for *STX1A*. Y. Q. Wu and colleagues (2002) searched for alterations in the STX1A gene that might account for the symptoms seen in patients with WBS-like features and no deletion, but they did not find any.

It is possible that STX1A does contribute to the WBS clinical spectrum but that its role is not in the brain. The basic components of the insulin exocytotic machinery in pancreatic islet beta cells closely resemble those that mediate neurotransmitter release, and several lines of evidence point toward a major role for STX1A in insulin secretion and glucose tolerance. First, rat models of diabetes (*fa/fa* and GK) have reduced levels of STX1A and other SNARE proteins, rendering them unable to enhance insulin secretion during high glycemic demand (such as glucose challenge) (Chan et al. 1999; Nagamatsu et al. 1999). Second, as discussed in chapter 6, there have been several reported cases of diabetes in adults with WBS, and recent studies have shown that adults with WBS have an increased frequency of elevated glucose levels on glucose challenge (Cherniske et al. 2004). Third, mouse models with altered levels of STX1A also exhibit impaired glucose tolerance and impaired insulin secretion (Lam et al. 2005). Finally, a *STX1A* genetic polymorphism was found to correlate with an earlier age at onset and with insulin requirement in type 2 diabetes (Tsunoda et al. 2001). Together these observations suggest that hemizygosity for *STX1A* may be causing impaired glucose tolerance in WBS by altering insulin secretion and the beta-cell response to hyperglycemia.

General Transcription Factor 2 I Gene Family (GTF2I and GTF2IRD1)

GTF2I is interrupted by the common telomeric deletion breakpoint and has at least two accompanying pseudogenes present in the WBS duplicons (Pérez Jurado et al. 1998). *GTF2I* codes for TFII-I, a protein with six HLH motifs termed I-repeats (R1 through R6), which mediate protein interactions, and an N-terminal leucine zipper and basic region, both of which are essential for DNA binding (Cheriyath and Roy 2001). TFII-I can act both as a basal transcription factor, which binds and functions through a core promoter element called initiator (Inr), and as an activator, which binds an unrelated upstream element called the E-box (Roy et al. 1991). TFII-I requires activation by phosphorylation, and this phosphorylation event can be mediated by extracellular signals through cell surface receptors, which implies that TFII-I participates in receptor-mediated signal transduction events (Novina et al. 1998). Indeed, this is exactly the case in B cells, where TFII-I—which was originally identified as BAP-135 (*B*runo's tyrosine kinase (Btk) *a*ssociated *p*rotein *135* kDa) (W. Yang and Desiderio 1997)—is tyrosine phosphorylated by Btk on immunoglobulin receptor cross-linking (Novina et al. 1999).

TFII-I exists in at least four isoforms generated by alternative splicing of two exons (A and B) between R1 and R2 (Cheriyath and Roy 2000). These isoforms have been termed α, β, γ, and Δ, and two additional, unpublished isoforms have also been reported (Roy 2001). The expression of each isoform is different, with the γ-isoform predominantly in neurons (Pérez Jurado et al. 1998), the β-isoform expressed at higher levels in mice than in humans (Cheriyath and Roy 2000), and the α-isoform not expressed at all in mice (Y. K. Wang et al. 1998). These isoform-specific expression patterns suggest that, although the isoforms are structurally similar, their functions may be nonredundant. This is supported by the observation that the isoforms participate in both homomeric and heteromeric interactions, providing an attractive model for a sophisticated system of gene regulation (Cheriyath and Roy 2000). The combination of TFII-I isoforms may be determined by different extracellular signals, may be spatially and temporally controlled, and may regulate the entry of TFII-I complexes into the nucleus, allowing differential gene expression (for a review, see Roy 2001). Interestingly, the expression of TFII-I in the mouse brain is widespread during development but is restricted to neurons in adulthood, with highest levels of expression observed in cerebellar Purkinje cells and in hippocampal interneurons (Danoff et al. 2004).

GTF2IRD1 (*GTF2I* repeat *d*omain protein *1*) was identified by three groups through use of positional cloning (*WBSCR11*, Osborne et al. 1999; *GTF2IRD1*, Franke et al. 1999; *GTF3*, Tassabehji et al. 1999), as an activator of troponin I in muscle (MusTRD1, O'Mahoney et al. 1998), as a retinoblastoma protein associated nuclear factor (CREAM1, Yan et al. 2000), and as a protein that binds the *Hoxc8* early enhancer in mouse (BEN, Bayarsaihan and Ruddle 2000). It is structurally similar to TFII-I, with five I-repeats in the human and six in the mouse protein, a leucine zipper domain, and a basic region. It is presumed that these two genes—*GTF2I* and *GTF2IRD1*—arose by duplication of a common ancestor, although the exact time of this event is unclear. Interestingly, a search of the available DNA sequences revealed that *GTF2IRD1* exists in human, mouse, rat, *Xenopus*, zebrafish, and fugu, but that *GTF2I* is found only in humans and rodents.

The *Xenopus* GTF2IRD1 gene (*XWBSCR11*) is well conserved between frog and mammals, and the repeat regions are highly conserved, ranging from 65% for R1 to 96% for R4. XWBSCR11 was identified as a protein that binds to the *Xenopus goosecoid* (*gsc*) promoter (Ring et al. 2002). *Gsc* is a target gene for the activin/nodal signaling pathway that is responsible for mesoderm initiation and patterning in the early embryo and is highly conserved through frogs, fish, and mammals (Schier 2003). Activin and nodal, which are members of the TGF-β superfamily of ligands, signal through a transmembrane serine/threonine kinase receptor complex and phosphorylate several Smads, which in turn form a complex and translocate into the nucleus to regulate transcription of responsive genes. *Gsc* contains a distal control element that binds to XWBSCR11 and a proximal control element that binds another transcription factor, FoxH1. The model generated from experiments in *Xenopus* proposes that XWBSCR11 binds the activated Smads and the *gsc* distal control element, while FoxH1 binds the *gsc* proximal control element and then XWBSCR11, forming a large transcriptional complex that promotes *gsc* expression. The distal control element is highly conserved in *Xenopus*, zebrafish, and mouse, suggesting that GTF2IRD1 may be performing a similar role in early development in mammals.

Haploinsufficiency of transcriptional activators is well known as a cause of developmental disorders, such as the genes *CBP* in Rubinstein-Taybi syndrome (Petrij et al. 1995), *TWIST* in Saethre-Chotzen syndrome (Howard et al. 1997; el Ghouzzi et al. 1997), and the TBX genes in Holt-Oram syndrome (*TBX5*, Basson et al. 1997; Q. Y. Li et al. 1997), ulnar-mammary syndrome (*TBX3*, Bamshad et al. 1997), and DiGeorge/velocardiofacial syndrome (*TBX1*, Lindsay et al. 2001; Merscher et al. 2001; Jerome and Papaioannou 2001). The widespread expression pattern and interaction of gene products makes the GTF2I family members tantalizing candidates for involvement in a multisystem disorder such as WBS. A mouse with greatly reduced *Gtf2ird1* expression was generated through the random insertion of a c-*myc* transgene, which resulted in a deletion of ~40 kb, including the transcriptional start site and exon 1 of *Gtf2ird1* (Durkin et al. 2001). These mice did not display any obvious phenotypic features, although comprehensive morphologic and behavioral studies may yet reveal subtle abnormalities. Although even the homozygous mutants showed no WBS-like features, the role of this gene in WBS is still unresolved, because the differential expression of TFII-I, and possibly GTF2IRD1, isoforms is quite different between mice and humans. GTF2IRD1 has been proposed as an activator in muscle and in one hybrid assay (O'Mahoney et al. 1998; Yan et al. 2000) but has also been shown to act as a repressor of TFII-I (Tussie-Luna et al. 2001). In the latter case, GTF2IRD1 excluded TFII-I from the nucleus and so prevented its functioning as an activator. It is possible, therefore, that the functions of TFII-I and GTF2IRD1 are inextricably linked and that in WBS there is a combinatorial effect of hemizygosity for both genes. In addition, the third member of the family, GTF2IRD2, is still uncharacterized but promises to add yet more complexity to the interactions and functions of this protein family.

Inversion of the WBS Chromosome Region

Analysis of the WBS duplicons has shown that homologous blocks of sequence are arranged in both direct and inverted orientation with respect to each other (Valero et al. 2000; Osborne et al. 2001) (see fig. 2.1). Blocks arranged in a direct orientation would be expected to mediate nonallelic recombination resulting in deletion or duplication, as is seen in WBS and other disorders discussed at the beginning of this chapter. Blocks arranged in an inverted orientation would be expected to mediate inversions of the region between the breakpoints, and this has been detected in WBS (Osborne et al. 2001).

Using three-color FISH to visualize the order of probes along the chromosome, investigators found that a third of parents who had transmitted the subsequently deleted chromosome to their child with WBS carried an inversion of the WBS region on one chromosome 7, WBSinv-1. The WBSinv-1 inversion was not identified on nontransmitting parental chromosomes or on chromosomes from a limited number of unrelated control individuals. These results suggest that inversion of the region may predispose the chromosome to deletion of the WBS region during meiotic recombination, presumably through the disruption of proper chromatid pairing. This finding was surprising because the WBS deletion was previously thought to be stochastic in nature, with no predisposing factors except the duplicons themselves, which are present on all chromosomes 7. The majority (~67%) of WBS interstitial deletions have been shown to be due to unbalanced recombination during meiosis (interchromosomal rearrangement), and fewer (~33%) seem to result from intrachromosomal recombination. Whether the inversion polymorphism is associated with one or both of these events is unknown, but recent data suggest that deletions on an inverted chromosome are associated only with interchromosomal recombination (Bayés et al. 2003). If the inversion truly disrupts proper meiotic recombination, then other rearrangements of chromosome 7 might also be expected, and at least six WBS families have now been identified that have other chromosome 7 rearrangements and a transmitting parent who has a WBS inversion (Osborne et al. 2001; Scherer et al. 2005; L. R. Osborne and S. W. Scherer, unpublished results).

Further experiments are needed to determine the frequency of the inversion in the general population before any risk value can be assigned, but the inversion may confer a slightly higher risk for having a child with a rearrangement of chromosome 7. Any increased risk will be very small: multiple-affected WBS families are not common, although they do exist (Kara-Mostefa et al. 1999; Scherer et al. 2005). In two affected sibships studied, one was shown to be due to parental germ-line mosaicism for the WBS deletion, whereas the other family carried an inversion of the region (Scherer et al., in press).

Inversion polymorphism may be a widespread phenomenon in the genome—certainly, many other regions flanked by duplicated segments have the potential to undergo inversion as well as deletion/duplication (Ji et al. 2000)—and this may be a common mechanism for recurrent chromosome rearrangements. Evidence supporting this has come from several studies. The distal region of chromosome 8p is subject to recurrent rearrangements, including inverted duplication, interstitial deletion, and translocation. Inversion of 8p between clusters of highly homologous olfactory receptor genes was found in mothers of individuals with 8p rearrangements and in a quarter of the general population (Giglio et al. 2001). In addition, the same researchers have shown that the t(4;8)(p16;p23) is also mediated by inversion polymorphisms on each of the participating chromosomes, again between clusters of olfactory receptor genes (Giglio et al. 2002). An inversion of the Angelman syndrome deletion region at 15q11–q13 was identified in four of six mothers of probands with this syndrome, in which the deletion was of maternal origin and the breakpoints were in the medial and telomeric LCRs (Gimelli et al. 2003). A survey of twenty-two sets of parents of children with velocardiofacial syndrome, however, did not reveal any evidence of predisposing inversions of 22q11.2 (Saitta et al. 2004).

An inversion of the 7q11.23 WBS region was also identified in three individuals who showed some symptoms of WBS but did not harbor a deletion of the region as evidenced by extensive FISH analysis (Osborne et al. 2001). Two of these individuals also had a second chromosome rearrangement, in one case an apparently balanced (6;7) translocation (von Dadelszen et al. 2000) and in the other a second, paracentric inversion. The third individual had no evidence of any chromosome abnormality except inversion of the WBS region. Some WBS facial features, developmental delay, strabismus, hyperacusis, musculoskeletal problems, and overfriendliness were seen in two of the patients (the third died shortly after birth), and hyperactivity and dental abnormalities in only one.

The presence of some symptoms overlapping with the WBS phenotype in these individuals suggests that the inversion could be related, although the majority of people carrying the inversion were parents with no phenotypic features. The inversion breakpoints for all individuals were mapped to the duplicons, but because of the repetitive nature of the sequence it was not possible to define their exact location. However, pulsed-field gel electrophoresis revealed a different inversion fragment in one individual with atypical WBS carrying WBSinv-1, compared with unaffected parents with inversions. This hints at different inversion breakpoints and presents a possible explanation for affected and unaffected individuals carrying what appears, at a gross level, to be the same inversion.

Inversions of small regions have been found to directly cause clinical symptoms by the interruption of specific disease genes, such as Hunter syndrome, in which an inversion occurs between the iduronate-2-sulfatase (IDS-2) gene and a neighboring pseudogene (Bondeson et al. 1995). If the WBS inversion can directly cause symptoms, one or both of the breakpoints must disrupt gene(s). These genes must be near or in the duplicons, making genes at the deletion boundaries good candidates for involvement in the symptoms seen in patients with atypical WBS who have WBSinv-1.

A second inversion of the WBS region has been found in several individuals with some symptoms of WBS: WBSinv-2 (Scherer et al. 2003). This inversion spans an interval between *WBSCR1* and *HIP1* (see fig. 2.2), with breakpoints that do not lie in known repetitive DNA sequence and may directly interrupt genes. Because these inversion breakpoints lie in an apparently unique sequence, the mechanism that leads to this chromosome rearrangement remains unclear.

Clinical Implications

At the present time, no gene except *ELN* has been shown to directly cause any symptoms of Williams-Beuren syndrome when one copy is missing. As a consequence, we have not gained extensive insight into the pathogenesis or mechanism of the disease from the study of genes in the deleted region. Some progress has been made: for example, the implication of STX1A in diabetes in WBS may offer routes for novel therapies, and the role of STX1A and associated proteins in insulin secretion is an active area of research. However, clinical management and treatment of people with WBS will not change significantly based on our current knowledge of gene function in the WBS region.

In contrast, the genetic counseling of families with WBS may change, based on the identification of predisposing inversions in parents of individuals with WBS. Indeed, many parents are already requesting inversion testing, initially for themselves but then for children without WBS if one parent is found to carry an inversion. Although the WBSinv-1 inversion was found in approximately one-third of WBS parents, the risk of recurrence in a family is still unknown. Further research is needed to provide accurate estimates of recurrence risk for siblings, even though this risk is likely to be very small.

The identification of individuals with WBS-like symptoms and inversions of the WBS region may also affect the diagnosis of WBS. Although the majority of individuals with WBS carry the common deletion, a small number do not, and some of these people may have a pathogenic inversion of the WBS region. Detection of the WBSinv-2 inversion may be valuable in assisting in clinical diagnosis of WBS in these families, although the frequency of such rearrangements in symptomatic individuals remains to be determined.

Future Directions

The molecular basis of Williams-Beuren syndrome is still somewhat of a mystery, but considerable progress has been made, and the next few years promise to reveal many of the secrets that surround this disorder. Over the next five years, knockout mouse models will be developed for many, if not all, of the genes in the WBS deletion region, and these models will teach us much about the normal function of each gene and its potential role in WBS. The emergence of techniques to mimic microdeletion disorders in mice raises the prospect of genetically re-creating the WBS deletion. Several laboratories are currently in the process of generating mice with large deletions of the WBS region, and these will provide a wealth of information on how the deletion of different genes in combination can lead to WBS phenotypes. Mouse models are clearly of extreme importance in achieving this goal, but they cannot tell us everything, and human studies will remain a top priority for WBS researchers.

The identification of inversions of the WBS region also opens up a fascinating avenue of research into chromosome structure, and future studies will address the importance of such rearrangements in both human disease and genome evolution. As our analysis of the genomic structure of the WBS region progresses, further rearrangements may be discovered and additional clues will emerge about the maintenance of this highly unstable region of the genome.

Williams-Beuren syndrome offers a unique entry point into genes that control human emotion, personality, and cognition. To date, few genes have been linked to mental function (for a review, see Chelly and Mandel 2001) and even fewer to behavior. Although most neurologic disorders are likely to be complex, involving both genetic and environmental factors, the genes that cause mental retardation in WBS may also do so in the general population. As researchers narrow in on the genes causing mental retardation, anxiety, and hyperactivity in WBS, they will be able to address the broader effects of such gene mutations.

REFERENCES

Allen, K. M., Gleeson, J. G., Bagrodia, S., Partington, M. W., MacMillan, J. C., Cerione, R. A., Mulley, J. C., and Walsh, C. A. 1998. *PAK3* mutation in nonsyndromic X-linked mental retardation. *Nature Genetics* 20:25–30.

Amir, R. E., Van den Veyver, I. B., Wan, M., Tran, C. Q., Francke, U., and Zoghbi, H. Y. 1999. Rett syndrome is caused by mutations in X-linked *MECP2*, encoding methyl-CpG-binding protein 2. *Nature Genetics* 23:185–188.

Amos-Landgraf, J. M., Ji, Y., Gottlieb, W., Depinet, T., Wandstrat, A. E., Cassidy, S. B., Driscoll, D. J., Rogan, P. K., Schwartz, S., and Nicholls, R. D. 1999. Chromosome breakage in the Prader-Willi and Angelman syndromes involves recombination between large, transcribed repeats at proximal and distal breakpoints. *American Journal of Human Genetics* 65:370–386.

Arber, S., Barbayannis, F. A., Hanser, H., Schneider, C., Stanyon, C. A., Bernard, O., and Caroni, P. 1998. Regulation of actin dynamics through phosphorylation of cofilin by LIM-kinase. *Nature* 393:805–809.

Bailey, J. A., Yavor, A. M., Massa, H. F., Trask, B. J., and Eichler, E. E. 2001. Segmental duplications: Organization and impact in the current human genome project assembly. *Genome Research* 11:1005–1017.

Bamshad, M., Lin, R. C., Law, D. J., Watkins, W. C., Krakowiak, P. A., Moore, M. E., Franceschini, P., Lala, R., Holmes, L. B., Gebuhr, T. C., Bruneau, B. G., Schinzel, A., Seidman, J. G., Seidman, C. E., and Jorde, L. B. 1997. Mutations in human *TBX3* alter limb, apocrine and genital development in ulnar-mammary syndrome. *Nature Genetics* 16:311–315.

Barr, C. L., Feng, Y., Wigg, K., Bloom, S., Roberts, W., Malone, M., Schachar, R., Tannock, R., and Kennedy, J. L. 2000. Identification of DNA variants in the SNAP-25 gene and linkage study of these polymorphisms and attention-deficit hyperactivity disorder. *Molecular Psychiatry* 5:405–409.

Basson, C. T., Bachinsky, D. R., Lin, R. C., Levi, T., Elkins, J. A., Soults, J., Grayzel, D., Kroumpouzou, E., Traill, T. A., Leblanc-Straceski, J., Renault, B., Kucherlapati, R., Seidman, J. G., and Seidman, C. E. 1997. Mutations in human *TBX5* cause limb and cardiac malformation in Holt-Oram syndrome. *Nature Genetics* 15:30–35.

Baumer, A., Dutly, F., Balmer, D., Riegel, M., Tukel, T., Krajewska-Walasek, M., and Schinzel, A. A. 1998. High level of unequal meiotic crossovers at the origin of the 22q11. 2 and 7q11.23 deletions. *Human Molecular Genetics* 7:887–894.

Bayarsaihan, D., and Ruddle, F. H. 2000. Isolation and characterization of BEN, a member of the TFII-I family of DNA-binding proteins containing distinct helix-loop-helix domains. *Proceedings of the National Academy of Sciences U S A* 97:7342–7347.

Bayarsaihan, D., Dunai, J., Greally, J. M., Kawasaki, K., Sumiyama, K., Enkhmandakh, B., Shimizu, N., and Ruddle, F. H. 2002. Genomic organization of the genes *Gtf2ird1*, *Gtf2i*, and *Ncf1* at the mouse chromosome 5 region syntenic to human chromosome 7q11.23 Williams syndrome critical region. *Genomics* 79:137–143.

Bayés, M., Prieto, I., Noguchi, J., Barbero, J. L., and Perez Jurado, L. A. 2001. Evaluation of the *Stag3* gene and the synaptonemal complex in a rat model (as/as) for male infertility. *Molecular Reproduction and Development* 60:414–417.

Bayés, M., Magano, L. F., Rivera, N., Flores, R., and Pérez Jurado, L. A. 2003. Mutational mechanisms of Williams-Beuren syndrome deletions. *American Journal of Human Genetics* 73:131–151.

Bennett, M. K., Calakos, N., and Scheller, R. H. 1992. Syntaxin: A synaptic protein implicated in docking of synaptic vesicles at presynaptic active zones. *Science* 257:255–259.

Billin, A. N., Eilers, A. L., Queva, C., and Ayer, D. E. 1999. Mlx, a novel Max-like BHLHZip protein that interacts with the Max network of transcription factors. *Journal of Biological Chemistry* 274:36344–36350.

Billuart, P., Bienvenu, T., Ronce, N., des Portes, V., Vinet, M. C., Zemni, R., Roest Crollius, H., Carrie, A., Fauchereau, F., Cherry, M., Briault, S., Hamel, B., Fryns, J. P., Beldjord, C., Kahn, A., Moraine, C., and Chelly, J. 1998. Oligophrenin-1 encodes a rhoGAP protein involved in X-linked mental retardation. *Nature* 392:923–926.

Bondeson, M. L., Dahl, N., Malmgren, H., Kleijer, W. J., Tonnesen, T., Carlberg, B. M., and Pettersson, U. 1995. Inversion of the IDS gene resulting from recombination with IDS-related sequences is a common cause of the Hunter syndrome. *Human Molecular Genetics* 4:615–621.

Bozhenok, L., Wade, P. A., and Varga-Weisz, P. 2002. WSTF-ISWI chromatin remodeling complex targets heterochromatic replication foci. *EMBO Journal* 21:2231–2241.

Brdicka, T., Imrich, M., Angelisova, P., Brdickova, N., Horvath, O., Spicka, J., Hilgert, I., Luskova, P., Draber, P., Novak, P., Engels, N., Wienands, J., Simeoni, L., Osterreicher, J., Aguado, E., Malissen, M., Schraven, B., and Horejsi, V. 2002. Non-T cell activation linker (NTAL): A transmembrane adaptor protein involved in immunoreceptor signaling. *Journal of Experimental Medicine*. 196:1617–1626.

Cairo, S., Merla, G., Urbinati, F., Ballabio, A., and Reymond, A. 2001. *WBSCR14*, a gene mapping to the Williams-Beuren syndrome deleted region, is a new member of the Mlx transcription factor network. *Human Molecular Genetics* 10:617–627.

Chan, C. B., MacPhail, R. M., Sheu, L., Wheeler, M., and Gaisano, H. Y. 1999. Beta cell hypertrophy in *fa/fa* rats is associated with basal glucose hypersensitivity and reduced SNARE protein expression. *Diabetes* 48:997–1005.

Chance, P. F., Abbas, N., Lensch, M. W., Pentao, L., Roa, B. B., Patel, P. I., and Lupski, J. R. 1994. Two autosomal dominant neuropathies result from reciprocal DNA duplication/deletion of a region on chromosome 17. *Human Molecular Genetics* 3:223–228.

Chelly, J., and Mandel, J. L. 2001. Monogenic causes of X-linked mental retardation. *Nature Reviews in Genetics* 2:669–680.

Chen, K. S., Manian, P., Koeuth, T., Potocki, L., Zhao, Q., Chinault, A. C., Lee, C. C., and Lupski, J. R. 1997. Homologous recombination of a flanking repeat gene cluster is a mechanism for a common contiguous gene deletion syndrome. *Nature Genetics* 17:154–163.

Cheng, A. K., and Robertson, E. J. 1995. The murine LIM-kinase gene (limk) encodes a novel serine threonine kinase expressed predominantly in trophoblast giant cells and the developing nervous system. *Mechanisms in Development* 52:187–197.

Cheriyath, V., and Roy, A. L. 2000. Alternatively spliced isoforms of TFII-I: Complex formation, nuclear translocation, and differential gene regulation. *Journal of Biological Chemistry* 275:26300–26308.

———. 2001. Structure-function analysis of TFII-I:. Roles of the N-terminal end, basic region, and I-repeats. *Journal of Biological Chemistry* 276:8377–8383.

Cherniske, E. M., Carpenter, T. O., Klaiman, C., Young, E., Bregman, J., Insogna, K., Schultz, R. T., and Pober, B. R. 2004. Multisystem study of 20 older adults with Williams syndrome. *American Journal of Medical Genetics A* 131:255–264.

Coquelle, F. M., Caspi, M., Cordelieres, F. P., Dompierre, J. P., Dujardin, D. L., Koifman, C., Martin, P., Hoogenraad, C. C., Akhmanova, A., Galjart, N., De Mey, J. R., and Reiner, O. 2002. LIS1, CLIP-170's key to the dynein/dynactin pathway. *Molecular and Cellular Biology* 22:3089–3102.

Crackower, M. A., Kolas, N. K., Noguchi, J., Sarao, R., Kikuchi, K., Kaneko, H., Kobayashi, E., Kawai, Y., Kozieradzki, I., Landers, R., Mo, R., Hui, C.-C., Nieves, E., Cohen, P. E., Osborne, L. R., Wada, T., Kunieda, T., Moens, P. B., and Penninger, J. M. 2003. Essential role of Fkbp6 in male fertility and homologous chromosome pairing in meiosis. *Science* 300:1291–1295.

Curran, M. E., Atkinson, D. L., Ewart, A. K., Morris, C. A., Leppert, M. F., and Keating, M. T. 1993. The elastin gene is disrupted by a translocation associated with supravalvular aortic stenosis. *Cell* 73:159–168.

D'Adamo, P., Menegon, A., Lo Nigro, C., Grasso, M., Gulisano, M., Tamanini, F., Bienvenu, T., Gedeon, A. K., Oostra, B., Wu, S. K., Tandon, A., Valtorta, F., Balch, W. E., Chelly, J., and Toniolo, D. 1998. Mutations in *GDI1* are responsible for X-linked non-specific mental retardation. *Nature Genetics* 19:134–139.

Danoff, S. K., Taylor, H. E., Blackshaw, S., and Desiderio, S. 2004. TFII-I, a candidate gene for Williams syndrome cognitive profile: Parallels between regional expression in mouse brain and human phenotype. *Neuroscience* 123:931–938.

de Luis, O., Valero, M. C., and Jurado, L. A. 2000. *WBSCR14,* a putative transcription factor gene deleted in Williams-Beuren syndrome: Complete characterisation of the human gene and the mouse ortholog. *European Journal of Human Genetics* 8:215–222.

DeSilva, U., Massa, H., Trask, B. J., and Green, E. D. 1999. Comparative mapping of the region of human chromosome 7 deleted in Williams syndrome. *Genome Research* 9:428–436.

DeSilva, U., Elnitski, L., Idol, J. R., Doyle, J. L., Gan, W., Thomas, J. W., Schwartz, S., Dietrich, N. L., Beckstrom-Sternberg, S. M., McDowell, J. C., Blakesley, R. W., Bouffard, G. G., Thomas, P. J., Touchman, J. W., Miller, W., and Green, E. D. 2002. Generation and comparative analysis of approximately 3.3 Mb of mouse genomic sequence orthologous to the region of human chromosome 7q11.23 implicated in Williams syndrome. *Genome Research* 12:3–15.

De Zeeuw, C. I., Hertzberg, E. L., and Mugnaini, E. 1995. The dendritic lamellar body: A new neuronal organelle putatively associated with dendrodendritic gap junctions. *Journal of Neuroscience* 15:1587–1604.

De Zeeuw, C. I., Hoogenraad, C. C., Goedknegt, E., Hertzberg, E., Neubauer, A., Grosveld, F., and Galjart, N. 1997. CLIP-115, a novel brain-specific cytoplasmic linker protein, mediates the localization of dendritic lamellar bodies. *Neuron* 19:1187–1199.

Doll, A., and Grzeschik, K. H. 2001. Characterization of two novel genes, WBSCR20 and WBSCR22, deleted in Williams-Beuren syndrome. *Cytogenetics and Cell Genetics* 95:20–27.

Doyle, J. L., DeSilva, U., Miller, W., and Green, E. D. 2000. Divergent human and mouse orthologs of a novel gene (WBSCR15/ *Wbscr15*) reside in the genomic interval commonly deleted in Williams syndrome. *Cytogenetics and Cell Genetics* 90:285–290.

Dujardin, D., Wacker, U. I., Moreau, A., Schroer, T. A., Rickard, J. E., and De Mey, J. R. 1998. Evidence for a role of CLIP-170 in the establishment of metaphase chromosome alignment. *Journal of Cell Biology* 141:849–862.

Durkin, M. E., Keck-Waggoner, C. L., Popescu, N. C., and Thorgeirsson, S. S. 2001. Integration of a c-*myc* transgene results in disruption of the mouse *Gtf2ird1* gene, the homologue of the human GTF2IRD1 gene hemizygously deleted in Williams-Beuren syndrome. *Genomics* 73:20–27.

Dutly, F., and Schinzel, A. 1996. Unequal interchromosomal rearrangements may result in elastin gene deletions causing the Williams-Beuren syndrome. *Human Molecular Genetics* 5:1893–1898.

Edelmann, L., Pandita, R. K., and Morrow, B. E. 1999a. Low-copy repeats mediate the common 3-Mb deletion in patients with velo-cardio-facial syndrome. *American Journal of Human Genetics* 64:1076–1086.

Edelmann, L., Pandita, R. K., Spiteri, E., Funke, B., Goldberg, R., Palanisamy, N., Chaganti, R. S., Magenis, E., Shprintzen, R. J., and Morrow, B. E. 1999b. A common molecular basis for rearrangement disorders on chromosome 22q11. *Human Molecular Genetics* 8:1157–1167.

Eichler, E. E. 2001. Segmental duplications: What's missing, misassigned, and misassembled—and should we care? *Genome Research* 11:653–656.

el Ghouzzi, V., Le Merrer, M., Perrin-Schmitt, F., Lajeunie, E., Benit, P., Renier, D., Bourgeois, P., Bolcato-Bellemin, A. L., Munnich, A., and Bonaventure, J. 1997. Mutations of the *TWIST* gene in the Saethre-Chotzen syndrome. *Nature Genetics* 15:42–46.

Ensenauer, R. E., Adeyinka, A., Flynn, H. C., Michels, V. V., Lindor, N. M., Dawson, D. B., Thorland, E. C., Lorentz, C. P., Goldstein, J. L., McDonald, M. T., Smith, W. E., Simon-Fayard, E., Alexander, A. A., Kulharya, A. S., Ketterling, R. P., Clark, R. D., and Jalal, S. M. 2003. Microduplication 22q11.2, an emerging syndrome: Clinical, cytogenetic, and molecular analysis of thirteen patients. *American Journal of Human Genetics* 73:1027–1040.

Everly, D. N., Jr., Feng, P., Mian, I. S., and Read, G. S. 2002. mRNA degradation by the virion host shutoff (Vhs) protein of herpes simplex virus: Genetic and biochemical evidence that Vhs is a nuclease. *Journal of Virology* 76:8560–8571.

Ewart, A. K., Morris, C. A., Atkinson, D., Jin, W., Sternes, K., Spallone, P., Stock, A. D., Leppert, M., and Keating, M. T. 1993. Hemizygosity at the elastin locus in a developmental disorder, Williams syndrome. *Nature Genetics* 5:11–16.

Feng, P., Everly, D. N., Jr., and Read, G. S. 2001. mRNA decay during herpesvirus infections: Interaction between a putative viral nuclease and a cellular translation factor. *Journal of Virology* 75:10272–10280.

Ferre-D'Amare, A. R., Prendergast, G. C., Ziff, E. B., and Burley, S. K. 1993. Recognition by Max of its cognate DNA through a dimeric b/HLH/Z domain. *Nature* 363:38–45.

Fink, A. L. 1999. Chaperone-mediated protein folding. *Physiology Reviews* 79:425–449.

Fonagy, A., Swiderski, C., Wilson, A., Bolton, W., Kenyon, N., and Freeman, J. W. 1993.

Cell cycle regulated expression of nucleolar antigen P120 in normal and transformed human fibroblasts. *Journal of Cellular Physiology* 154:16–27.

Frangiskakis, J. M., Ewart, A. K., Morris, C. A., Mervis, C. B., Bertrand, J., Robinson, B. F., Klein, B. P., Ensing, G. J., Everett, L. A., Green, E. D., Pröschel, C., Gutowski, N. J., Noble, M., Atkinson, D. L., Odelberg, S. J., and Keating, M. T. 1996. *LIM-kinase 1* hemizygosity implicated in impaired visuospatial constructive cognition. *Cell* 86:59–69.

Franke, Y., Peoples, R. J., and Francke, U. 1999. Identification of GTF2IRD1, a putative transcription factor in the Williams-Beuren syndrome deletion at 7q11.23. *Cytogenetics and Cell Genetics* 86:296–304.

Gibbons, R. J., Picketts, D. J., Villard, L., and Higgs, D. R. 1995. Mutations in a putative global transcriptional regulator cause X-linked mental retardation with alpha-thalassemia (ATR-X syndrome). *Cell* 80:837–845.

Giglio, S., Broman, K. W., Matsumoto, N., Calvari, V., Gimelli, G., Neumann, T., Ohashi, H., Voullaire, L., Larizza, D., Giorda, R., Weber, J. L., Ledbetter, D. H., and Zuffardi, O. 2001. Olfactory receptor-gene clusters, genomic-inversion polymorphisms, and common chromosome rearrangements. *American Journal of Human Genetics* 68:874–883.

Giglio, S., Calvari, V., Gregato, G., Gimelli, G., Camanini, S., Giorda, R., Ragusa, A., Guerneri, S., Selicorni, A., Stumm, M., Tonnies, H., Ventura, M., Zollino, M., Neri, G., Barber, J., Wieczorek, D., Rocchi, M., and Zuffardi, O. 2002. Heterozygous submicroscopic inversions involving olfactory receptor-gene clusters mediate the recurrent t(4;8)(p16;p23) translocation. *American Journal of Human Genetics* 71:276–285.

Gimelli, G., Pujana, M. A., Patricelli, M. G., Russo, S., Giardino, D., Larizza, L., Cheung, J., Armengol, L., Schinzel, A., Estivill, X., and Zuffardi, O. 2003. Genomic inversions of human chromosome 15q11–q13 in mothers of Angelman syndrome patients with class II (BP2/3) deletions. *Human Molecular Genetics* 12:849–858.

Görlach, A., Lee, P. L., Roesler, J., Hopkins, P. J., Christensen, B., Green, E. D., Chanock, S. J., and Curnutte, J. T. 1997. A p47-phox pseudogene carries the most common mutation causing p47-phox-deficient chronic granulomatous disease. *Journal of Clinical Investigation* 100:1907–1918.

Hess, E. J., Collins, K. A., and Wilson, M. C. 1996. Mouse model of hyperkinesis implicates SNAP-25 in behavioural regulation. *Journal of Neuroscience* 16:3104–3111.

Holzbaur, E. L., Hammarback, J. A., Paschal, B. M., Kravit, N. G., Pfister, K. K., and Vallee, R. B. 1991. Homology of a 150K cytoplasmic dynein-associated polypeptide with the *Drosophila* gene Glued. *Nature* 351:579–583.

Hoogenraad, C. C., Eussen, B. H., Langeveld, A., van Haperen, R., Winterberg, S., Wouters, C. H., Grosveld, F., De Zeeuw, C. I., and Galjart, N. 1998. The murine *CYLN2* gene: Genomic organization, chromosome localization, and comparison to the human gene that is located within the 7q11.23 Williams syndrome critical region. *Genomics* 53:348–358.

Hoogenraad, C. C., Koekkoek, B., Akhmanova, A., Krugers, H., Dortland, B., Miedema, M., Van Alphen, A., Kistler, W. M., Jaegle, M., Koutsourakis, M., Van Camp, N., Verhoye, M., Van Der Linden, A., Kaverina, I., Grosveld, F., De Zeeuw, C. I., and Galjart, N. 2002. Targeted mutation of *Cyln2* in the Williams syndrome critical region links CLIP-115 haplo-insufficiency to neurodevelopmental abnormalities in mice. *Nature Genetics* 32:116–127.

Horii, A., Han, H.-J., Sasaki, S., Shimada, M., and Nakamura, Y. 1994. Cloning, characterization and chromosomal assignment of the human genes homologous to yeast *PMS1*, a member of mismatch repair genes. *Biochemical and Biophysical Research Communications* 204:1257–1264.

Howard, T. D., Paznekas, W. A., Green, E. D., Chiang, L. C., Ma, N., Ortiz de Luna, R. I., Garcia Delgado, C., Gonzalez-Ramos, M., Kline, A. D., and Jabs, E. W. 1997. Mutations in *TWIST*, a basic helix-loop-helix transcription factor, in Saethre-Chotzen syndrome. *Nature Genetics* 15:36–41.

Ikadai, H., Noguchi, J., Yoshida, M., and Imamichi, T. 1992. An aspermia rat mutant (as/as) with spermatogenic failure at meiosis. *Journal of Veterinary Medical Science* 54:745–749.

Jadayel, D., Osborne, L. R., Zani, V. J., Coignet, L. F. A., Tsui, L.-C., Scherer, S. W., and Dyer, M. J. S. 1998. The BCL7 gene family: Deletion of the BCL7B gene in Williams syndrome. *Gene* 224:35–44.

Jerome, L. A., and Papaioannou, V. E. 2001. DiGeorge syndrome phenotype in mice mutant for the T-box gene, *Tbx1*. *Nature Genetics* 27:286–291.

Ji, Y., Eichler, E. E., Schwartz, S., and Nicholls, R. D. 2000. Structure of chromosomal duplicons and their role in mediating human genomic disorders. *Genome Research* 10:597–610.

Kabuki, T., Kawai, T., Kin, Y., Joh, K., Ohashi, H., Kosho, T., Yachie, A., Kanegane, H., Miyawaki, T., and Oh-ishi, T. 2003. A case of Williams syndrome with p47-phox-deficient chronic granulomatous disease. *Nihon Rinsho Meneki Gakkai Kaishi—Japanese Journal of Clinical Immunology* 26:299–303.

Kalchman, M. A., Koide, H. B., McCutcheon, K., Graham, R. K., Nichol, K., Nishiyama, K., Kazemi-Esfarjani, P., Lynn, F. C., Wellington, C., Metzler, M., Goldberg, Y. P., Kanazawa, I., Gietz, R. D., and Hayden, M. R. 1997. HIP1, a human homologue of *S. cerevisiae* Sla2p, interacts with membrane-associated huntingtin in the brain. *Nature Genetics* 16:44–53.

Kara-Mostefa, A., Raoul, O., Lyonnet, S., Amiel, J., Munnich, A., Vekemans, M., Magnier, S., Ossareh, B., and Bonnefont, J. P. 1999. Recurrent Williams-Beuren syndrome in a sibship suggestive of maternal germ-line mosaicism. *American Journal of Human Genetics* 64:1475–1478.

Kaufmann, W. E., and Moser, H. W. 2000. Dendritic anomalies in disorders associated with mental retardation. *Cerebral Cortex* 10:981–991.

Kipersztok, S., Osawa, G. A., Liang, L. F., Modi, W. S., and Dean, J. 1995. POM-ZP3, a bipartite transcript derived from human ZP3 and a POM121 homologue. *Genomics* 25:354–359.

Kitagawa, H., Fujiki, R., Yoshimura, K., Mezaki, Y., Uematsu, Y., Matsui, D., Ogawa, S., Unno, K., Okubo, M., Tokita, A., Nakagawa, T., Ito, T., Ishimi, Y., Nagasawa, H., Matsumoto, T., Yanagisawa, J., and Kato, S. 2003. The chromatin-remodeling complex WINAC targets a nuclear receptor to promoters and is impaired in Williams syndrome. *Cell* 113:905–917.

Kotzot, D., Bernasconi, F., Brecevic, L., Robinson, W. P., Kiss, P., Kosztolanyi, G., Lurie, I. W., Superti-Furga, A., and Schinzel, A. 1995. Phenotype of the Williams-Beuren syndrome associated with hemizygosity at the elastin locus. *European Journal of Pediatrics* 154:477–482.

Kretzner, L., Blackwood, E. M., and Eisenman, R. N. 1992. Myc and Max proteins possess distinct transcriptional activities. *Nature* 359:426–429.

Kutsche, K., Yntema, H., Brandt, A., Jantke, I., Nothwang, H. G., Orth, U., Boavida, M. G., David, D., Chelly, J., Fryns, J. P., Moraine, C., Ropers, H. H., Hamel, B. C., van Bokhoven, H., and Gal, A. 2000. Mutations in *ARHGEF6*, encoding a guanine nucleotide exchange factor for Rho GTPases, in patients with X-linked mental retardation. *Nature Genetics* 26:247–250.

Lam, P. P. L., Leung, Y.-M., Sheu, L., Ellis, J., Tsushima, R. G., Osborne, L. R., and

Gaisano, H. Y. 2005. Transgenic mouse over-expressing Syntaxin-1A as a diabetes model. *Diabetes* 54:2744–2754.

Lantz, V. A., and Miller, K. G. 1998. A class VI unconventional myosin is associated with a homologue of a microtubule-binding protein, cytoplasmic linker protein-170, in neurons and at the posterior pole of *Drosophila* embryos. *Journal of Cell Biology* 140:897–910.

Li, D. Y., Toland, A. E., Boak, B. B., Atkinson, D. L., Ensing, G. J., Morris, C. A., and Keating, M. T. 1997. Elastin point mutations cause an obstructive vascular disease, supravalvular aortic stenosis. *Human Molecular Genetics* 6:1021–1028.

Li, D. Y., Brooke, B., Davis, E. C., Mecham, R. P., Sorensen, L. K., Boak, B. B., Eichwald, E., and Keating, M. T. 1998a. Elastin is an essential determinant of arterial morphogenesis. *Nature* 393:276–280.

Li, D. Y., Faury, G., Taylor, D. G., Davis, E. C., Boyle, W. A., Mecham, R. P., Stenzel, P., Boak, B. B., and Keating, M. T. 1998b. Novel arterial pathology in mice and humans hemizygous for elastin. *Journal of Clinical Investigation* 102:1783–1787.

Li, Q. Y., Newbury-Ecob, R. A., Terrett, J. A., Wilson, D. I., Curtis, A. R., Yi, C. H., Gebuhr, T., Bullen, P. J., Robson, S. C., Strachan, T., Bonnet, D., Lyonnet, S., Young, I. D., Raeburn, J. A., Buckler, A. J., Law, D. J., and Brook, J. D. 1997. Holt-Oram syndrome is caused by mutations in *TBX5*, a member of the Brachyury (T) gene family. *Nature Genetics* 15:21–29.

Lindsay, E. A., Vitelli, F., Su, H., Morishima, M., Huynh, T., Pramparo, T., Jurecic, V., Ogunrinu, G., Sutherland, H. F., Scambler, P. J., Bradley, A., and Baldini, A. 2001. *Tbx1* haploinsufficiency in the DiGeorge syndrome region causes aortic arch defects in mice. *Nature* 410:97–101.

López-Correa, C., Dorschner, M., Brems, H., Lazaro, C., Clementi, M., Upadhyaya, M., Dooijes, D., Moog, U., Kehrer-Sawatzki, H., Rutkowski, J. L., Fryns, J. P., Marynen, P., Stephens, K., and Legius, E. 2001. Recombination hotspot in *NF1* microdeletion patients. *Human Molecular Genetics* 10:1387–1392.

Lowery, M. C., Morris, C. A., Ewart, A., Brothman, L. J., Zhu, X. L., Leonard, C. O., Carey, J. C., Keating, M., and Brothman, A. R. 1995. Strong correlation of elastin deletions, detected by FISH, with Williams syndrome: Evaluation of 235 patients. *American Journal of Human Genetics* 57:49–53.

Lu, X., Meng, X., Morris, C. A., and Keating, M. T. 1998. A novel human gene, *WSTF*, is deleted in Williams syndrome. *Genomics* 54:241–249.

Makeyev, A. V., Erdenechimeg, L., Mungunsukh, O., Roth, J. J., Enkhmandakh, B., Ruddle, F. H., and Bayarsaihan, D. 2004. GTF2IRD2 is located in the Williams-Beuren syndrome critical region 7q11.23 and encodes a protein with two TFII-I-like helix-loop-helix repeats. *Proceedings of the National Academy of Sciences U S A* 101:11052–11057.

Mari, A., Amati, F., Mingarelli, R., Giannotti, A., Sebastio, G., Colloridi, V., Novelli, G., and Dallapiccola, B. 1995. Analysis of the elastin gene in 60 patients with clinical diagnosis of Williams syndrome. *Human Genetics* 96:444–448.

Martindale, D. W., Wilson, M. D., Wang, D., Burke, R. D., Chen, X., Duronio, V., and Koop, B. F. 2000. Comparative genomic sequence analysis of the Williams syndrome region (LIMK1-RFC2) of human chromosome 7q11.23. *Mammalian Genome* 11:890–898.

Meng, X., Lu, X., Li, Z., Green, E. D., Massa, H., Trask, B. J., Morris, C. A., and Keating, M. T. 1998a. Complete physical map of the common deletion region in Williams syndrome and identification and characterization of three novel genes. *Human Genetics* 103:590–599.

Meng, X., Lu, X., Morris, C. A., and Keating, M. T. 1998b. A novel human gene *FKBP6* is deleted in Williams syndrome. *Genomics* 52:130–137.

Meng, Y., Zhang, Y., Tregoubov, V., Janus, C., Cruz, L., Jackson, M., Lu, W. Y., MacDonald, J. F., Wang, J. Y., Falls, D. L., and Jia, Z. 2002. Abnormal spine morphology and enhanced LTP in LIMK-1 knockout mice. *Neuron* 35:121–133.

Merla, G., Ucla, C., Guipponi, M., and Reymond, A. 2002. Identification of additional transcripts in the Williams-Beuren syndrome critical region. *Human Genetics* 110:429–38.

Merla, G., Howald, C., Antonarakis, S. E., and Reymond, A. 2004. The subcellular localization of the ChoRE-binding protein, encoded by the Williams-Beuren syndrome critical region gene 14, is regulated by 14-3-3. *Human Molecular Genetics* 13:1505–1514.

Merscher, S., Funke, B., Epstein, J. A., Heyer, J., Puech, A., Lu, M. M., Xavier, R. J., Demay, M. B., Russell, R. G., Factor, S., Tokooya, K., Jore, B. S., Lopez, M., Pandita, R. K., Lia, M., Carrion, D., Xu, H., Schorle, H., Kobler, J. B., Scambler, P., Wynshaw-Boris, A., Skoultchi, A. I., Morrow, B. E., and Kucherlapati, R. 2001. *TBX1* is responsible for cardiovascular defects in velo-cardio-facial/DiGeorge syndrome. *Cell* 104:619–629.

Metcalfe, K., Simeonov, E., Beckett, W., Donnai, D., and Tassabehji, M. 2005. Autosomal dominant inheritance of Williams-Beuren syndrome in a father and son with haploinsufficiency for FKBP6. *Clinical Dysmorphology* 14:61–65.

Metzler, M., Li, B., Gan, L., Georgiou, J., Gutekunst, C. A., Wang, Y., Torre, E., Devon, R. S., Oh, R., Legendre-Guillemin, V., Rich, M., Alvarez, C., Gertsenstein, M., McPherson, P. S., Nagy, A., Wang, Y. T., Roder, J. C., Raymond, L. A., and Hayden, M. R. 2003. Disruption of the endocytic protein HIP1 results in neurological deficits and decreased AMPA receptor trafficking. *EMBO Journal* 22:3254–3266.

Mill, J., Curran, S., Kent, L., Gould, A., Huckett, L., Richards, S., Taylor, E., and Asherson, P. 2002. Association study of a SNAP-25 microsatellite and attention deficit hyperactivity disorder. *American Journal of Medical Genetics* 114:269–271.

Mizugishi, K., Yamanaka, K., Kuwajima, K., and Kondo, I. 1998. Interstitial deletion of chromosome 7q in a patient with Williams syndrome and infantile spasms. *Journal of Human Genetics* 43:178–181.

Mizuno, K., Okano, I., Ohashi, K., Nunoue, K., Kuma, K., Miyata, T., and Nakamura, T. 1994. Identification of a human cDNA encoding a novel protein kinase with two repeats of the LIM/double zinc finger motif. *Oncogene* 9:1605–1612.

Mori, T., Okano, I., Mizuno, K., Tohyama, M., and Wanaka, A. 1997. Comparison of tissue distribution of two novel serine/threonine kinase genes containing the LIM motif (LIMK-1 and LIMK-2) in the developing rat. *Brain Research Molecular Brain Research* 45:247–254.

Morita, K., Furuse, M., Fujimoto, K., and Tsukita, S. 1999. Claudin multigene family encoding four-transmembrane domain protein components of tight junction strands. *Proceedings of the National Academy of Sciences USA* 96:511–516.

Nagamatsu, S., Nakamichi, Y., Yamamura, C., Matsushima, S., Watanabe, T., Ozawa, S., Furukawa, H., and Ishida, H. 1999. Decreased expression of t-SNARE, syntaxin-1 and SNAP-25 in pancreatic beta cells is involved in impaired insulin secretion from diabetic GK rat islets, restoration of decreased t-SNARE proteins improves impaired insulin secretion. *Diabetes* 48:2367–2373.

Nair, S. C., Rimerman, R. A., Toran, E. J., Chen, S., Prapapanich, V., Butts, R. N., and

Smith, D. F. 1997. Molecular cloning of human FKBP51 and comparisons of immunophilin interactions with Hsp90 and progesterone receptor. *Molecular and Cellular Biology* 17:594–603.

Nesbit, C. E., Tersak, J. M., and Prochownik, E. V. 1999. *MYC* oncogenes and human neoplastic disease. *Oncogene* 18:3004–3016.

Nickerson, E., Greenberg, F., Keating, M. T., McCaskill, C., and Shaffer, L. G. 1995. Deletions of the elastin gene at 7q11.23 occur in ~90% of patients with Williams syndrome. *American Journal of Human Genetics* 56:1156–1161.

Nicolaides, N. C., Carter, K. C., Shell, B. K., Papadopoulos, N., Vogelstein, B., and Kinzler, K. 1995. Genomic organization of the human *PMS2* gene family. *Genomics* 30:195–206.

Nishiyama, K., Sakaguchi, H., Hu, J. G., Bok, D., and Hollyfield, J. G. 2002. Claudin localization in cilia of the retinal pigment epithelium. *Anatomical Record* 267:196–203.

Noguchi, J., Kobayashi, E., Shimada, A., Kikuchi, K., Kaneko, H., Takahashi, H., Ikadai, H., and Kunieda, T. 1999. A locus responsible for arrest of spermatogenesis is located on rat chromosome 12. *Mammalian Genome* 10:189–190.

Novina, C. D., Cheriyath, V., and Roy, A. L. 1998. Regulation of TFII-I activity by phosphorylation. *Journal of Biological Chemistry* 273:33443–33448.

Novina, C. D., Kumar, S., Bajpai, U., Cheriyath, V., Zhang, K., Pillai, S., Wortis, H. H., and Roy, A. L. 1999. Regulation of nuclear localization and transcriptional activity of TFII-I by Bruton's tyrosine kinase. *Molecular and Cellular Biology* 19:5014–5024.

O'Mahoney, J. V., Guven, K. L., Lin, J., Joya, J. E., Robinson, C. S., Wade, R. P., and Hardeman, E. C. 1998. Identification of a novel slow-muscle-fiber enhancer binding protein, MusTRD1. *Molecular and Cellular Biology* 18:6641–6652.

Oravecz-Wilson, K. I., Kiel, M. J., Li, L., Rao, D. S., Saint-Dic, D., Kumar, P. D., Provot, M. M., Hankenson, K. D., Reddy, V. N., Lieberman, A. P., Morrison, S. J., and Ross, T. S. 2004. Huntingtin Interacting Protein 1 mutations lead to abnormal hematopoiesis, spinal defects and cataracts. *Human Molecular Genetics* 13:851–867.

Osborne, L. R., Martindale, D., Scherer, S. W., Shi, X.-M., Huizenga, J., Heng, H. H., Costa, T., Pober, B., Lew, L., Brinkman, J., Rommens, J., Koop, B., and Tsui, L.-C. 1996. Identification of genes from a 500-kb region at 7q11.23 that is commonly deleted in Williams syndrome patients. *Genomics* 36:328–336.

Osborne, L. R., Herbrick, J. A., Greavette, T., Heng, H. H., Tsui, L. C., and Scherer, S. W. 1997a. PMS2-related genes flank the rearrangement breakpoints associated with Williams syndrome and other disease on human chromosome 7. *Genomics* 45:402–406.

Osborne, L. R., Soder, S., Shi, X.-M., Pober, B., Costa, T., Scherer, S. W., and Tsui, L.-C. 1997b. Hemizygous deletion of syntaxin 1A gene in individuals with Williams syndrome. *American Journal of Human Genetics* 61:449–452.

Osborne, L. R., Campbell, T. L., Daradich, A., Scherer, S. W., and Tsui, L.-C. 1999. Identification of a putative transcription factor gene (*WBSCR11*) that is commonly deleted in Williams-Beuren syndrome. *Genomics* 57:279–284.

Osborne, L. R., Li, M., Pober, B., Chitayat, D., Bodurtha, J., Mandel, A., Costa, T., Grebe, T., Cox, S., Tsui, L. C., and Scherer, S. W. 2001. A 1.5 million–base pair inversion polymorphism in families with Williams-Beuren syndrome. *Nature Genetics* 29:321–325.

Ota, T., Suzuki, Y., Nishikawa, T., Otsuki, T., Sugiyama, T., Irie, R., et al. 2004. Complete sequencing and characterization of 21,243 full-length human cDNAs. *Nature Genetics.* 36:40–45.

Pan, Z. Q., Chen, M., and Hurwitz, J. 1993. The subunits of activator 1 (replication factor C) carry out multiple functions essential for proliferating-cell nuclear antigen-dependent DNA synthesis. *Proceedings of the National Academy of Sciences USA* 90:6–10.

Paperna, T., Peoples, R., Wang, Y.-K., Kaplan, P., and Francke, U. 1998. Genes for the CPE receptor (*CPETR1*) and the human homolog of RVP1 (*CPETR2*) are localized in the Williams-Beuren syndrome deletion. *Genomics* 54:453–459.

Pentao, L., Wise, C. A., Chinault, A. C., Patel, P. I., and Lupski, J. R. 1992. Charcot-Marie-Tooth type 1A duplication appears to arise from recombination at repeat sequences flanking the 1.5 Mb monomer unit. *Nature Genetics* 2:292–300.

Peoples, R., Perez-Jurado, L. A., Wang, Y.-K., Kaplan, P., and Francke, U. 1996. The gene for replication factor C subunit 2 (*RFC2*) is in the 7q11.23 Williams syndrome deletion. *American Journal of Human Genetics* 58:1370–1373.

Peoples, R., Cisco, M. J., Kaplan, P., and Francke, U. 1998. Identification of the WB-SCR9 gene, encoding a novel transcriptional regulator, in the Williams-Beuren syndrome deletion at 7q11.23. *Cytogenetics and Cell Genetics* 82:238–246.

Peoples, R., Franke, Y., Wang, Y. K., Perez-Jurado, L., Paperna, T., Cisco, M., and Francke, U. 2000. A physical map, including a BAC/PAC clone contig, of the Williams-Beuren syndrome–deletion region at 7q11.23. *American Journal of Human Genetics* 66:47–68.

Perez, F., Pernet-Gallay, K., Nizak, C., Goodson, H. V., Kreis, T. E., and Goud, B. 2002. CLIPR-59, a new trans-Golgi/TGN cytoplasmic linker protein belonging to the CLIP-170 family. *Journal of Cell Biology* 156:631–642.

Pérez Jurado, L. A., Peoples, R., Kaplan, P., Hamel, B. C. J., and Francke, U. 1996. Molecular definition of the chromosome 7 deletion in Williams syndrome and parent-of-origin effects on growth. *American Journal of Human Genetics* 59:781–792.

Pérez Jurado, L. A., Wang, Y.-K., Peoples, R., Coloma, A., Cruces, J., and Francke, U. 1998. A duplicated gene in the breakpoint regions of the 7q11.23 Williams-Beuren syndrome deletion encodes the initiator binding protein TFII-I and BAP-135, a phosphorylation target of BTK. *Human Molecular Genetics* 7:325–334.

Pérez Jurado, L. A., Wang, Y. K., Francke, U., and Cruces, J. 1999. TBL2, a novel transducin family member in the WBS deletion. *Cytogenetics and Cell Genetics* 86:277–284.

Petrij, F., Giles, R. H., Dauwerse, H. G., Saris, J. J., Hennekam, R. C., Masuno, M., Tommerup, N., van Ommen, G. J., Goodman, R. H., Peters, D. J., and Breuning, M. H. 1995. Rubinstein-Taybi syndrome caused by mutations in the transcriptional co-activator CBP. *Nature* 376:348–351.

Pezzi, N., Prieto, I., Kremer, L., Perez Jurado, L. A., Valero, C., Del Mazo, J., Martinez, A. C., and Barbero, J. L. 2000. *STAG3*, a novel gene encoding a protein involved in meiotic chromosome pairing and location of *STAG3*-related genes flanking the Williams-Beuren syndrome deletion. *FASEB Journal* 14:581–592.

Pober, B. R., and Dykens, E. M. 1996. Williams syndrome: An overview of medical, cognitive, and behavioural features. *Child and Adolescent Psychiatric Clinics of North America* 5:929–943.

Potocki, L., Chen, K. S., Park, S. S., Osterholm, D. E., Withers, M. A., Kimonis, V., Summers, A. M., Meschino, W. S., Anyane-Yeboa, K., Kashork, C. D., Shaffer, L. G., and Lupski, J. R. 2000. Molecular mechanism for duplication 17p11.2. *Nature Genetics* 24:84–87.

Pröschel, C., Blouin, M.-J., Gutowski, N. J., Ludwig, R., and Noble, M. 1995. Limk1 is predominantly expressed in neural tissues and phosphorylates serine, threonine and tyrosine residues in vitro. *Oncogene* 11:1271–1281.

Ranheim, E. A., Kuan, H. C., Reya, T., Wang, Y. K., Weissman, I. L, and Francke, U. 2005. Frizzled 9 knock-out mice have abnormal B-cell development. *Blood* 105:2487–2494.

Rao, D. S., Hyun, T. S., Kumar, P. D., Mizukami, I. F., Rubin, M. A., Lucas, P. C., Sanda, M. G., and Ross, T. S. 2002. Huntingtin-interacting protein 1 is overexpressed in prostate and colon cancer and is critical for cellular survival. *Journal of Clinical Investigation* 110:351–360.

Reiner, O., Carrozzo, R., Shen, Y., Wehnert, M., Faustinella, F., Dobyns, W. B., Caskey, C. T., and Ledbetter, D. H. 1993. Isolation of a Miller-Dieker lissencephaly gene containing G protein beta-subunit-like repeats. *Nature* 364:717–721.

Reiter, L. T., Hastings, P. J., Nelis, E., De Jonghe, P., Van Broeckhoven, C., and Lupski, J. R. 1998. Human meiotic recombination products revealed by sequencing a hotspot for homologous strand exchange in multiple *HNPP* deletion patients. *American Journal of Human Genetics* 62:1023–1033.

Reymond, A., Meroni, G., Fantozzi, A., Merla, G., Cairo, S., Luzi, L., Riganelli, D., Zanaria, E., Messali, S., Cainarca, S., Guffanti, A., Minucci, S., Pelicci, P. G., and Ballabio, A. 2001. The tripartite motif family identifies cell compartments. *EMBO Journal* 20:2140–2151.

Richter, N. J., Rogers, G. W., Jr., Hensold, J. O., and Merrick, W. C. 1999. Further biochemical and kinetic characterization of human eukaryotic initiation factor 4H. *Journal of Biological Chemistry* 274:35415–35424.

Ring, C., Ogata, S., Meek, L., Song, J., Ohta, T., Miyazono, K., and Cho, K. W. 2002. The role of a Williams-Beuren syndrome-associated helix-loop-helix domain-containing transcription factor in activin/nodal signaling. *Genes and Development* 16:820–835.

Robinson, W. P., Waslynka, J., Bernasconi, F., Wang, M., Clark, S., Kotzot, D., and Schinzel, A. 1996. Delineation of 7q11.2 deletions associated with Williams-Beuren syndrome and mapping of a repetitive sequence to in and to either side of the common deletion. *Genomics* 34:17–23.

Roesler, J., Curnutte, J. T., Rae, J., Barrett, D., Patino, P., Chanock, S. J., and Görlach, A. 2000. Recombination events between the p47-phox gene and its highly homologous pseudogenes are the main cause of autosomal recessive chronic granulomatous disease. *Blood* 95:2150–2156.

Rogers, G. W., Jr., Richter, N. J., Lima, W. F., and Merrick, W. C. 2001. Modulation of the helicase activity of eIF4A by eIF4B, eIF4H, and eIF4F. *Journal of Biological Chemistry* 276:30914–30922.

Roy, A. L. 2001. Biochemistry and biology of the inducible multifunctional transcription factor TFII-I. *Gene* 274:1–13.

Roy, A. L., Meisterernst, M., Pognonec, P., and Roeder, R. G. 1991. Cooperative interaction of an initiator-binding transcription initiation factor and the helix-loop-helix activator USF. *Nature* 354:245–248.

Saitta, S. C., Harris, S. E., Gaeth, A. P., Driscoll, D. A., McDonald-McGinn, D. M., Maisenbacher, M. K., Yersak, J. M., Chakraborty, P. K., Hacker, A. M., Zackai, E. H., Ashley, T., and Emanuel, B. S. 2004. Aberrant interchromosomal exchanges are the predominant cause of the 22q11.2 deletion. *Human Molecular Genetics* 13:417–428.

Samonte, R. V., and Eichler, E. E. 2002. Segmental duplications and the evolution of the primate genome. *Nature Reviews in Genetics* 3:65–72.

Schenck, A., Bardoni, B., Langmann, C., Harden, N., Mandel, J. L., and Giangrande,

A. 2003. CYFIP/Sra-1 controls neuronal connectivity in *Drosophila* and links the Rac1 GTPase pathway to the fragile X protein. *Neuron* 38:887–898.

Scherer, S. W., Cheung, J., MacDonald, J. R., Osborne, L. R., Nakabayashi, K., Herbrick, J. A., et al. 2003. Human chromosome 7: DNA sequence and biology. *Science* 300:767–772.

Scherer, S. W., Gripp, K. W., Lucena, J., Nicholson, L., Bonnefont, J.-P., Pérez-Jurado, L. A., and Osborne, L. R. 2005. Observation of a parental inversion variant in a rare Williams-Beuren syndrome family with two affected children. *Human Genetics* 117:383–388.

Schier, A. F. 2003. Nodal signaling in vertebrate development. *Annual Reviews of Cell Developmental Biology* 19:589–621.

Schmidt, S. L., Pautz, A. L., and Burgers, P. M. 2001. ATP utilization by yeast replication factor C. IV. RFC ATP-binding mutants show defects in DNA replication, DNA repair, and checkpoint regulation. *Journal of Biological Chemistry* 276:34792–34800.

Schulze, K. L., Broadie, K., Perin, M. S., and Bellen, H. J. 1995. Genetic and electrophysiological studies of *Drosophila* syntaxin-1A demonstrate its role in nonneuronal secretion and neurotransmission. *Cell* 80:311–320.

Sollner, T., Bennett, M. K., Whiteheart, S. W., Scheller, R. H., and Rothman, J. E. 1993. A protein assembly-disassembly pathway in vitro that may correspond to sequential steps of synaptic vesicle docking, activation, and fusion. *Cell* 75:409–418.

Sonoda, N., Furuse, M., Sasaki, H., Yonemura, S., Katahira, J., Horiguchi, Y., and Tsukita, S. 1999. *Clostridium perfringens* enterotoxin fragment removes specific claudins from tight junction strands: Evidence for direct involvement of claudins in tight junction barrier. *Journal of Cell Biology* 147:195–204.

Stankiewicz, P., and Lupski, J. R. 2002. Genome architecture, rearrangements and genomic disorders. *Trends in Genetics* 18:74–82.

Stock, A. D., Spallone, P. A., Dennis, T. R., Netski, D., Morris, C. A., Mervis, C. B., and Hobart, H. H. 2003. Heat shock protein 27 gene: Chromosomal and molecular location and relationship to Williams syndrome. *American Journal of Medical Genetics.* 120A:320–325.

Stoeckman, A. K., Ma, L., and Towle, H. C. 2004. Mlx is the functional heteromeric partner of ChREBP in glucose regulation of lipogenic enzyme genes. *Journal of Biological Chemistry* 279:15662–15669.

Strausberg, R. L., and the Mammalian Gene Collection Program Team. 2002. Generation and initial analysis of more than 15,000 full-length human and mouse cDNA sequences. *Proceedings of the National Academy of Sciences USA* 99:16899–16903.

Tai, C. Y., Dujardin, D. L., Faulkner, N. E., and Vallee, R. B. 2002. Role of dynein, dynactin, and CLIP-170 interactions in LIS1 kinetochore function. *Journal of Cell Biology* 156:959–968.

Tassabehji, M., Metcalfe, K., Fergusson, W. D., Carette, M. J., Dore, J. K., Donnai, D., Read, A. P., Proschel, C., Gutowski, N. J., Mao, X., and Sheer, D. 1996. LIM-kinase deleted in Williams syndrome. *Nature Genetics* 13:272–273.

Tassabehji, M., Metcalfe, K., Donnai, D., Hurst, J., Reardon, W., Burch, M., and Read, A. P. 1997. Elastin: Genomic structure and point mutations in patients with supravalvular aortic stenosis. *Human Molecular Genetics* 6:1029–1036.

Tassabehji, M., Carette, M., Wilmot, C., Donnai, D., Read, A. P., and Metcalfe, K. 1999. A transcription factor involved in skeletal muscle gene expression is deleted in patients with Williams syndrome. *European Journal of Human Genetics* 7:737–747.

Tebbe, B., Mankertz, J., Schwarz, C., Amasheh, S., Fromm, M., Assaf, C., Schultz-Ehrenburg, U., Sanchez Ruderish, H., Schulzke, J. D., and Orfanos, C. E. 2002. Light junction proteins: A novel class of integral membrane proteins. Expression in human epidermis and in HaCaT keratinocytes. *Archives of Dermatology Research* 294:14–18.

Tipney, H. J., Hinsley, T. A., Brass, A., Metcalfe, K., Donnai, D., and Tassabehji, M. 2004. Isolation and characterisation of *GTF2IRD2*, a novel fusion gene and member of the TFII-I family of transcription factors, deleted in Williams-Beuren syndrome. *European Journal of Human Genetics* 12:551–560.

Tsunoda, K., Sanke, T., Nakagawa, T., Furuta, H., and Nanjo, K. 2001. Single nucleotide polymorphism (D68D, T to C) in the syntaxin 1A gene correlates to age at onset and insulin requirement in type II diabetic patients. *Diabetologia* 44:2092–2097.

Tussie-Luna, M. I., Bayarsaihan, D., Ruddle, F. H., and Roy, A. L. 2001. Repression of TFII-I-dependent transcription by nuclear exclusion. *Proceedings of the National Academy of Sciences USA* 98:7789–7794.

Uitto, J., Christiano, A. M., Kähäri, V.-M., Bashir, M. M., and Rosenbloom, J. 1991. Molecular biology and pathology of human elastin. *Biochemical Society Transactions* 19:824–829.

Urban, Z., Helms, C., Fekete, G., Csiszar, K., Bonnet, D., Munnich, A., Donis-Keller, H., and Boyd, C. 1996. 7q11.23 deletions in Williams syndrome arise as a consequence of unequal meiotic crossover. *American Journal of Human Genetics* 59:958–962.

Urban, Z., Riazi, S., Seidl, T. L., Katahira, J., Smoot, L. B., Chitayat, D., Boyd, C. D., and Hinek, A. 2002. Connection between elastin haploinsufficiency and increased cell proliferation in patients with supravalvular aortic stenosis and Williams-Beuren syndrome. *American Journal of Human Genetics* 71:30–44.

Uyeda, K., Yamashita, H., and Kawaguchi, T. 2002. Carbohydrate responsive element-binding protein (ChREBP): A key regulator of glucose metabolism and fat storage. *Biochemical Pharmacology* 63:2075–2080.

Valero, M. C., de Luis, O., Cruces, J., and Perez Jurado, L. A. 2000. Fine-scale comparative mapping of the human 7q11.23 region and the orthologous region on mouse chromosome 5G: The low-copy repeats that flank the Williams-Beuren syndrome deletion arose at breakpoint sites of an evolutionary inversion(s). *Genomics* 69:1–13.

Vazquez, N., Lehrnbecher, T., Chen, R., Christensen, B. L., Gallin, J. I., Malech, H., Holland, S., Zhu, S., and Chanock, S. J. 2001. Mutational analysis of patients with p47-phox-deficient chronic granulomatous disease: The significance of recombination events between the p47-phox gene (*NCF1*) and its highly homologous pseudogenes. *Experimental Hematology* 29:234–243.

von Dadelszen, P., Chitayat, D., Winsor, E. J., Cohen, H., MacDonald, C., Taylor, G., Rose, T., and Hornberger, L. K. 2000. De novo 46,XX,t(6;7)(q27;q11;23) associated with severe cardiovascular manifestations characteristic of supravalvular aortic stenosis and Williams syndrome. *American Journal of Medical Genetics* 90:270–275.

Wang, M. S., Schinzel, A., Kotzot, D., Balmer, D., Casey, R., Chodirker, B. N., Gyftodimou, J., Petersen, M. B., Lopez-Rangel, E., and Robinson, W. P. 1999. Molecular and clinical correlation study of Williams-Beuren syndrome: No evidence of molecular factors in the deletion region or imprinting affecting clinical outcome. *American Journal of Medical Genetics* 86:34–43.

Wang, Y. K., Samos, C. H., Peoples, R., Perez-Jurado, L. A., Nusse, R., and Francke, U. 1997. A novel human homologue of the *Drosophila frizzled* wnt receptor gene binds wingless protein and is in the Williams syndrome deletion at 7q11.23. *Human Molecular Genetics* 6:465–472.

Wang, Y. K., Perez-Jurado, L. A., and Francke, U. 1998. A mouse single-copy gene, Gtf2i, the homolog of human *GTF2I,* that is duplicated in the Williams-Beuren syndrome deletion region. *Genomics* 48:163–170.

Wang, Y. K., Sporle, R., Paperna, T., Schughart, K., and Francke, U. 1999. Characterization and expression pattern of the *frizzled* gene *Fzd9,* the mouse homolog of *FZD9* which is deleted in Williams-Beuren syndrome. *Genomics* 57:235–248.

Wang, Y., Horvath, O., Hamm-Baarke, A., Richelme, M., Gregoire, C., Guinamard, R., Horejsi, V., Angelisova, P., Spicka, J., Schraven, B., Malissen, B., and Malissen, M. 2005. Single and combined deletions of the NTAL/LAB and LAT adaptors minimally affect B-cell development and function. *Molecular and Cellular Biology* 25:4455–4465

Wanker, E. E., Rovira, C., Scherzinger, E., Hasenbank, R., Walter, S., Tait, D., Colicelli, J., and Lehrach, H. 1997. HIP-I: A huntingtin interacting protein isolated by the yeast two-hybrid system. *Human Molecular Genetics* 6:487–495.

Weber, T., Zemelman, B. V., McNew, J. A., Westerman, B., Gmachl, M., Parlati, F., Sollner, T. H., and Rothman, J. E. 1998. SNAREpins: Minimal machinery for membrane fusion. *Cell* 92:759–772.

Wu, T. C., and Lichten, M. 1994. Meiosis-induced double-strand break sites determined by yeast chromatin structure. *Science* 263:515–518.

Wu, Y. Q., Sutton, V. R., Nickerson, E., Lupski, J. R., Potocki, L., Korenberg, J. R., Greenberg, F., Tassabehji, M., and Shaffer, L. G. 1998. Delineation of the common critical region in Williams syndrome and clinical correlation of growth, heart, ethnicity, and parental origin. *American Journal of Human Genetics* 78:82–89.

Wu, Y. Q., Nickerson, E., Shaffer, L. G., Keppler-Noreuil, K., and Muilenburg, A. 1999. A case of Williams syndrome with a large, visible cytogenetic deletion. *Journal of Medical Genetics* 36:928–932.

Wu, Y. Q., Lin, X., Liu, C. M., Jamrich, M., and Shaffer, L. G. 2001. Identification of a human brain-specific gene, calneuron 1, a new member of the calmodulin superfamily. *Molecular Genetics and Metabolism* 72:343–350.

Wu, Y. Q., Bejjani, B. A., Tsui, L. C., Mandel, A., Osborne, L. R., and Shaffer, L. G. 2002. Refinement of the genomic structure of *STX1A* and mutation analysis in nondeletion Williams syndrome patients. *American Journal of Medical Genetics* 109:121–124.

Wydner, K. S., Sechler, J. L., Boyd, C. D., and Passmore, H. C. 1994. Use of an intron polymorphism to localize the tropoelastin gene to mouse chromosome 5 in a region of linkage conservation with human chromosome 7. *Genomics* 23:125–131.

Yan, X., Zhao, X., Qian, M., Guo, N., Gong, X., and Zhu, X. 2000. Characterization and gene structure of a novel retinoblastoma-protein-associated protein similar to the transcription regulator TFII-I. *Biochemical Journal* 345:749–757.

Yang, N., Higuchi, O., Ohashi, K., Nagata, K., Wada, A., Kangawa, K., Nishida, E., and Mizuno, K. 1998. Cofilin phosphorylation by LIM-kinase 1 and its role in Rac-mediated actin reorganization. *Nature* 393:809–812.

Yang, W., and Desiderio, S. 1997. BAP-135, a target for Bruton's tyrosine kinase in response to B cell receptor engagement. *Proceedings of the National Academy of Sciences U S A* 94:604–609.

Zhu, M., Liu, Y., Koonpaew, S., Granillo, O., and Zhang, W. 2004. Positive and negative regulation of FcepsilonRI-mediated signaling by the adaptor protein LAB/NTAL. *Journal of Experimental Medicine* 200:991–1000.

Genotype-Phenotype Correlations in Williams-Beuren Syndrome

3

Colleen A. Morris, M.D.

A *phenotype* is an observable, measurable trait in an individual that is the result of interaction between the *genotype* (the inherited DNA code) and the environment. Genotype-phenotype correlation studies attempt to link the action of a specific gene with a particular structural or functional outcome in an individual. Before considering the results of investigations of this type, it is important to understand the role that variability plays on each side of the genotype-phenotype equation.

Genes are located on the paired chromosomes and are composed of sequences of nucleotide pairs of DNA that are organized into coding regions (exons) separated by noncoding regions (introns). For a particular gene, the sequence is often conserved evolutionarily, resulting in few differences among species. A single nucleotide that is different from the usual sequence is termed a polymorphism. The polymorphism may be neutral, not altering the function of the gene, or it may represent a mutation that causes a change in the phenotype. In medicine, observation of the negative effect of a deleterious mutation on the phenotype has traditionally yielded the most insight into normal function and development. The site and type of mutation in the gene determines the way in which gene expression is altered. For instance, a premature termination (stop) codon will result in a null allele, so that one of the gene pair is not expressed (haploinsufficiency). Alternatively, a missense mutation may result in the production of a protein with a structural abnormalities that prevent or interfere with the normal function of the protein in the cell or tissue. Different mutations in the same gene can thus result in clinically distinct syndromes. For example, various genetic alterations affecting the elastin gene (*ELN*) result in the following overlapping yet distinct phenotypes: cutis laxa (OMIM [Online Mendelian Inheritance in Man catalogue number] 123700), supravalvular aortic stenosis (OMIM 185500), and Williams-Beuren syndrome (OMIM 194050). In addition, because genes are often expressed differently in different tissues (pleiotropy), a given mutation may affect one tissue but not have a significant effect on another. Another type of genetic variability, genetic or nonallelic (locus) heterogeneity, occurs when a mutation in a different gene results in the same clinical phenotype. Often, the mutated genes that result in the same clinical syndrome are part of the same metabolic pathway or developmental cascade.

Variability also characterizes the phenotype, with each individual's expression of the genetic mutation being influenced by several factors. Environmental modifiers include prenatal exposures, socioeconomic background, educational opportunity, nutritional status, and medical treatment. Most phenotypic features also vary with time due to the effects of developmental processes and aging. Interpretation of the genotype-phenotype correlation for a particular mutation may be clearer in experimental animals with a uniform genetic background than in humans, in which the mutation of interest occurs in the setting of the individual's unique and uncharacterized genetic background. Finally, epigenetic factors may influence gene expression. For instance, for some traits expression varies with the gender of the affected individual. Imprinted genes that most commonly affect growth or behavior provide another example, because the expression of a particular allele depends on whether it was inherited from the mother or the father.

In this chapter I describe both the variability of reported genotypes in the Williams-Beuren syndrome chromosome region (WBSCR) of chromosome 7 and the resultant diverse phenotypes and discuss the current understanding of human genotype-phenotype correlations.

Clinical Phenotypes Associated with *ELN* Mutation

The elastin gene (*ELN*), located on chromosome 7, encodes the protein elastin, which is produced by fibroblasts, smooth muscle cells, and endothelial cells. Elastin is the major component of the elastic fibers found in many connective tissues. Elastic fibers supply stretchiness to tissues that must expand and contract with movement, such as the skin, cartilage, ligaments, lungs, and arteries. The fibers can deform with little applied force and store mechanical energy that is released on the recoil (Gosline et al. 2002).

The precursor protein, tropoelastin, is a soluble monomer that is transported to the extracellular matrix by elastin binding protein. In the matrix, it polymerizes by cross-linking, mediated by the enzyme lysyl oxidase, to form insoluble hydrophobic elastin. The mature elastic fibers are composed of the amorphous component, elastin, on a scaffold of microfibrils, which are assembled from several glycoproteins, including the fibrillins (Urban and Boyd 2000). Most elastic fibers are produced in the late prenatal period and in the first year of life. The organization of the elastic fibers varies with the tissue type. In skin, the fibrillar network is perpendicular to the dermoepi-

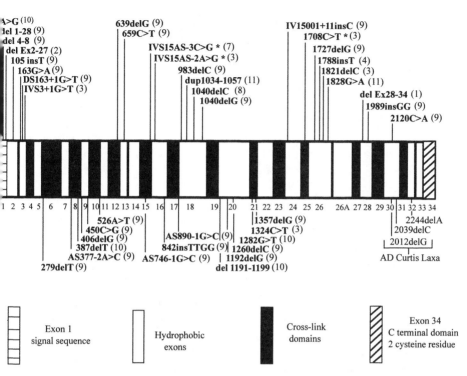

Fig. 3.1. Mutations of *ELN*. Asterisks designate mutation hotspots found in more than one family. The numbers in parentheses refer to sources: (1) Ewart et al. 1994; (2) Olson et al. 1995; (3) Li et al. 1997; (4) Tassabehji et al. 1997; (5) Tassabehji et al. 1998; (6) Zhang et al. 1999; (7) Urban et al. 1999; (8) Boeckel et al. 1999; (9) Metcalfe et al. 2000; (10) Urban et al. 2000; (11) Urban et al. 2001.

dermal junction, with the associated elastic fibers oriented parallel to the junction (Ghomrasseni et al. 2001). In the media of arteries, the elastic fibers are arranged in concentric rings called lamellae that alternate with rings of smooth muscle cells. Hollow organs such as bowel, bladder, and lung have networks of elastic fibers.

The human elastin gene has thirty-four exons, which alternate between coding for the hydrophobic domains that confer elasticity and for the lysine-rich cross-linking domains that provide stability (fig. 3.1). This structure allows alternative splice sites without changing the reading frame. Up-regulators of *ELN* expression include transforming growth factor β (TGF-β), insulinlike growth factor I (IGF1), and glucocorticoids. Down-regulators include tumor necrosis factor α, interferon γ, and vitamin D_3 (Milewicz et al. 2000).

Clinical abnormalities involving elastin can result from a mutation in *ELN* leading to an abnormal protein product, deletion of the *ELN* gene causing haploinsufficiency, or mutations in other genes that are involved in the biosynthesis, transport, or degradation of elastin (Urban and Boyd 2000).

Supravalvular Aortic Stenosis

Supravalvular aortic stenosis (SVAS) can be a familial condition inherited as an autosomal dominant or can be part of a broader pattern of malformation, Williams-Beuren syndrome (WBS). Most families with SVAS have point mutations in *ELN*, have normal intelligence, and do not fit the WBS cognitive profile (Frangiskakis et al. 1996). However, the arterial pathology and the variability in severity of the cardiovascular disease is the same for both disorders. SVAS is named for the narrowing of the aorta above the aortic valve, which results in the most significant symptoms, morbidity, and mortality of the disorder. The condition would more appropriately be termed an elastin arteriopathy: any artery can be clinically affected by the disease, and, histologically, all arteries demonstrate the pathology. In SVAS, the arterial media is thicker than normal because there is an increased number of lamellar units (Li et al. 1998b). Discrete areas of stenosis tend to occur where there is greater hemodynamic stress or turbulence, such as above the semilunar valves of the heart or at the bifurcation or origins of large arteries. If obstruction of the aortic outflow tract is untreated, the result is left ventricular hypertrophy, cardiac failure, and death. The most common forms of aortic involvement are an hourglass stenosis above the aortic valve in ~75% of cases and diffuse aortic narrowing in ~25%. The nonstenotic regions of the artery have an increased number of elastic lamellae; in the stenotic regions, the media is disorganized, with smooth muscle cell hypertrophy and absence of the usual parallel orientation of the elastic fibers (Perou 1961; O'Connor et al. 1985). Hypertension is common both in familial SVAS and in WBS. In addition to the cardiovascular effects of SVAS, individuals with nonsyndromic SVAS often have other connective tissue abnormalities including hoarse voice and hernias (Grimm and Wesselhoeft 1980; Morris and Moore 1991). The diagnosis of SVAS is most often suspected when a pathologic systolic murmur is heard in the aortic area and radiates to the carotids. Other common signs may include a thrill in the suprasternal notch, a systolic murmur in the lung fields that is due to peripheral pulmonic stenosis, or blood pressure that is higher in the right arm than the left, which is due to the Coanda effect (French and Guntheroth 1970). The diagnosis can be confirmed by Doppler echocardiography to measure pressure gradients and flow velocities across the stenotic regions (Ensing et al. 1989). The aortic lesion may worsen over time (Ino et al. 1988; Morris et al. 1990), but the peripheral pulmonic stenosis is more likely to improve (Giddens et al. 1989; Wren et al. 1990). As in most dominant conditions, there is a great deal of variability among affected individuals; the SVAS pressure gradients can range from 0 to 110 mm Hg in

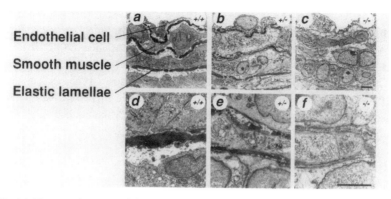

Endothelial cell

Smooth muscle

Elastic lamellae

Fig. 3.2. Electron microscopy of the aortic media in mice. $+/+$ (*a* and *d*) is the wild type (normal); $+/-$ (*b* and *e*) is hemizygous for *ELN*, and $-/-$ (*c* and *f*) is the homozygous *ELN* knockout. Compared with the wild type (normal), mice hemizygous for *ELN* show thin elastic lamellae. The bar (in *f*) is 3.0 μm. *Source:* Li et al. 1998b. Novel Arterial Pathology in Mice and Humans Hemizygous for Elastin, *Journal of Clinical Investigation* 102:1784. Reprinted with permission.

those with the mutant gene. Approximately 30% of affected individuals have significant outflow tract obstruction requiring surgery. For a detailed discussion of the diagnosis and treatment of SVAS, see chapter 5.

Several mutations in *ELN* have been described that result in SVAS (fig. 3.1). The mutations that cause SVAS occur in the region between exons 1 and 30 (Metcalfe et al. 2000). Splice site mutations have been found, but mutations that result in a premature termination (stop) codon are the most common. Both nonsense and frameshift mutations leading to a premature termination codon have been reported; Urban et al. (2000) demonstrated that a premature termination resulted in degradation of mutant mRNA (nonsense-mediated decay), resulting in production of 50% of the normal amount of tropoelastin in fibroblasts. Thus, SVAS is typically the result of a functionally null allele.

Studies of elastin gene (*Eln*) knockout mice have provided clues to the pathogenesis of the obstructive vascular disease in SVAS. Mice that were homozygous for the *Eln* deletion died by postnatal day 4.5, following obliteration of the aortic lumen by smooth muscle (Li et al. 1998a). Mice that were hemizygous for *Eln* produced 50% of the normal amount of Eln mRNA and elastin protein, resulting in thin elastic lamellae (Li et al. 1998b) (fig. 3.2). In the hemizygous mice, there was a significant increase in the number of lamellar units in the aorta, corresponding to the observed 2.5-fold increase in the number of lamellar units in the aorta of humans with SVAS. The increased lamellar units allowed the normal extensibility of the arteries to be maintained at physiologic pressures, and the authors proposed that the number of smooth muscle cells increased during arterial development in response to arterial wall stress (Li et al. 1998b). They also suggested that the resultant thickened media of the arterial wall could outstrip its blood supply, leading to fibrosis and subsequent stenosis. Urban and colleagues (2002) studied elastin production in cultured smooth muscle cells from people with SVAS. These cells produced ~50% of the elastin made by normal cells and, as a result, the proliferation rate of the smooth muscle cells increased. Adding exogenous elastin to the cultures reversed the effect (Urban et al. 2002).

Cutis Laxa

The phenotype of cutis laxa is primarily observed in the skin. One of the forms of congenital cutis laxa is inherited as an autosomal dominant disorder. It is characterized by soft, loose skin that is not hyperextensible or fragile. The skin hangs in redundant folds and has decreased recoil. Histologic examination of elastic fibers in the skin shows a decreased number and fragmentation of fibers, but the diameters of the mature fibers are normal (Ghomrasseni et al. 2001). The ligaments are lax, and craniofacial features may include iris hypoplasia, a hoarse/deep voice, and long earlobes (Beighton 1972). Less frequent complications may include hernias and bowel diverticula, and peripheral pulmonic stenosis has occasionally been reported (Damkier et al. 1991). Intelligence and behavior are normal. Frameshift mutations in exons 30 and 32 have been associated with cutis laxa (Tassabehji et al. 1998; Zhang et al. 1999) (see fig. 3.1). Tassabehji and colleagues (1999) demonstrated expression of the mutant allele in skin, which results in abnormal elastic fibers through a dominant-negative effect. These mutations damage the C-terminus of elastin, which is required for deposition of elastin on microfibrils during assembly of elastic fibers.

Williams-Beuren Syndrome

Williams-Beuren syndrome is a congenital multisystem disorder with a prevalence of 1 in 7,500 (Strømme et al. 2002). It is characterized by mild to moderate mental retardation or learning difficulties, an unusual cognitive profile, a distinctive personality, dysmorphic facial features, infantile hypercalcemia, and SVAS (Morris et al. 1988). The WBS cognitive profile consists of a relative strength in verbal short-term memory and language and a severe deficit in visuospatial constructive cognition (Mervis et al. 2000). The characteristic personality of WBS includes anxiety, empathy, attention deficit hyperactivity disorder, and sociability (Morris and Mervis 2000). The genetic etiology of WBS is a submicroscopic deletion of ~1.6 Mb of the long arm of chromosome 7 encompassing the elastin gene (Ewart et al. 1993). Haploinsufficiency of elastin accounts for the connective tissue abnormalities of WBS, including the cardiovascular disease, but does not readily explain the other features of the condition, such as hypercalcemia or impaired visuospatial construction. WBS is a contiguous gene disorder; there are more than twenty genes, including *ELN*, in the commonly deleted region. It is likely that deletion of other genes in the region contributes to the phenotype. As we attempt to ascribe particular WBS traits to haploinsufficiency for a specific gene, it is important to note that every phenotypic feature of WBS demonstrates variability in the WBS population. For example, some children with WBS require lifesaving cardiovascular surgery in infancy, but others have only a mild peripheral pulmonic stenosis that resolves spontaneously. Similarly, the mean IQ for WBS on the Kaufman Brief Intelligence Test (K-BIT; Kaufman and Kaufman 1990), which measures verbal ability and non-verbal reasoning ability but not visuospatial construction ability, is 68. However, the range is 40 (the lowest possible IQ on this measure) to 104 (Morris and Mervis 2000). The phenotypic features of WBS are summarized in table 3.1. Details of these phenotypic characteristics are described in chapter 1 and the medical complications in chapters 4 and 6.

The role of *ELN* in the WBS phenotype is well established. Haploinsufficiency for the elastin gene results in decreased production of elastin protein. A study of cultured smooth muscle cells from patients with familial non-syndromic SVAS showed ELN mRNA levels at 50% of normal, but the ELN mRNA levels were only 15% of normal in cells from individuals with WBS (Urban et al. 2002). The etiology of this reduced expression relative to non-syndromic SVAS is unknown, although the *ELN* expression might be altered by the haploinsufficiency of one of the other genes deleted in the WBSCR. Microscopic examination of the skin of patients with WBS shows a decreased number of both pre-elastic and elastic fibers and a decreased diameter of mature elastic fibers (Ghomrasseni et al. 2001). This abnormality results in the soft, loose skin seen in individuals with WBS. Elastic fibers are found in the middle layer of the vocal cords, accounting for the hoarse voice in WBS (Hammond et al. 1998; Vaux et al. 2003). It is likely that the periorbital fullness seen in WBS is also related to elastin haploinsufficiency, because elastin is a major component of the dense connective tissue of the anterior orbit that supports the orbital fat (Sires et al. 1998). *ELN* insufficiency has been shown to account for the cardiovascular phenotype in both SVAS and WBS. Other connective tissue abnormalities (inguinal and umbilical hernias, bowel and bladder diverticula, and lax joints) are found both in nonsyndromic SVAS and in WBS and are thus likely the result of a reduced amount of elastin protein.

Epigenetic and Genomic Factors

One potential cause of phenotypic variability in WBS is the influence of epigenetic factors, such as imprinting. The expression of imprinted genes in the individual depends on the parent of origin. The sporadic deletion of chro-

Table 3.1.
WBS Phenotypic Features by Organ System and Prevalence (%)

Cognitive	Cardiovascular
Developmental delay (95%)	Any abnormality (total) (80%)
Mental retardation (75%)	SVAS (75%)
Borderline intellectual functioning (20%)	SVPS (25%)
Normal intelligence (5%)	PPS (50%)
WBS Cognitive Profile (90%)	VSD (10%)
Behavioral	Renal artery stenosis (45%)
Attention deficit hyperactivity disorder (17%)	Other arterial stenosis (20%)
Anxiety disorder (80%)	Aortic insufficiency[b] (10%)
Neurologic	Mitral valve prolapse[b] (15%)
Hyperactive deep tendon reflexes (75%)	Hypertension[b] (50%)
Chiari malformation (10%)	*Genitourinary*
Hypotonia (central) (80%)	Structural anomaly (20%)
Hypertonia (peripheral) (50%)	Enuresis (50%)
Facial Features (100%)[a]	Nephrocalcinosis (<5%)
Broad brow	Bladder diverticula (75%)
Bitemporal narrowing	Recurrent urinary tract infections[b] (30%)
Epicanthal folds	*Gastrointestinal*
Periorbital fullness	Feeding difficulties (70%)
Strabismus	Constipation (40%)
Stellate/lacy iris pattern	Colon diverticula[b] (30%)
Short nose or anteversion of nares	Rectal prolapse (15%)
Bulbous or full nasal tip	*Integument*
Malar hypoplasia	Soft lax skin (90%)
Full cheeks	Inguinal hernia (40%)
Long philtrum	Umbilical hernia (50%)
Full prominent lips	Prematurely gray hair[b] (90%)
Small, widely spaced teeth	Sacral crease (50%)
Wide mouth	*Musculoskeletal*
Malocclusion	Joint hypermobility (90%)
Small jaw	Joint contractures (50%)
Prominent earlobes	Radioulnar synostosis (20%)
Growth	Kyphosis (20%)
Prenatal growth deficiency (50%)	Lordosis (40%)
Postnatal short stature (70%)	Awkward gait (60%)
Ocular and visual	Hallux valgus (70%)
Esotropia (50%)	*Calcium*
Hyperopia (50%)	Hypercalcemia (15%)
Auditory	Hypercalciuria (30%)
Chronic otitis media (50%)	*Endocrine*
Hypersensitivity to sound (90%)	Hypothyroidism (10%)
Dental/Voice	Early puberty (50%)
Malocclusion (85%)	Diabetes mellitus[b] (15%)
Microdontia (95%)	Obesity[b] (30%)
Hoarse voice (95%)	

Abbreviations: SVAS, supravalvular aortic stenosis; SVPS, supravalvular pulmonic stenosis; PPS, peripheral pulmonary artery stenosis; VSD, ventricular septal defect.
[a]100% of individuals with WBS have 9 or more of these 17 facial features.
[b]A feature most commonly observed in adults.

mosome 7q11.23 that causes WBS can be of maternal or paternal origin, and multiple series have shown an even distribution (Ewart et al. 1993; Pérez Jurado et al. 1996; Wu et al. 1998; Wang et al. 1999). The first study to suggest there could be a parent-of-origin effect in WBS evaluated thirty-eight individuals with WBS and reported a more severe postnatal growth deficiency in those with a maternal origin of deletion (Pérez Jurado et al. 1996). A subsequent study of fifty-one individuals with WBS failed to show a parent-of-origin effect on growth or any evidence for imprinting (Wu et al. 1998). A third study, including eighty-five individuals with WBS, showed no phenotypic effect related to gender or parent of origin (Wang et al. 1999).

One retrospective study of variable expression of the cardiovascular phenotype in 127 individuals with WBS reported increased prevalence and severity of cardiovascular disease in males (Sadler et al. 2001). Another study, of fifty-three patients, found that males with WBS presented earlier with cardiovascular disease than females (Bruno et al. 2003).

Most individuals with WBS have the same sized chromosomal deletion, because the breakpoints typically occur in the region of low-copy repeats (LCRs) on either side of the common deletion region. The LCRs, consisting of gene clusters and pseudogenes, predispose to nonallelic homologous recombination in meiosis. This unequal crossing over may result in deletion (in WBS), duplication (unpublished data), or inversion. Conditions that arise through this mechanism are termed genomic disorders. Osborne and colleagues (2001) found that four of twelve parents who transmitted the deleted chromosome had an inversion. Bayés and colleagues (2003) found that twenty-one of seventy-one individuals with WBS showed molecular evidence of a parental rearrangement; an inversion was confirmed in nine. Neither of these studies evaluated the frequency of the inversion in the general population or investigated genotype-phenotype correlation. A third study, a series of 266 parents of individuals with WBS, showed that 25% of the transmitting parents had an inversion and the population prevalence of the inversion was 7% (Hobart et al. 2004). No phenotypic effect of the parental inversion on the individual with WBS has been reported, though further study is needed. (*Note:* Despite the presence of paracentric inversions in 25% of transmitting parents, the empiric recurrence risk for WBS is low [<1%], and, other than identical twins, few siblings with WBS have been reported [Kara-Mostefa et al. 1999]. Individuals with WBS have a 50% risk of transmitting the deletion to offspring, and dominant inheritance has been reported [Morris et al. 1993; Ounap et al. 1998; Sadler et al. 1993].)

Two developmentally delayed individuals with "atypical WBS" were found to have the inversion polymorphism; one also had a second, larger inversion and had inattention, strabismus, ectrodactyly, lordosis, and dysmorphic facial features, and the other had strabismus, joint contractures, and hypersensitivity to sound (Osborne et al. 2001). Although both of these individuals had some nonspecific features that occur in WBS, photographs were not published and the genotype-phenotype correlation is not clear. In a study of sixty-five individuals who were referred with a previous clinical diagnosis of WBS but had no deletion demonstrated by FISH (fluorescent in situ hybridization) for *ELN*, no gene deletion was detected in the WBSCR (Morris et al. 1998). Overlapping phenotypic features in the group included mental retardation /

developmental delay (92%), attention deficit hyperactivity disorder (50%), short stature (30%), and congenital heart defects (25%).

Translocations that involve the WBSCR have also been reported. One large family with a 6;7 translocation had SVAS cosegregating with the translocation; the translocation was found to disrupt the elastin gene in exon 28 (Morris et al. 1993; Curran et al. 1993). A child with a de novo 6;7 translocation died shortly after birth as a result of complications of severe SVAS with hydrops fetalis; both the child and the father had the inversion polymorphism (Osborne et al. 2001). In a family with SVAS, a 7;16 translocation was found to disrupt the elastin gene between exons 4 and 5 (Duba et al. 2002). One of the affected family members had a clinical diagnosis of WBS and had dysmorphic facial features, mild mental retardation, and anxiety; all other affected family members had phenotypic features consistent with familial SVAS, such as hoarse voice and joint hypermobility. The authors suggested that the occurrence of the WBS features could be related to a position effect. An alternative explanation would be a second undetected genetic abnormality resulting in the mild mental retardation in the family member who had been clinically diagnosed with WBS, given that the facial features could be part of the SVAS phenotype.

In summary, there is evidence that the gender of the individual with WBS affects the expression of the cardiovascular disease, with males more severely affected than females. Other factors that could potentially affect the phenotype have been proposed, but more study is required to resolve the issue.

Long Deletions

Although most individuals with Williams-Beuren syndrome have the standard chromosomal deletion length, some individuals with longer or shorter deletions have been reported. Cytogenetically visible (>2–4 Mb) interstitial deletions of 7q11.23 result in a more severe phenotype than typical WBS, though there are overlapping features such as dysmorphic facial features, short stature, developmental delay, obstructive cardiovascular disease, and hernias (Morris et al. 1993; Zackowski et al. 1990). An association has been noted between seizures/infantile spasm/severe mental retardation and deletions that extend telomeric to the WBS region (Crawfurd et al. 1979; Mizugishi et al. 1998; Young et al. 1984; Wu et al. 1999). In the series of individuals reported by Wang and colleagues (1999), two had deletions distal to the usual telomeric breakpoint.

We determined the size of the deletion in 256 individuals with classic WBS; 248 had a deletion of ~1.6 Mb (classic deletion), 6 had a longer deletion, and 2 had a shorter deletion (Stock et al. 2003; Morris et al. 2004). Individuals with longer deletions fit the WBS cognitive profile but had lower cognitive ability than those with classic deletions, suggesting that genes telomeric to the WBS region are important for cognitive development. In three of six individuals with long deletions, the gene *HSP27* was deleted (Stock et al. 2003); these individuals had the lowest IQs. Interestingly, *HSP27* is important in actin dynamics, as is a gene in the commonly deleted region, *LIMK1*. It is possible that neuronal migration, which depends on normal actin function, is more severely disturbed when *both* genes are deleted. In summary, there is evidence to suggest that long deletions are associated with greater cognitive impairment than is found in the average person with WBS.

Short Deletions

Short deletions in the WBSCR occur in two clinical settings. The first is in a family with autosomal dominant SVAS. Seven such families have been reported in the world literature (see the discussion of deletion mapping later in this chapter). The other circumstance is that of individuals with sporadic occurrence of the phenotype. The phenotypes of individuals with short deletions have been variable; some have a clinical diagnosis of SVAS, and some have a diagnosis of WBS. The sporadic deletions can be subdivided into two major genotypic categories: those that include the classic WBS telomeric breakpoint and those that do not (fig. 3.3).

Short Deletions Including the Usual WBSCR Telomeric Breakpoint

Botta and colleagues (1999) reported on two developmentally delayed children with WBS who had the proximal breakpoint between *STX1A* and *ELN* and the usual telomeric breakpoint. Both children had SVAS and classic facial features of WBS. The thirty-month-old boy reported by Heller et al. (2003) had a proximal breakpoint between *STX1A* and *ELN* and the usual distal breakpoint at D7S489A (fig. 3.3). His physical findings included dysmorphic facial features (broad forehead, bitemporal narrowness, periorbital fullness, broad nasal tip, full cheeks, wide mouth, and prominent earlobes). He had SVAS, pulmonic valve stenosis, hypersensitivity to sound, developmental delay, and a history of one slightly elevated serum calcium level. Another report described a man with WBS who had a deletion that extended from *ELN* through *GTF2I* (Morris et al. 2004). He had an IQ of 60 (mild mental retardation), the WBS cognitive profile, anxiety, the WBS facial features, hoarse voice, SVAS, hypertension, inguinal hernia, colon diverticula, and joint contractures. Thus, individuals with short deletions that include the usual WBS telomeric breakpoint, including deletion of *GTF2I*, have developmental delay or mental retardation.

These four individuals with deletions spanning the region between *STX1* and *GTF2I* have a classic WBS phenotype, suggesting that deletion of the

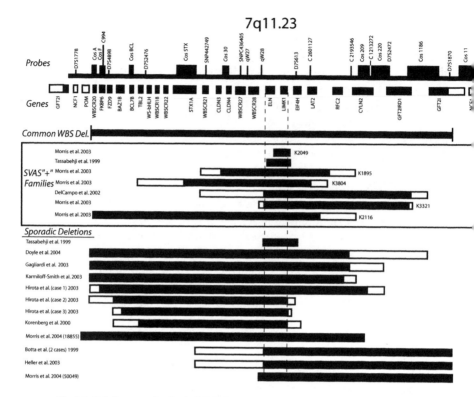

Fig. 3.3. Deletion mapping in the WBS chromosome region (WBSCR) of chromosome 7q11.23. The common WBS deletion is ~1.6 Mb and extends from *WBSCR20* through *GTF2I* (telomeric). The probes are shown above the line, and the genes in the region are represented by boxes below the line. The extent of the reported deletion is shown: the minimum extent is shown as a black bar; the white bar indicates the breakpoint region. Seven families with SVAS have been reported with deletions in the WBSCR. The sporadic short deletions in the WBSCR region in the thirteen individuals reported are shown at the bottom of the figure. Some were diagnosed with sporadic SVAS; others have a diagnosis of WBS.

more centromeric genes is not required for the WBS phenotype. However, some of these centromeric genes might be involved in WBS traits that occur at a lower frequency, such as the hypercalcemia (Tassabehji 2003).

Short Deletions Not Including the Telomeric Breakpoint

In contrast to those with a short deletion that includes the telomeric region, individuals whose deletions do not include the most telomeric genes usually have normal intelligence. Tassabehji and colleagues (1999) described an engineering student who had a short deletion (170 kb) including *ELN* and *LIMK1;* his primary symptom was SVAS. The same paper described a girl with normal height, normal facial features, and an IQ of 117 who had an

800 kb deletion from the centromeric breakpoint through *RFC2* (see also Karmiloff-Smith et al. 2003). She did not fit the WBS cognitive profile, but because of her higher cognitive ability she may have been able to employ compensatory strategies (Mervis et al. 1999).

Gagliardi et al. (2003) reported on a five-year-old boy with an IQ of 83 who had a deletion from the centromeric breakpoint through a portion of *CYLN2*. The boy was noted to have SVAS, vesicoureteral reflux, and the facial features of mild bitemporal narrowness, prominent cheeks, and a long philtrum that underwent "gradual reduction" with aging.

A man with WBS was found to have a deletion that extended from the centromeric breakpoint through *CYLN2;* he did not have a deletion of *GTF2I* (Morris et al. 2004). His IQ was 94, and he had typical WBS facies, normal stature, a hoarse voice, SVAS, the WBS cognitive profile, anxiety, hypertension, inguinal hernia, colon diverticula, and joint contractures. An eight-year-old with a diagnosis of WBS, who reportedly had mild mental retardation, had a deletion from the centromeric breakpoint that did not include genes telomeric to *RFC2*, but further clinical details including a photograph and IQ data were not available (Korenberg et al. 2000). A two-and-a-half-year-old girl was reported to have a short deletion starting from the usual centromeric breakpoint, but *GTF2I* was not deleted; the exact telomeric breakpoint was not reported (Doyle et al. 2004). That child had short stature, facial features of WBS, and SVAS but did not have hypersociability; her IQ was not reported.

In a series published by Hirota and colleagues (2003), three of sixty individuals with a clinical diagnosis of WBS had short deletions, none extending to the telomeric breakpoint. In case 1, a twenty-three-year-old woman had a deletion that spanned *FKBP6* through *CYLN2*. She did not have a history of facial features of WBS; she did have SVAS. She was reported to have a full-scale IQ of 64 as measured on the WAIS-R (Wechsler Adult Intelligence Scale–Revised), but she also was a graduate of junior high school and was working in a factory. In case 2, a seventeen-year-old girl had a smaller deletion that extended from *FKBP6* through *LIMK1*, did not have WBS facial features, but did have SVAS, peripheral pulmonic stenosis, and hoarse voice. Her full-scale IQ on the WAIS-R was reported to be 55, but she attended nursing school and attained formal certification. The third case in the series was that of a ten-year-old girl with a deletion that included *BAZ1B* through *LIMK1*. She had SVAS but did not have facial features of WBS. When tested on the WISC III (Wechsler Intelligence Scale for Children–III), her full-scale IQ was 54. Photographs were not published. From the descriptions, these individuals would be more appropriately diagnosed with SVAS than with WBS. The reported IQs in the range of mental retardation are puzzling, at least for the two older individuals, because they had occupations that require higher functioning, such as nursing.

In summary, other than the cases reported by Hirota and colleagues, individuals with short deletions that did not include *GTF2I* did not have mental retardation, but deletion of *GTF2I* was associated with decreased cognitive ability. Unfortunately, it is difficult to draw firm conclusions about genotype-phenotype relations from the few published cases because the methods of phenotype evaluation varied widely, precise breakpoints were not defined, and photographs were not published for all cases. Figure 3.3 shows the overlapping deletions in the region.

Deletion Mapping in the WBS Critical Region

A rare, but important group to study with deletion mapping strategies is families with SVAS who have deletions in the WBS region. Seven such families have been reported, five by our group (Morris et al. 2003) and two by others (see fig. 3.3). Tassabehji et al. (1999) reported on two adult brothers with SVAS who had deletion of *LIMK1* and *ELN;* the two men had normal facial features, normal intelligence, and did not fit the WBS cognitive profile. Del Campo and colleagues (2002) described a family with a deletion that included *ELN* through *GTF2IRD1*. Affected family members reportedly had borderline IQ and the WBS personality; detailed cognitive and behavioral data were not published.

We characterized five such families and discovered that affected members had the WBS cognitive profile and cardiovascular disease but lacked many other features of WBS (Frangiskakis et al. 1996; Mervis et al. 1999; Morris et al. 1996, 2003). None of the affected family members had mental retardation. As commonly occurs in autosomal dominant conditions, variability of the phenotype was noted in affected family members. All but two of the twenty-one affected individuals fit the WBS cognitive profile. Cardiovascular disease was documented in 86%, hoarse voice in 50%, mitral valve prolapse in 10%, hernia in 32%, spine abnormality in 18%, and joint laxity or contractures in 23%. It is likely that these connective tissue abnormalities, which are also part of the WBS phenotype, are due to haploinsufficiency of *ELN*. Most affected family members showed some aspect of the WBS facial features at some point in their life, but none had the classic WBS facies (score > 9 for facial features) (fig. 3.4). The most common WBS facial features observed in the SVAS kindreds were periorbital fullness and full cheeks in infancy and a long philtrum and wide mouth in adulthood. The appearance of the soft tissues of the face in infancy resembles that of WBS, but as the child ages, the WBS features become less prominent (fig. 3.5).

The overlapping deletions for the five families we have studied are shown in figure 3.3. Probes consisting of cosmids, BACs, and PACs (artificial chromosomes) were used in FISH experiments to define the deletion breakpoints (Frangiskakis et al. 1996; Morris et al. 2003). SNP (single nucleotide poly-

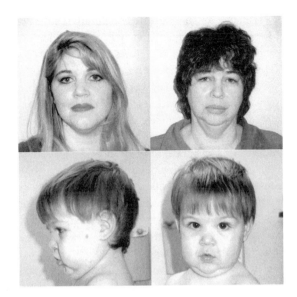

Fig. 3.4. Individuals with SVAS (Morris et al. 2003, K3804). Note the full cheeks, long philtrum, and full lips.

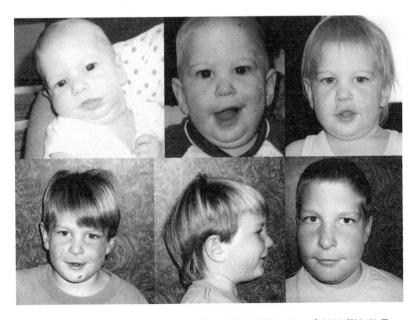

Fig. 3.5. Facial features shown over time in a boy with SVAS (Morris et al. 2003, K2049). Top row (left to right): 2 months, 9 months, 2 years. Bottom row (left to right): 4 years, 4 years (profile), 10 years. Note that in the two youngest pictures, the face has the characteristics most similar to WBS. *Source:* Morris et al. 2003. Reprinted with permission.

morphism) analysis was informative for more precisely defining the breakpoints in three of the five families. DNA sequence analysis of the region affected by the smallest deletion revealed only two genes, *ELN* and *LIMK1* (Frangiskakis et al. 1996). The latter encodes a novel protein kinase with LIM domains and is strongly expressed in the brain. Because *ELN* mutations cause vascular disease but not cognitive abnormalities, these data implicate *LIMK1* hemizygosity in impaired visuospatial constructive cognition. Visuospatial construction ability is a heritable trait that varies in the general population, likely following a quantitative trait loci model (Mervis et al. 1999). Thus, *LIMK1* is probably one of the genes contributing to visuospatial ability.

The LIM kinase 1 protein phosphorylates cofilin, a protein important in actin mechanics necessary for growth of neuronal axons. *LIMK1* knockout mice have abnormal neuronal dendritic spines in the hippocampus, and homozygous knockouts have impaired spatial learning as demonstrated by their performance in the Morris water maze (Meng et al. 2002).

Affected and unaffected members of the five families had similar IQs when tested with the K-BIT. Mean K-BIT IQ for affected members of these kindreds was twenty-seven points higher than the mean for individuals with classic WBS deletions (Morris et al. 2003). Taken together, the deletions in these five families nearly span the entire WBS deletion region but do not include the most centromeric gene, *FKBP6*, or the most telomeric gene, *GTF2I*. Evidence from other rare families and individuals with short deletions indicates that those with deletions that include *FKBP6* have normal intelligence whereas those who have deletions of *GTF2I* have mental retardation or lowered IQ (Botta et al. 1999; Heller et al. 2003; Karmiloff-Smith et al. 2003). The contrasting performance of two individuals with WBS who have short deletions (one including *GFT2I*) provides further support for the hypothesis that *GTF2I* is important for intellectual ability (Morris et al. 2004).

GTF2I codes for a transcription factor that regulates gene expression both by activating other genes and repressing transcription (Hakimi et al. 2003). Alternative splicing of the gene results in four isoforms of the protein TFII-I; the γ form is predominantly expressed in neurons and is strongly expressed in fetal brain (Pérez Jurado et al. 1998). A similar expression pattern is found in mice, suggesting evolutionary conservation of function. In embryonic mice, *Gtf2i* is expressed throughout the brain, and in adult mice it is present only in neurons, with the highest levels of expression in cerebellar cells and hippocampal interneurons (Danoff et al. 2004).

Clinical Implications

In addition to the research goals of learning more about the pathophysiology of Williams-Beuren syndrome and determining the individual genetic contributions to cognition and behavior, there are practical outcomes of genotype-phenotype correlation studies. Today, some information can be provided to families about prognosis for individuals with WBS—based on the size of the deletion, for instance. Continued analysis should begin to illuminate the cause for variability of the phenotypic features. For example, if a predisposing gene that contributes to hypercalcemia were to be discovered, then only those children at risk would need to undergo periodic monitoring of calcium status, instead of the entire population of children with WBS. Moreover, because WBS treatment strategies alter the phenotype (outcome), the efficacy of various therapies can be studied. In the past few years, there has been significant progress in our understanding of the structure and function of the genes located in the WBSCR. Advances in our knowledge about their role in development may lead to new, innovative treatments for individuals with WBS. It will be possible to investigate the role of genes in the WBSCR in the general population as well (e.g., evaluating individuals with nonspecific mental retardation for mutations in *GTF2I*).

Future Directions

In addition to analysis of individuals with rare deletions, clues about genotype-phenotype correlation come from expression studies of genes in the WBSCR and from knockout mouse models (discussed in more detail in chapter 2). Only those genes that are dosage sensitive would be expected to play a role in the WBS phenotype. The currently proposed genotype-phenotype relations are summarized in table 3.2. The role of *ELN* in the WBS phenotype is well known; its hemizygosity accounts for the cardiovascular and connective tissue abnormalities associated with this syndrome. Haploinsufficiency for *LIMK1* is strongly implicated in the impairment of visuospatial construction ability in WBS, and there is compelling evidence that deletion of *GTF2I* results in the diminished overall cognitive ability. Additional study of mouse knockouts for those two genes may yield insight into their neurodevelopmental expression. Further study of rare individuals with short deletions in the WBS region may provide additional evidence for the role of deletions of these genes in WBS cognition.

Table 3.2.
Genotype-Phenotype Correlation in Williams-Beuren Syndrome

Phenotype	Gene(s)
Supravalvular aortic stenosis	*ELN*
Williams-Beuren syndrome	Contiguous gene deletion syndrome
Vascular disease	*ELN*
Connective tissue abnormalities	*ELN*
Dysmorphic facial features	*ELN* + ?
Infantile hypercalcemia	? *BAZ1B*
Visuospatial construction impairment	*LIMK1*
Mental retardation	*GTF2I*
WBS personality characteristics	?

Prime candidate genes for other WBS phenotypic features include *BAZ1B*, *CYLN2*, and *GTF2IRD1*. Studies suggest *BAZ1B* is important in heterochromatin remodeling (Lu et al. 1998). Kitagawa and colleagues (2003) have shown that this gene interacts with the vitamin D receptor, suggesting a potential role in calcium metabolism, perhaps causing the infantile hypercalcemia of WBS. *CYLN2* is strongly expressed in the brain, especially in the hippocampus, amygdala, and cerebellum, all areas adversely affected in WBS (Hoogenraad et al. 2002). The protein product is important in organization of microtubules in cells; *Cyln2* knockout mice showed both impaired motor coordination and impaired hippocampal function. *GTF2IRD1* is expressed in muscle and thus could potentially have a role in the easy fatigability common in WBS (O'Mahoney et al. 1998; Osborne et al. 1999; Tassabehji 2003.) Continued genotype-phenotype studies, both in experimental animals and in rare families with partial deletions, are required to determine the potential role of these genes in the phenotype of WBS. Of special interest are the potential genetic contributors to the WBS personality and behavior; genes in the WBSCR are most likely involved in problems with attention and anxiety.

ACKNOWLEDGMENTS

The author's research is supported by grant NS35102 from the National Institute of Neurological Disorders and Stroke. I am thankful to the Williams Syndrome Association and its Medical Advisory Board, to the Williams Syndrome Foundation, and to the individuals with WBS and their families who have given generously of their time in support of research. I am grateful for the expert collaboration of researchers Dr. Carolyn Mervis, Dr. Holly Hobart, Dr. Mark Keating, Dr. Dean Stock, and Dr. Ron Gregg and for the assistance of Michelle Perez, our research coordinator, and of Steven LoMastro.

REFERENCES

Bayés, M., Magano, L. F., Rivera, N., Flores, R., and Perez Jurado, L. A. 2003. Mutational mechanisms of Williams-Beuren syndrome deletions. *American Journal of Human Genetics* 73:131–151.

Beighton, P. 1972. The dominant and recessive forms of cutis laxa. *Journal of Medical Genetics* 9:216–221.

Boeckel, T., Dierks, A., Vergopoulos, A., Bahring, S., Knoblauch, H., Muller-Myhsok, B., Baron, H., Aydin, A., Bein, G., Luft, F. C., and Schuster, H. 1999. A new mutation in the elastin gene causing supravalvular aortic stenosis. *American Journal of Cardiology* 83:1141–1143.

Botta, A., Novelli, G., Mari, A., Novelli, A., Sabini, M., Korenberg, J., Osborne, L. R., Digilio, M. C., Giannotti, A., and Dallapiccola, B. 1999. Detection of an atypical 7q11.2 deletion in Williams syndrome patients which does not include the STX1A and FZD genes. *Journal of Medical Genetics* 36:478–480.

Bruno, E., Rossi, N., Thuer, O., Cordoba, R., and Alday, L. E. 2003. Cardiovascular findings, and clinical course, in patients with Williams syndrome. *Cardiology in the Young* 13:532–536.

Crawfurd, M. D., Kessel, I., Liberman, M., McKeown, J. A., Mandalia, P. Y., and Ridler, M. A. 1979. Partial monosomy 7 with interstitial deletions in two infants with differing congenital abnormalities. *Journal of Medical Genetics* 16:453–460.

Curran, M. E., Atkinson, D. L., Ewart, A. K., Morris, C. A., Leppert, M. F., and Keating, M. T. 1993. The elastin gene is disrupted by a translocation associated with supravalvular aortic stenosis. *Cell* 73:159–168.

Damkier, A., Brandrup, F., and Starklint, H. 1991. Cutis laxa: Autosomal dominant inheritance in five generations. *Clinical Genetics* 39:321–329.

Danoff, S. K., Taylor, H. E., Blackshaw, S., and Desiderio, S. 2004. TFII-I, a candidate gene for Williams syndrome cognitive profile: Parallels between regional expression in mouse brain and human phenotype. *Neuroscience* 123:931–938.

Del Campo, M., Magano, L., Martinez Iglesias, J., and Perez Jurado, L. 2002. Partial features of Williams-Beuren syndrome in a family with a novel 700 KB 7q11.23 deletion. *Proceedings of the Greenwood Genetic Center* 21:169.

Doyle, T. F., Bellugi, U., Korenberg, J. R., and Graham, J. 2004. "Everybody in the world is my friend": Hypersociability in young children with Williams syndrome. *American Journal of Medical Genetics* 124A:263–273.

Duba, H. C., Doll, A., Neyer, M., Erdel, M., Mann, C., Hammerer, I., Utermann, G., and Grzeschik, K. H. 2002. The elastin gene is disrupted in a family with a balanced translocation t(7;16)(q11.23;q13) associated with a variable expression of the Williams-Beuren syndrome. *European Journal of Human Genetics* 10:351–361.

Ensing, G. J., Schmidt, M. A., Hagler, D. J., Michels, V. V., Carter, G. A., and Felt, R. H. 1989. Spectrum of findings in a family with nonsyndromatic autosomal dominant supravalvular aortic stenosis: A Doppler echocardiographic study. *Journal of the American College of Cardiology* 13:413–419.

Ewart, A. K., Morris, C. A., Ensing, G. J., Loker, J., Moore, C., Leppert, M., Keating, M. 1993. A human vascular disorder, supravalvular aortic stenosis, maps to chromosome 7. *Proceedings of the National Academy of Sciences U S A* 90:3226–3230.

Ewart, A. K., Jin, W., Atkinson, D., Morris, C. A., and Keating, M. T. 1994. Supravalvular aortic stenosis associated with a deletion disrupting the elastin gene. *Journal of Clinical Investigation* 93:1071–1077.

Frangiskakis, J. M., Ewart, A. K., Morris, C. A., Mervis, C. B., Bertrand, J., Robinson, B. F., Klein, B. P., Ensing, G. J., Everett, L. A., Green, E. D., Pröschel, C., Gutowski, N., Noble, M., Atkinson, D. L., Odelberg, S., and Keating, M. T. 1996. *LIM-Kinase1* hemizygosity implicated in impaired visuospatial constructive cognition. *Cell* 86:59–69.

French, J. W., and Guntheroth, W. G. 1970. An explanation of asymmetric upper extremity blood pressures in supravalvular aortic stenosis. *Circulation* 42:31–36.

Gagliardi, C., Bonaglia, M. C., Selicorni, A., Borgatti, R., and Giorda, R. 2003. Unusual cognitive and behavioural profile in a Williams syndrome patient with atypical 7q11.23 deletion. *Journal of Medical Genetics* 40:526–530.

Ghomrasseni, S., Dridi, M., Bonnefoix, M., Septier, D., Gogly, G., Pellat, B., and Godeau, G. 2001. Morphometric analysis of elastic skin fibres from patients with: Cutis laxa, antoderma, pseudoxanthoma elasticum, and Buschke-Ollendorff and Williams-Beuren syndromes. *Journal of the European Academy of Dermatology and Venereology* 15:305–311.

Giddens, N. G., Finley, J. P., Nanton, M. A., and Roy, D. L. 1989. The natural course of supravalvular aortic stenosis and peripheral pulmonary artery stenosis in Williams syndrome. *British Heart Journal* 62:315–319.

Gosline, J., Lillie, M., Carrington, E., Guerette, P., Ortlepp, C., and Savage, K. 2002. Elastic proteins: Biological roles and mechanical properties. *Philosophical Transactions of the Royal Society of London. Series B, Biological Science* 357(1418):121–132.

Grimm, T., and Wesselhoeft, H. 1980. Zur Genetik des Williams-Beuren-Syndroms und der Isolierten Form der Supravalvularen Aortenstenose Untersuchungen von 128 Familien. *Zeitschrift fur Kardiologie* 69:168–172.

Hakimi, M. A., Dong, Y., Lane, W. S., Speicher, D. W., and Shiekhattar, R. 2003. A candidate X-linked mental retardation gene is a component of a new family of histone deacetylase-containing complexes. *Journal of Biological Chemistry* 278:7234–7239.

Hammond, T. H., Gray, S. D., Butler, J., Zhou, R., and Hammond, E. 1998. Age- and gender-related elastin distribution changes in human vocal folds. *Otolaryngology—Head and Neck Surgery* 119:314–322.

Heller, R., Rauch, A., Luttgen, S., Schroder, B., and Winterpacht, A. 2003. Partial deletion of the critical 1.5 MB interval in Williams-Beuren syndrome. *Journal of Medical Genetics* 40(8):e99.

Hirota, H., Matsuoka, R., Chen, X. N., Salandanan, L. S., Lincoln, A., Rose, F. E., Sunahara, M., Osawa, M., Bellugi, U., and Korenberg, J. R. 2003. Williams syndrome deficits in visual spatial processing linked to GTF2IRD1 and GTF2I on chromosome 7q11.23. *Genetics in Medicine* 5:311–321.

Hobart, H. H., Gregg, R. G., Mervis, C. B., Kimberley, K. K., Rios, C. M., and Morris, C. A. 2004. Frequency of the inversion encompassing the Williams-Beuren syndrome region in parents and in the population. *Genetics in Medicine* 6:320.

Hoogenraad, C. C., Koekkoek, B., Akhmanova, A., Krugers, H., Dortland, B., Miedema, M., Van Alphen, A., Kistler, W. M., Jaegle, M., Koutsourakis, M., Van Camp, N., Verhoye, M., Van Der Linden, A., Kaverina, I., Grosveld, F., De Zeeuw, C. I., and Galjart, N. 2002. Targeted mutation of *Cyln2* in the Williams syndrome critical region links CLIP-115 haploinsufficiency to neurodevelopmental abnormalities in mice. *Nature Genetics* 32:116–127.

Ino, T., Nishimoto, K., Iwahara, M., Akimoto, K., Boku, H., Daneko, K., Tokita, A., Yabuta, K., and Tanaka, J. 1988. Progressive vascular lesions in Williams-Beuren syndrome. *Pediatric Cardiology* 9:55–58.

Kara-Mostefa, A., Raoul, O., Lyonnet, S., Amiel, J., Munnich, A., Vekemans, M., Magnier, S., Ossareh, B., Bonnefont, J. P. 1999. Recurrent Williams-Beuren syndrome in a sibship suggestive of maternal germ-line mosaicism. *American Journal of Human Genetics* 64:1475–1478.

Karmiloff-Smith, A., Grant, J., Ewing, S., Carette, M. J., Metcalfe, K., Donnai, D., Read, A. P., and Tassabehji, M. 2003. Using case study comparisons to explore genotype-phenotype correlations in Williams-Beuren syndrome. *Journal of Medical Genetics* 40:136–140.

Kaufman, A. S., and Kaufman, N. L. 1990. *Kaufman Brief Intelligence Test.* Circle Pines, MN: American Guidance Service.

Kitagawa, H., Fujiki, R., Yoshimura, K., Mezaki, Y., Uematsu, Y., Matsui, D., Ogawa, S., Unno, K., Okubo, M., Tokita, A., Nakagawa, T., Ito, T., Ishimi, Y., Nagasawa, H., Matsumoto, T., Yanagisawa, J., and Kato, S. 2003. The chromatin-remodeling complex WINAC targets a nuclear receptor to promoters and is impaired in Williams syndrome. *Cell* 113:905–917.

Korenberg, J. R., Chen, X. N., Hirota, H., Lai, Z., Bellugi, U., Burian, D., Roe, B., and Matsuoka, R. 2000. VI. Genome structure and cognitive map of Williams syndrome. *Journal of Cognitive Neuroscience* 1:89–107.

Li, D. Y., Toland, A. E., Boak, B. B., Atkinson, D., Ensing, G. J., Morris, C. A., and Keating, M. T. 1997. Elastin point mutations cause an obstructive vascular disease, supravalvular aortic stenosis. *Human Molecular Genetics* 6:1021–1028.

Li, D. Y., Brooke, B., Davis, E. C., Mecham, R. P., Sorensen, L. K., Boak, B. B., Eichwald, E., and Keating, M. T. 1998a. Elastin is an essential determinant of arterial morphogenesis. *Nature* 393:276–280.

Li, D. Y., Faury, G., Taylor, D. G., Davis, E. C., Boyle, W. A., Mecham, R. P., Stenzel, P., Boak, B. B., and Keating, M. T. 1998b. Novel arterial pathology in mice and humans hemizygous for elastin. *Journal of Clinical Investigation* 102:1783–1787.

Lu, X., Meng, X., Morris, C. A., and Keating, M. T. 1998. A novel human gene *WSTF* is deleted in Williams syndrome. *Genomics* 54:241–249.

Meng, Y., Zhang, Y., Tregoubov, V., Janus, C., Cruz, L., Jackson, M., Lu, W. Y., MacDonald, J. F., Wang, J. Y., Falls, D. L., and Jia, Z. 2002. Abnormal spine morphology and enhanced LTP in LIMK-1 knockout mice. *Neuron* 35:121–133.

Mervis, C. B., Robinson, B. F., and Pani, J. R. 1999. Visuospatial construction. *American Journal of Human Genetics* 65:1222–1229.

Mervis, C. B., Robinson, B. F., Bertrand, J., Morris, C. A., Klein-Tasman, B. P., and Armstrong, S. C. 2000. The Williams syndrome cognitive profile. *Brain and Cognition* 44:604–628.

Metcalfe, K., Rucka, A. K., Smoot, L., Hofstadler, G., Tuzler, G., McKeown, P., Siu, V., Rauch, A., Dean, J., Dennis, N., Ellis, I., Reardon, W., Cytrynbaum, C., Osborne, L., Yates, J. R., Read, A. P., Donnai, D., and Tassabehji, M. 2000. Elastin: Mutational spectrum in supravalvular aortic stenosis. *European Journal of Human Genetics* 8:955–963.

Milewicz, D. M., Urban, Z., and Boyd, C. 2000. Genetic disorders of the elastic fiber system. *Matrix Biology* 19:471–480.

Mizugishi, K., Yamanaka, K., Kuwajima, K., and Kondo, I. 1998. Interstitial deletion of chromosome 7q in a patient with Williams syndrome and infantile spasms. *Journal of Human Genetics* 43:178–181.

Morris, C. A., and Mervis, C. B. 2000. Williams syndrome and related disorders. *Annual Review of Genomics and Human Genetics* 1:461–484.

Morris, C. A., and Moore, C. A. 1991. The inheritance of Williams syndrome. *Proceedings of the Greenwood Genetics Center* 10:81–82.

Morris, C. A., Dilts, C., Demsey, S. A., Leonard, C. O., and Blackburn, B. 1988. The natural history of Williams syndrome: Physical characteristics. *Journal of Pediatrics* 113:318–326.

Morris, C. A., Leonard, C. O., Dilts, C., and Demsey, S. A. 1990. Adults with Williams syndrome. *American Journal of Medical Genetics Supplement* 6:102–107.

Morris, C. A., Thomas, I. T., and Greenberg, F. 1993. Williams syndrome: Autosomal dominance. *American Journal of Medical Genetics* 47:478–481.

Morris, C. A., Mervis, C. B., Bertrand, J., Robinson, B. F., Klein, B. P., Ensing, G., Keating, M., and Ewart, A. 1996. Lumping vs. splitting in Williams syndrome: Supravalvar aortic stenosis families with a phenotype overlapping WS. *Proceedings of the Greenwood Genetics Center* 15:154–155.

Morris, C. A., Lu, X., and Greenberg, F. 1998. Syndromes identified in patients with a previous diagnosis of Williams syndrome who do not have elastin deletion. *Proceedings of the Greenwood Genetics Center* 17:116.

Morris, C. A., Mervis, C. B., Hobart, H. H., Gregg, R. G., Bertrand, J., Ensing, G. J., Sommer, A., Moore, C. A., Hopkin, R. J., Spallone, P., Keating, M. T., Osborne, L., Kimberley, K. W., and Stock, A. D. 2003. GTF2I hemizygosity implicated in mental retardation in Williams syndrome: Genotype-phenotype analysis of five families with deletions in the Williams syndrome region. *American Journal of Medical Genetics* 123A:45–59.

Morris, C. A., Mervis, C. B., Rowe, M. L., Fricke, J. S., Hobart, H. H., Gregg, R. G., Rios, C., Kimberley, K. K., Toland, A. E., and Stone, N. I. 2004. Haplo-insufficiency of *GTF2I* implicated in mental retardation in Williams syndrome. *Genetics in Medicine* 6:264.

O'Connor, W. N., Davis, J. B., Jr., Geissler, R., Cottrill, C. M., Noonan, J. A., and Todd, E. P. 1985. Supravalvular aortic stenosis: Clinical and pathologic observations in six patients. *Archives of Pathology and Laboratory Medicine* 109:179–185.

Olson, T. M., Michels, V. V., Urban, Z., Csiszar, K., Christiano, A. M., Driscoll, D. J., Feldt, R. H., Boyd, C. D., and Thibodeau, S. N. 1995. A 30kb deletion in the elastin gene results in familial supravalvular aortic stenosis. *Human Molecular Genetics* 4:1677–1679.

O'Mahoney, J. V., Guven, K. L., Lin, J., Joya, J. E., Robinson, C. S., Wade, R. P., and Hardeman, E. C. 1998. Identification of a novel slow-muscle-fiber enhancer binding protein, MusTRD1. *Molecular and Cellular Biology* 18:6641–6652.

Osborne, L. R., Campbell, T., Daradich, A., Scherer, S. W., and Tsui, L.-C. 1999. Identification of a putative transcription factor gene (WBSCR11) that is commonly deleted in Williams-Beuren syndrome. *Genomics* 57:279–284.

Osborne, L. R., Li, M., Pober, B., Chitayat, D., Bodurtha, J., Mandel, A., Costa, T., Grebe, T., Cox, S., Tsui, L. C., and Scherer, S. W. 2001. A 1.5 million-base pair inversion polymorphism in families with Williams-Beuren syndrome. *Nature Genetics* 29:321–325.

Ounap, K., Laidre, P., Bartsch, O., Rein, R., and Lipping-Sitska, M. 1998. Familial Williams-Beuren syndrome. *American Journal of Medical Genetics* 80:491–493.

Pérez Jurado, L. A., Peoples, R., Kaplan, P., Hamel, B. C., and Francke, U. 1996. Molecular definition of the chromosome 7 deletions in Williams syndrome and parent-of-origin effects on growth. *American Journal of Human Genetics* 59:781–792.

Pérez Jurado, L. A., Wang, Y. K., Peoples, R., Coloma, A., Cruces, J., and Francke, U. 1998. A duplicated gene in the breakpoint regions of the 7q11.23 Williams-Beuren syndrome deletion encodes the initiator binding protein TFII-I and BAP-135, a phosphorylation target of BTK. *Human Molecular Genetics* 7:325–334.

Perou, M. L. 1961. Congenital supravalvular aortic stenosis: A morphological study with attempt at classification. *Archives of Pathology* 71:453–466.

Sadler, L. S., Robinson, L. K., Verdaasdonk, K. R., and Gingell, R. 1993. The Williams syndrome: Evidence for possible autosomal dominant inheritance. *American Journal of Medical Genetics* 47:468–470.

Sadler, L. S., Pober, B. R., Grandinetti, A., Scheiber, D., Fekete, G., Sharma, A. N., and Urban, Z. 2001. Differences by sex in cardiovascular disease in Williams syndrome. *Journal of Pediatrics* 139:849–853.

Sires, B. S., Lemke, B. N., Dortzbach, R. K., and Gonnering, R. S. 1998. Characterization of human orbital fat and connective tissue. *Ophthalmic Plastic and Reconstructive Surgery* 14:403–414.

Stock, A. D., Spallone, P. A., Dennis, T. R., Netski, D., Morris, C. A., Mervis, C. B., and Hobart, H. H. 2003. *Heat Shock Protein 27* gene: Chromosomal and molecular location and relationship to Williams syndrome. *American Journal of Medical Genetics* 120A:320–325.

Strømme, P., Bjørnstad, P. G., and Ramstad, K. 2002. Prevalence estimation of Williams syndrome. *Journal of Child Neurology* 17:269–271.

Tassabehji, M. 2003. Williams-Beuren syndrome: A challenge for genotype-phenotype correlations. *Human Molecular Genetics* 12 (rev. issue 2): R227–R237.

Tassabehji, M., Metcalfe, K., Donnai, D., Hurst, J., Reardon, W., Burch, M., and Read, A. P. 1997. Elastin: Genomic structure and point mutations in patients with supravalvular aortic stenosis. *Human Molecular Genetics* 6:1029–1036.

Tassabehji, M., Metcalfe, K., Hurst, J., Ashcroft, G. S., Kielty, C., Wilmot, C., Donnai, D., Read, A. P., and Jones, C. J. 1998. An *elastin* gene mutation producing abnormal tropoelastin and abnormal elastic fibres in a patient with autosomal dominant cutis laxa. *Human Molecular Genetics* 7:1021–1028.

Tassabehji, M., Metcalfe, K., Karmiloff-Smith, A., Carette, M. J., Grant, J., Dennis, N., Reardon, W., Splitt, M., Read, A. P., and Donnai, D. 1999. Williams syndrome: Use of chromosomal microdeletions as a tool to dissect cognitive and physical phenotypes. *American Journal of Human Genetics* 64:118–125.

Urban, Z., and Boyd, C. D. 2000. Elastic-fiber pathologies: Primary defects in assembly and secondary disorders in transport and delivery. *American Journal of Human Genetics* 67:4–7.

Urban, Z., Michels, V. V., Thibodeau, S. N., Donis-Keller, H., Csiszar, K., and Boyd, C. D. 1999. Supravalvular aortic stenosis: A splice site mutation in the elastin gene results in reduced expression of two aberrantly spliced transcripts. *Human Genetics* 104:135–142.

Urban, Z., Michels, V. V., Thibodeau, S. N., Davis, E. C., Bonnefont, J.-P., Munnich, A., Eyskens, B., Gewillig, M., Devriendt, K., and Boyd, C. D. 2000. Isolated supravalvular aortic stenosis: Functional haploinsufficiency of the elastin gene as a result of nonsense-mediated decay. *Human Genetics* 106:577–588.

Urban, Z., Zhang, J., Davis, E. C., Maeda, G. K., Kumar, A., Stalker, H., Belmont, J. W., Boyd, C. D., and Wallace, M. R. 2001. Supravalvular aortic stenosis: Genetic and molecular dissection of a complex mutation in the elastin gene. *Human Genetics* 109:512–520.

Urban, Z., Riazi, S., Seidl, T. L., Katahira, J., Smoot, L. B., Chitayat, D., Boyd, C. D., and Hinek, A. 2002. Connection between elastin haploinsufficiency and increased cell proliferation in patients with supravalvular aortic stenosis and Williams-Beuren syndrome. *American Journal of Human Genetics* 71:30–44.

Vaux, K. K., Wojtczak, H., Benirschke, K., and Jones, K. L. 2003. Vocal cord abnormalities in Williams syndrome: A further manifestation of elastin deficiency. *American Journal of Medical Genetics* 119A:302–304.

Wang, M. S., Schinzel, A., Kotzot, D., Balmer, D., Casey, R., Chodirker, B. N., Gyftodimou, J., Petersen, M. B., Lopez-Rangel, E., and Robinson, W. P. 1999. Molecular and clinical correlation study of Williams-Beuren Syndrome: No evidence of molecular factors in the deletion region or imprinting affecting clinical outcome. *American Journal of Medical Genetics* 86:34–43.

Wren, C., Oslizlok, P., and Bull, C. 1990. Natural history of supravalvular aortic stenosis and pulmonary artery stenosis. *Journal of the American College of Cardiology* 15:1625–1630.

Wu, Y.-Q., Sutton, V. R., Nickerson, E., Lupski, J. R., Potocki, L., Korenberg, J. R., Greenberg, F., Tassabehji, M., and Shaffer, L. G. 1998. Delineation of the common critical region in Williams syndrome and clinical correlation of growth, heart defects, ethnicity, and parental origin. *American Journal of Medical Genetics* 78:82–89.

Wu,Y.-Q., Nickerson, E., Shaffer, L. G., Keppler-Noreuil, K., and Muilenburg, A. 1999. A case of Williams syndrome with a large, visible cytogenetic deletion. *Journal of Medical Genetics* 36:928–932.

Young, R. S., Weaver, D. D., Kukolich, M. K., Heerema, N. A., Palmer, C. G., Kawira, E. L., and Bender, H. A. 1984. Terminal and interstitial deletions of the long arm of chromosome 7: A review with five new cases. *American Journal of Medical Genetics* 17:437–450.

Zackowski, J. L., Raffel, L. J., Blank, C. A., and Schwartz, S. 1990. Proximal interstitial deletion of 7q: A case report and review of the literature. *American Journal of Medical Genetics* 36:328–332.

Zhang, M.-C., He, L., Giro, M., Yong, S. L., Tiller, G. E., and Davidson, J. M. 1999. Cutis laxa arising from frameshift mutations in exon 30 of the elastin gene (*ELN*). *Journal of Biological Chemistry* 274:981–986.

The Medical Management of Children with Williams-Beuren Syndrome

4

Paige Kaplan, M.B.B.Ch.

For children with Williams-Beuren syndrome (WBS), early diagnosis and management will improve their quality of life and long-term prognosis (American Academy of Pediatrics Committee on Genetics 2001) and have a positive effect on their families and society. Optimal medical, educational, and community support can help the child with WBS lead a fulfilling life. Acute and anticipatory management should begin at the moment of diagnosis. Relatively few primary care physicians have any experience in managing the many complex aspects of WBS, and the American Academy of Pediatrics has published a set of guidelines compiled by a group of experienced physicians to assist the pediatrician caring for children with Williams-Beuren syndrome (American Academy of Pediatrics 2001). Physicians and parents may also consult specialists in multidisciplinary clinics for WBS that have been established at several centers in North America. A multispecialty WBS clinic, staffed by medical personnel with expertise in cardiology, genetics, developmental pediatrics, nephrology, urology, nutrition and feeding, behavioral pediatrics, ophthalmology, orthopedics, dentistry, psychiatry, gynecology, neurology, neuroradiology, and physical, occupational, and speech therapies can give integrated, acute, and anticipatory care and advice. Appropriate evaluations are done at one- to three-year intervals, depending on age and medical needs, during a one- to two-day outpatient visit. Close links between WBS specialists and the child's caregivers and primary care pediatrician will optimize the outcome for these children (P. Kaplan et al., unpublished observations).

Gastrointestinal System, Feeding, and Diet

Feeding difficulties manifest in the first days and months of life in a high proportion of infants with WBS. Several factors contribute to the problem, and recognizing these will help with management: (1) sucking may be weak because of hypotonia; (2) swallowing may be uncoordinated; (3) gastroesoph-ageal reflux may produce profuse vomiting; and (4) the infant may be irrita-ble, crying constantly and inconsolably, and may refuse to feed. Refusal to feed can be due to (1) pain from esophagitis, caused by frequent gastroesoph-ageal reflux; (2) idiopathic hypercalcemia, which causes vomiting, constipa-tion, and irritability (and usually resolves after infancy); and/or (3) tactile defensiveness (irritability on being touched).

After the first year, when the irritability and vomiting improve or resolve, significant feeding problems may persist, with an inability to chew and swal-low coarser foods and (continuing) food avoidance. The narrow range of foods that most children will eat usually has minimal roughage. Constipa-tion due to the low-fiber diet and bowel hypotonia is common. If the child has chronic constipation, diverticula may develop in the colon (which has less elastin in the wall). Diverticulitis may develop, causing an "acute ab-domen" and necessitating abdominal surgery. Rectal prolapse may occur.

Celiac disease has been reported to affect a higher proportion of children with WBS than children in the general population. Giannotti et al. (2001) screened a consecutive series of sixty-three Italian children (mean age eleven years) for molecular and immunologic markers of celiac disease (IgA-antigliadin and IgA-antiendomysium antibodies). Seven children had abnor-mal levels, six (9.6%) of whom had a jejunal biopsy that showed characteris-tic histologic villous atrophy. In a general population of seventeen thousand Italians aged six to fifteen years the prevalence was 0.54%. All patients with confirmed celiac disease in the series responded well to a gluten-free diet.

Management

Radiologic investigations for gastroesophageal reflux are indicated in symp-tomatic individuals and should include an upper GI series, pH probe, and/or milk scan. When esophagitis is diagnosed, treatment with antireflux med-ications will help. Rarely, in recalcitrant cases, a gastrostomy tube should be placed.

Intervention by feeding specialists knowledgeable about WBS can be in-valuable. They can teach parents optimal positioning of the child's body, with support to the mandible; techniques for inserting the bottle nipple or spoon; and exercises to coordinate chewing and swallowing. Speech therapy is im-portant in overcoming oral-motor impairments and for stimulating speech. Behavior modification with relatively simple interventions such as denying escape (the child is not allowed to leave the table for specified periods) and positive reinforcement (praise) can improve both mealtime behavior and the amount of food consumed (O'Reilly and Lancioni 2001; Ahearn et al. 2001). Improvement requires persistence and patience.

To prevent constipation, the diet must include adequate roughage (fiber).

The child should be encouraged to develop a daily routine of going to the toilet at a specific time to defecate; the best times are after a meal and when sufficient time is available to prevent stress. Mineral oil may be helpful in difficult cases of constipation.

Antibody screening for celiac disease (IgA-antigliadin antibodies and IgA-antiendomysium antibodies) is recommended for patients with symptoms of celiac disease. Patients with positive test results may require a small-bowel biopsy.

Hypercalcemia

Calcium homeostasis causes problems mainly in the first year and is detected in a small number of infants with Williams-Beuren syndrome. The reports of irritability and/or constipation in many children who were not diagnosed and investigated in their first year suggest that the incidence of hypercalcemia may be higher. The pathogenesis is not understood. Hypercalcemia can result in vomiting, irritability, constipation, and/or polyuria and subsequent dehydration; occasionally there may be seizures. Mild hypercalcemia may be asymptomatic. Nephrocalcinosis and hypercalciuria sometimes develop. Data on a relationship between nephrocalcinosis and renal failure are insufficient (Cote et al. 1989).

Management

Tests. Blood calcium (preferably ionized), intact parathyroid hormone, 25-hydroxyvitamin D, 1,25-hydroxyvitamin D, phosphorus, blood urea nitrogen, and creatinine should be measured at the time of diagnosis (Rodd and Goodyer 1999). Ionized calcium is a more accurate test than total calcium; the latter may be normal when ionized calcium is elevated.

Urine calcium/creatinine is best measured in a twenty-four-hour sample; this may not be possible for an infant, in which case a single-void urine sample should be analyzed. Calcium/creatinine ratios in a single-void urine sample may be used as a *screening* test but may not be an accurate measure; normal values have been published (Sargent et al. 1993).

Treatment. Mild elevations of calcium can be treated by limiting calcium in the diet. In the first year, a low-calcium "milk" formula (Calcilo) can be substituted for regular formula. When solid foods are added, diets should be monitored to optimize the amount of calcium, which should be the recommended daily allowance. Excessively high or low blood calcium can cause disease, so calcium levels should be monitored. Severe limitation of dietary calcium can result in rickets (Mathias 2000). Vitamin supplements containing vitamin D must be avoided; multivitamin preparations lacking vitamin D are available. Sunscreen filters (ointments) should be applied whenever the child is exposed to sunlight, to prevent excessive formation of vitamin D.

Moderate to severe hypercalcemia requires immediate treatment. Vitamin D supplements should be stopped. Intravenous rehydration, with normal saline at 1.5- to 2.5-fold normal maintenance, 150 to 250 mL/kg /24 hr, followed by furosemide, 0.5 to 1.0 mg/kg /6 hr, will increase the renal excretion of calcium. High-dose glucocorticoids will decrease absorption of calcium from the gastrointestinal tract and bone. Intravenous methyl prednisolone, 1 mg/kg/24 hr, or hydrocortisone, 1 mg/kg /6 hr, are usually effective for more severe hypercalcemia. Blood ionized calcium, serum electrolytes, magnesium, and phosphorus should be monitored at approximately two- to four-hour intervals during acute treatment and less frequently when the levels have decreased, with continuous electrocardiographic monitoring. A low-calcium diet should be maintained until the hypercalcemia has resolved. If hypercalcemia is not present in early childhood, it is unlikely to develop later (P. Kaplan, unpublished data), so it is not necessary to measure blood calcium frequently in older children who have not been hypercalcemic.

Central Nervous System and Connective Tissues
Tone and Joints

Hypotonia affects most infants with WBS and is probably present in utero. Hypotonia contributes to the motor delays, feeding difficulties, constipation, and joint laxity. Most joints are hypermobile, with the exception of the Achilles tendons (heel cords), which are invariably tight. Deep tendon reflexes are brisk. There is some improvement of the hypotonia and joint laxity during childhood (Chapman et al. 1995).

Hypertonia develops in about one-third of children and is more prevalent (85%) in adults (Chapman et al. 1995). Mild, moderate, or severe contractures develop in childhood in almost half of individuals with WBS; large and small joints may be affected (P. Kaplan et al. 1989) (figs. 4.1 and 4.2). Contractures interfere with activities of daily living such as buttoning garments, writing, and walking, and they can cause pain. Muscle mass is prominent, especially in the thighs. The gait is "clumsy," characterized by a wide base, with the upper part of the body leaning forward and a tendency to toe-walk, even in the absence of joint contractures. Inguinal and umbilical hernias develop in about 50% of individuals with WBS, mainly in childhood but also in adults.

Management

Physical therapy should be started as soon as the WBS is diagnosed, even in early infancy. It should be continued over the long term to improve tone and gait and to prevent or treat contractures. Occupational therapy will improve fine motor function, especially with tasks such as writing, fastening buttons, and tying shoelaces. Adaptive aids such as rubber bands around a pencil will

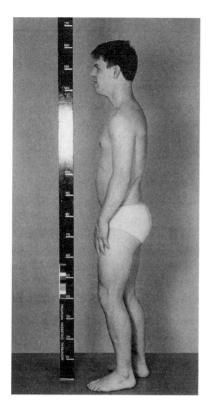

Fig. 4.1. An adolescent with WBS, showing contractures at the knees and elbows. Note the appearance of "large" muscle mass.

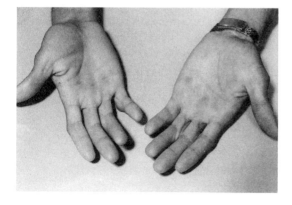

Fig. 4.2. Contractures of the fingers in an individual with WBS.

help the grip, improve writing, and diminish fatigue. If handwriting is too difficult, children can use computers. If joint contractures, particularly of heel cords, are severe despite physical therapy, they may require surgical release. The possibility of the Chiari I "sequence" should be investigated before surgery is done.

Chiari I "Malformation"

The Chiari I malformation is more appropriately named a "sequence" because of the herniation of a normal-sized neocerebellum through a small posterior fossa. Chiari I sequence has been reported in a small number of individuals with WBS (P. Kaplan et al. 1989; Wang et al. 1992; Jernigan and Bellugi 1990; Pober and Filiano 1995; Mercuri et al. 1997). It may be asymptomatic or manifest at any age with neurologic signs, including headaches, vertigo, tinnitus, diplopia, change in symmetry or degree of the hyperreflexia and/or contractures, and decreased muscle strength.

Management

Magnetic resonance imaging should be performed with the head in specific positions to detect whether the Chiari phenomenon is present and, if so, whether there is obstruction to outflow of cerebrospinal fluid. Surgical decompression may relieve symptoms. If the condition does not cause symptoms and does not seem to be worsening, six- to twelve-monthly reevaluations by a neurologist are recommended.

Learning, Education, and Independence

Learning, education, and independence of individuals with WBS are discussed in detail in chapters 10 and 12.

Management

Age-appropriate early intervention with education, physical therapy, occupational therapy, and speech/feeding therapy should be initiated as soon as the diagnosis has been made. Music therapy is thought to help children with WBS in learning and organizational skills, but a controlled prospective study has not yet been published. At five or six years, the child's parents can choose to educate the child in a regular school or in a school for children with special needs. Many parents choose a mainstream school so the child can have the opportunity to socialize with children who do not have special educational needs. In the regular school, the child usually is "mainstreamed" for art, gymnastics, and appropriate academic subjects; the other subjects are taught in small classes by special-education teachers. The child may need the constant help of a teacher's aide.

The adolescent should receive appropriate academic or vocational training. A work environment with routine assignments and minimal stress is the most satisfactory. A job in the regular work force is appropriate for some adults with WBS, but others need sheltered employment and some are not employable. Self-care and participation in household activities should be encouraged from as early an age as possible, with the aim of fostering maximal independence by adulthood

Temperament and Behavior

Attention deficit hyperactivity disorder (ADHD) affects many individuals with WBS.

Management

When treated with medication, school-aged children with WBS who have ADHD are calmer, more attentive, and learn more optimally. In two small placebo-controlled, double-blinded studies, treatment with methylphenidate was effective in modulating behavior in four of six children assessed by parents' and teachers' questionnaires and by objective psychometric measures (Power et al. 1997; Bawden et al. 1997). In these studies, a dose of 0.5 mg/kg or 10 mg twice daily produced better control of ADHD symptoms than lower doses. Many parents who are reluctant to treat the ADHD medically can be assured that the side effects are not common or permanent and that the benefits outweigh the risks. Whether the response is suboptimal if these medications are stopped during weekends and vacations is controversial; the decision to do this should be made on an individual case basis.

Sleep

Many children with WBS have difficulties initiating and maintaining sleep (Sarimski 1996; Einfeld et al. 1997). Sleep is discussed in more detail in chapter 13.

Management

Studies with polysomnography have shown that children with WBS may have significantly more periodic limb movements during sleep, called "restless legs syndrome," than children in the general population. There are associated arousals and awakenings and more time spent awake during "sleep" periods compared with controls (Arens et al. 1998). Consequently, the children do not have restful sleep and are tired the next day. The symptoms of ADHD may also be exacerbated. Periodic limb movement is more frequent in children with WBS than in non-WBS children with ADHD (Picchietti et al. 1998). In WBS, clonazepam significantly improves sleep, behavior, and learning (Arens et al. 1998).There are anecdotal reports of melatonin improving sleep but no data to support these claims.

Ears and Hearing

Otitis media affects ~60% of children with WBS and hyperacusis affects 95% (Klein et al. 1990). Older children report that hyperacusis is painful. The cause is not yet known. Children with WBS have abnormal responses to high-frequency auditory tones (Van Borsel et al. 1997), and a decreased refractory period to auditory stimuli has been reported (Bellugi et al. 1999). Loss of inhibitory control of efferent sensory input to the cochlea is a possible mechanism. In one study, seven of nine children with WBS, three with sensorineural hearing loss, had absent transient evoked otoacoustic emissions (Johnson et al. 2001).

There are isolated reports of hearing loss in WBS, but studies have not been done in a large group. Three of seven children with hyperacusis and absent transient evoked otoacoustic emissions had high-frequency sensorineural hearing loss (Johnson et al. 2001) that might have been overlooked in earlier childhood. Ruangdaraganon and colleagues (1999) reported on a child with bilateral sensorineural hearing loss. In my practice, I have encountered a few children with sensorineural hearing loss. Occasionally, bilateral conductive hearing loss unrelated to secretory otitis media has been reported (Miani et al. 2001).

Management

Audiogram, speech reception thresholds, acoustic reflexes, and impedance tests should be conducted. Chronic treatment of hyperacusis by acoustic training can alleviate distress. Strategies to accustom the child to noise include desensitization and masking, such as by wearing headphones connected to a portable cassette player to block distressing sounds. The child will benefit from a quiet classroom.

Seizures

Seizures are not common in WBS. Reports describe four children who had infantile spasms, hypsarrhythmia, and, in the three tested, severe mental retardation; two had microscopically visible interstitial deletions of 7q11.23–q21.11, larger than in "classic" WBS (Kahler et al. 1995; Tsao and Westman 1997; Mizugishi et al. 1998). Interstitial deletions of 7q11.2–q22 have been reported in children with retardation, hypotonia, and seizures (hypsarrhythmia) but not diagnosed with WBS (Crawfurd et al. 1979; Young et al. 1984; Zackowski et al. 1990).

Eyes

In Williams-Beuren syndrome, the iris stroma has a lacy or stellate pattern (74%), with absent or incomplete iris collarette, and is blue in 77% of children with WBS (Winter et al. 1996). The lacy pattern is detectable in brown irides by slit-lamp examination. Hyperopia occurs in 68% (Winter et al. 1996). Strabismus is common (27%–78%) (Pagon et al. 1987; Greenberg and Lewis 1988; Kapp et al. 1995; Winter et al. 1996; Sadler et al. 1996; Olitsky et al. 1997). In one series, 28% (7/25) had dissociated vertical deviation, 40% oblique dysfunction, and 24% amblyopia (Kapp et al. 1995); abnormal binocular vision is also evident. There are difficulties in depth perception (even in the absence of strabismus), possibly due to dysgenesis in the visual association cortex, which compounds motor and cognitive problems.

Congenital partial or complete nasolacrimal duct obstruction, with overflow of tears, is common in WBS (P. Kaplan, unpublished data). Most resolve spontaneously.

Management

Congenital esotropia should be treated as early as possible to ensure binocular vision and cosmetically straight eyes. After associated amblyopia has been treated, surgery may be performed to align the eyes. Various surgical techniques have been used for the correction of congenital esotropia. Most surgeons perform symmetric recession (weakening) of both medial rectus muscles or monocular medial rectus recession combined with a lateral rectus resection (tightening). Many children may redevelop strabismus and amblyopia; close monitoring is essential.

Nasolacrimal sac massage is effective in overcoming most obstructions. Probing of the nasolacrimal duct may be effective for unresolved blockage.

Cardiovascular System

Cardiovascular abnormalities in WBS are discussed in detail in chapter 5.

Arterial Narrowing

One of the well-known aspects of WBS is the narrowing (stenosis, hypoplasia, coarctation) of the great arteries, in the supravalvular region of the aorta and the peripheral pulmonic arteries. It is prevalent in WBS and is an important cause of morbidity and early death. However, many or all arteries may be narrowed in WBS without overt disease in all areas; Sadler et al. (1998) reported ultrasonographic evidence that the carotid arteries were narrowed without apparent effects. The supravalvular aortic and peripheral pulmonic artery stenoses are clinically apparent in ~50% to 75% of cases and cause murmurs in many neonates and infants. Most great vessel narrowing seems to develop before five years of age (Bockoven et al. 1996). The presence of supravalvular aortic stenosis (SVAS) and/or peripheral pulmonic stenoses (PPS) should always raise the suspicion of WBS, and this must be included in the differential diagnosis.

Less commonly recognized is diffuse or segmental narrowing of the aortic arch, descending thoracic and abdominal aorta, and renal and mesenteric arteries. Two studies of individuals with WBS (Radford and Pohlner 2000; Rose et al. 2001) found radiologic evidence of narrowing in these arteries in 55% (10/18) and 80% (20/25): thoracic aorta in 16% (3/18) and 36% (9/25), respectively, abdominal aorta in 11% and 28%, renal arteries in 38% and 44%, and visceral arteries in 33% (6/18) (Radford and Pohlner 2000). In one group (Rose et al. 2001), most WBS patients with renal stenoses also had aortic stenosis. The caliber of the aortic lumen did not increase with age in three males who had serial angiographic studies. One of them developed mesenteric arterial stenosis, with mild bilateral renal arterial stenoses, between the ages of nine and nineteen years. The narrowed great vessels and/or renal arteries caused hypertension in 58% to 68% of cases in the two studies.

Occasionally, narrowing of subclavian or cerebral arteries may manifest as disease even if there are no signs of SVAS/PPS (P. Kaplan et al. 1995) (see below). Intracardiac lesions are less common: mitral valve prolapse affects about 13% of individuals with WBS (Bockoven et al. 1996).

Hypertension

Hypertension is common, affecting ~40% of individuals with WBS (compared with 14% of controls; $P < 0.05$) (Broder et al. 1999), with significantly higher (10 mm Hg) mean day and night ambulatory pressures (Broder et al. 1999; Giordano et al. 2001) but normal diurnal variation. Systolic blood pressure in seventeen adolescents (eight male and nine female) with WBS was noted to be higher than in healthy controls when measured continuously for twenty-four hours (during day and night) and during exercise on a treadmill (146 ± 27 mm Hg, compared with 128 ± 12 mm Hg in healthy controls). The individuals with WBS also had increased heart rate (167 ± 19 beats/min vs. 145 ± 16 beats/min.; $P < 0.001$) with exercise and could tolerate it for half as long as the control subjects.

Severe hypertension and cardiac hypertrophy may culminate in cardiac failure. Sudden death may occur. Insufficient cardiac output, myocardial infarction, or arrhythmia due to coronary artery stenosis and severe cardiac biventricular outflow obstructions are probably responsible for these adverse events (Lacro et al. 1994; Bird et al. 1996; Bonnet et al. 1997). In these studies, one-third of the events occurred in children less than one year old, one-third between one and two years of age, and one-third between two and six years (with a single exception at fifteen years).

Strokes

Infrequently, stenoses of one or more of the cerebral arteries and/or carotid, vertebral, or basilar arteries can manifest as single or recurrent strokes (Ardinger et al. 1994; P. Kaplan et al. 1995; Kawai et al. 1993; Soper et al. 1995;

Wollack et al. 1996). The stroke may be heralded by irritability, headaches, difficulty walking, loss of consciousness, and/or seizures in young children or adults; hypertension may be a precipitating factor. Transient or permanent hemipareses or parapareses can aggravate cognitive problems and, occasionally, are fatal (Kawai et al. 1993). The cerebral arteriopathy can develop in the absence of significant SVAS and other arterial narrowing, as in the case of a four-year-old girl with two episodes of transient hemiparesis, in whom only the middle cerebral artery was narrowed (P. Kaplan and J. Hunter, unpublished data). Magnetic resonance angiography is used to demonstrate the stenoses. The extent of infarction is related to the acuteness and duration of ischemia. Collateral vessels can develop if there is chronic narrowing but may be insufficient to prevent severe neurologic sequelae (P. Kaplan et al. 1995).

Management of Cardiovascular Disease

Tests. Morbidity and mortality have been markedly reduced by early diagnosis, expectant management, and appropriate vascular surgery. Blood pressure should be measured in all four limbs at regular intervals. This is difficult to achieve in most infants and young children because of their anxiety. Twenty-four-hour continuous ambulatory monitoring at home may be required for accurate measurement. Electrocardiography and echocardiography should be performed at the time of diagnosis and at regular intervals thereafter, the frequency depending on the presence and severity of arterial narrowing. After mid to late childhood, patients without great vessel narrowing can be monitored at two- to three-year intervals unless they become symptomatic, which occurs infrequently (Bockoven et al. 1996).

If there is hypertension without an apparent cause, angiography of the aorta and its branches with measurement of aortic diameters should be performed. Doppler renal ultrasonography may not be sensitive enough to detect renal artery narrowing. Magnetic resonance arteriography can be used to study cerebral artery caliber in symptomatic patients; it is not appropriate for asymptomatic children because there is no proven preventive treatment.

Treatment. For great vessel and renal artery stenoses: balloon dilatation, surgical patch aortoplasty, and stenting are discussed in detail in chapter 5. For cerebral artery stenoses: acetylsalicylic acid (81 mg daily) has been used empirically to prevent recurrences of strokes, but its effectiveness has not been established. Physical, occupational, and speech therapy are important for rehabilitation after a stroke.

Renal Tract Abnormalities

There is an increased prevalence of renal abnormalities in WBS (Ingelfinger and Newburger 1991; Pober et al. 1993; Pankau et al. 1996; Sheih et al. 1989). The most common abnormalities are unilateral renal agenesis (3.8%, compared with 0.07% in the general population) (Wilson and Baird 1985), kidney duplication or ectopia (4%–7%), and small kidneys (1.5%). Renal failure has been reported in a few young adults (Biesecker et al. 1987; Steiger et al. 1988; Ichinose et al. 1996). Renal failure and diminished function do not seem to be common, affecting 2% in one WBS cohort and manifesting in young adults who had not been diagnosed with WBS and/or monitored in childhood (B. S. Kaplan and P. Kaplan, unpublished data). The pathogenesis is not understood, because no serial monitoring of renal function in childhood and no renal biopsies had been done for these patients. A few patients had narrowing of the descending aorta, suggesting insufficient renal blood flow. Several had renal cysts detected with ultrasonography or radiologic "nephrocalcinosis." However, most individuals with WBS who have radiologic "nephrocalcinosis" do not have renal dysfunction (Cote et al. 1989).

Nephrocalcinosis

The prevalence of "nephrocalcinosis" ranges from zero in a group of 130 children and adults (Sheih et al. 1989), to 5% (P. Kaplan, unpublished data), to 20% of 25 individuals in the first two decades (Cote et al. 1989), a variation possibly due to regional environmental differences. There may be an association between infantile hypercalcemia and "nephrocalcinosis," but the data are insufficient.

Urinary Continence

Children with WBS achieve daytime urinary continence / toilet training at an average of thirty-nine months of age (Schulman et al. 1996). Subsequent voiding problems can lead to social and medical problems. In a cohort of children with WBS (Schulman et al. 1996), 32% had urinary frequency ("urgency") and/or incontinence. In 10% it was due to uninhibited detrusor muscle contractions or bladder dyssynergy, with diverticula of the bladder. The elastin deficiency in WBS may predispose the bladder to diverticula. It is possible that both the elastin deficiency and central nervous system defects may contribute to the voiding dysfunction.

Management of Renal System
Tests. Anticipatory tests of renal function at baseline and every one to two years:
- Blood creatinine and urea nitrogen (BUN)
- Urine calcium/creatinine ratio—a twenty-four-hour specimen is optimal but, if this is not feasible, a single-void ("spot") specimen can be used; urinalysis
- Renal ultrasonography to check for malformations, calcinosis, and diverticula:

—annually if the patient has calcinosis and/or diverticula or if renal signs/
symptoms develop
—every two years until later childhood in the absence of calcinosis and/or diverticula
—every five years in adolescence and adulthood in the absence of calcinosis
and/or diverticula

A history of urinary tract infections, increased frequency, or daytime wetting
requires further study: urine culture, urodynamic studies, and voiding cys-
tourethrogram.

Treatment. Uninhibited detrusor contractions may resolve but generally
should be treated with bladder retraining by an experienced nephrologist/
urologist and anticholinergic medications such as oxybutynin or hyoscy-
amine (Schulman et al. 1996). This will help reduce the embarrassment associated with increased urinary frequency and daytime wetting and prevent
development of diverticula. Chronic hemodialysis and renal transplantation
have been successful in several adults.

Growth and Puberty
Weight

In a large proportion of individuals with WBS, body fat is lost in childhood
or adolescence, causing an appearance resembling lipodystrophy. This may
occur despite good appetites and well-balanced diets, normal physical activities, and absence of other disease. Parents are greatly concerned by their children's appearance because it connotes poor health and poor care to others.
Studies of resting energy expenditure in a small group of peripubertal children and adults showed significantly increased metabolic rates compared
with age- and height-matched control subjects, and this probably accounts
for the loss of fat stores (A. Kaplan et al. 1998). However, many children with
WBS do become obese from the second decade onward. Studies have not
been done to determine the cause, but one possible reason is inadequate exercise.

Linear Growth and Puberty

Growth charts have been compiled for height, weight, and head circumference
in males and females with Williams-Beuren syndrome and take into account
specific growth patterns of WBS. Short stature is common but is usually not
evident at birth. Mean birth length is 48.3 ± 3.1 cm (~5%–50%) in girls and
48.3 ± 2.9 cm (~5%–50%) in boys (Partsch et al. 1999). Short stature man-
ifests in early childhood, with a large proportion of children having heights
below the fifth percentile; however, some individuals grow in the normal range
compared with both the National Center for Health Statistics percentiles and

midparental height (Tanner et al. 1970). A premature pubertal growth spurt occurs in WBS and is greater in intensity than in a control group, but it has shorter duration. Overall final heights are in the low centiles: in German females with WBS, average heights were 152.4 ± 5.7 cm (n = 38) at maturity, 11 cm shorter than expected for their parents' heights and 14 cm less than average German females. In males, average adult heights were 165 ± 10.9 cm (n = 43), about 14.7 cm lower than for healthy control males (Partsch et al. 1999).

Precocious puberty, defined as onset of secondary sexual characteristics before eight years in girls and nine years in boys, is unusual in Williams-Beuren syndrome (Scothorn and Butler 1997; Douchi et al. 1999). However, early puberty is not uncommon in WBS for both girls and boys (Partsch et al. 1999). The average age for menarche in girls with WBS is 10.3 years in the United States (compared with 12.3 years in healthy control children) (Morris et al. 1993; Scothorn and Butler 1997; Cherniske et al. 1999), 11.2 ± 1.3 years in the United Kingdom (Martin et al. 1984), and 11.3 ± 1.6 years in Germany (13.5 years for controls) (Pankau et al. 1992). Partsch and colleagues (1999) noted an interesting correlation with mid-childhood growth spurts in German girls with WBS. In twenty girls it occurred between 4 and 5 years of age, and in five girls between 6 and 7 years. Four years later, each group had experienced onset of pubertal growth spurts (at 9 and 11 years, respectively) with menarche at 10.4 ± 1.4 years and 12.6 ± 1.3 years. Pubertal growth spurts occurred in thirty-four German boys with WBS at an average age of 10 years (two years earlier than in healthy control children) and peaked between 11 and 12 years. Hypergonadotropic hypogonadism has been reported (Ichinose et al. 1996)

Concomitant with accelerated growth during puberty, weight and bone age are advanced. The advanced bone maturation results in early closure of epiphyses, and final height is less than if puberty had occurred later.

Management

Referral of girls with WBS to a gynecologist, especially one specializing in adolescents and knowledgeable about WBS, is important.

Tests. The following tests should be done if precocious puberty is suspected:

- Boys
  —Serum testosterone
- Girls
  —Serum luteinizing hormone (LH) by immunofluorimetric assay, follicle stimulating hormone (FSH), and serum estradiol
  —Pelvic ultrasound to exclude an ovarian cyst or tumor; however, findings should be interpreted with caution because multiple small cysts are not uncommon in a prepubertal ovary
  —Bone age

In girls with precocious puberty, in addition to accelerated growth rate and bone age, increased uterine length and ovarian volume may be noted on pelvic ultrasound but are not diagnostic. Serum FSH, LH, and estradiol levels are generally in the pubertal age range, although there may be overlap between prepubertal and early puberty ranges.

Treatment. Because of the psychosocial impact, precocious puberty in girls with WBS should be treated with gonadotropin suppression. There are three routes of administration: intramuscular, subcutaneous, and intranasal spray. A long-acting ("depot preparation") gonadotropin-suppressive agent, a gonadotropin-releasing hormone (GnRH) agonist such as depot leuprolide (0.3 mg/kg), should be given every four weeks. In a study of non-WBS girls, GnRH agonist treatment prolonged puberty and delayed menarche significantly, compared with the accelerated course in untreated girls (4.7 ± 0.4 years vs. 2.45 ± 0.4 years) but did not change the total pubertal growth and the bone maturation rate (Lazar et al. 2002). The treated and untreated girls achieved a similar mean final height. The long-acting intramuscular form provides more gonadotropin suppression and is less dependent on patients' compliance, although clinical suppression of puberty can be achieved with daily intranasal spray or the subcutaneous preparation. In a study of forty-six non-WBS pubertal girls below the age of 9.5 years, the efficacy of buserelin, a GnRH agonist, given by intranasal spray was compared with that of the same compound given as a subcutaneous depot preparation (Tuvemo et al. 2002). During the first two years, 300 μg of buserelin acetate was given six times daily as a nasal spray. During the third year, 6.3 mg of subcutaneous buserelin, Suprefact Depot, was given every eight weeks. GnRH provocation tests showed greater suppression of gonadotropin secretion with the long-acting subcutaneous preparation.

Most girls with WBS, even with early-onset puberty, accommodate to menstruation without many problems. Irregular menses may be common during the first year or two after menarche, as in the general population. If excessive or prolonged bleeding occurs, referral to a gynecologist should be considered. Mood swings are as common as in the general population.

Sexual desires seem to be as prevalent in individuals with WBS as in the general population, and they are voiced more often by males than by females in our clinic. Females should be constantly supervised to protect them from malevolent sexual encounters. Nevertheless, contraception should be discussed with a gynecologist when the girl reaches menarche.

Thyroid Function

The prevalence of hypothyroidism and compensated hypothyroidism (elevated thyroid-stimulating hormone [TSH] with normal thyroxine level) may be higher in people with WBS than in the general population, especially in the early years. In a retrospective study of fifty-two patients with data on thyroid function and TSH, Breault et al. (2000) found that 11% (twelve patients) had clinical or compensated hypothyroidism, compared with 0.1% to 0.3% in the general population. Three children were diagnosed before one year of age. Compensated hypothyroidism was noted in six children. The prevalence of symptoms in the children, antithyroid antibodies, or familial hypothyroidism could not be determined. Cammareri and colleagues (1999) reported on a two-year-old girl with WBS who had thyroid hemiagenesis with compensated hypothyroidism, and they referred to two other children, each with an underdeveloped thyroid lobe. A 25% (19/78) incidence of clinical or compensated hypothyroidism was reported by Cappa et al. in 1994 (cited in Cammareri et al. 1999; Bini and Pela 2004).

Management

Thyroid function studies (TSH, T3 [triiodothyronine], and T4 [thyroxine] levels) should be performed in the first few years and then every four to five years in asymptomatic children. If the results of thyroid function studies are abnormal, measurement of thyroid antibodies and family history and data on thyroid disease should be obtained. Treatment with thyroxine may be warranted.

Teeth

Dental anomalies occur more frequently in people with WBS than in the general population. The more common problems affecting both primary and secondary teeth are small size, spaces between teeth, absence of some teeth, and malocclusion (Hertzberg et al. 1994). Enamel hypoplasia and caries are not more frequent than in the general population.

Management

Annual dental exams by a pediatric dentist familiar with WBS are important. At times it may be necessary to perform the exams with sedation or, if multiple caries or other problems are suspected, with general anesthesia because of the anxiety in WBS. Malocclusion often requires orthodontic treatment.

Response to Anesthesia

The perception that anesthesia carries greater risk for individuals with WBS because of an intrinsic abnormality (such as malignant hyperthermia) developed after published reports of isolated "muscle spasm" (Patel and Harrison 1991) or sudden death in eighteen cases. Only half the cases involved anesthesia and cardiac catheterization (Lacro et al. 1994; Bird et al. 1996; Bonnet et al. 1997). It is more likely that sudden death is related to cardiac and coronary artery status, as discussed above. Deering et al. (2000) conducted a retrospective review in one tertiary care hospital of twenty-five WBS patients with cardiovascular disease, aged six months to nineteen years, who had undergone seventy surgical and interventional catheterization procedures during a fourteen-year period (1987–2000). In some respects, this was a more severely affected WBS cohort than average, placing the children at a potentially higher risk for complications: a larger proportion (84%) suffered from cardiovascular disease, and a substantial portion had severe vascular narrowing. In 96% of the procedures, there were no problems. Two children, both with severe pulmonary hypertension, had adverse effects. In one case, an eighteen-month-old boy with severe distal branch pulmonary stenosis and pulmonary hypertension, resuscitation resulted in full recovery. The second child, with severe pulmonary hypertension and right ventricular hypertrophy, had two adverse reactions; on the second occasion, the child died of cardiac failure as the anesthesia was being initiated. The death rate for these seventy procedures was 1.42%. We can conclude that anesthesia may be an additional risk factor for patients with severe cardiac outflow tract obstruction and/or coronary artery narrowing. However, it can be administered safely to most other individuals with WBS. In the presence of severe outflow cardiovascular disease, anesthesia should be given under optimal circumstances by very experienced anesthesiologists, with careful monitoring and availability of resuscitation equipment.

Inheritance and Genetic Counseling

Williams-Beuren syndrome results from a deletion of the chromosome 7q11.23 region. It is a consequence of unequal crossing over between highly homologous sequences (low-copy repeat elements containing genes) that flank the commonly deleted region (see chapters 2 and 3). The frequencies of maternally and paternally inherited deletions are the same, without a parental age effect (Pérez Jurado et al. 1996). The majority of cases of WBS are sporadic occurrences in a family. Each child of an affected person has a 50% chance of inheriting the chromosome 7 deletion, and several families with affected parent and child of both genders have been reported (Morris et al. 1993). In almost all families with only one affected child, the risk of unaffected parents having another child with WBS is minimal. However, there are a few brother-sister pairs with WBS whose parents were not affected and whose deletions were derived from the same parental chromosome (Kara-Mostefa et al. 1999; K. Gripp et al., unpublished data). There are a few possible causes, including somatic or germ-line mosaicism in one parent or inversion of the critical chromosome 7q11.23 region in one parent, with subsequent loss of the region in one or more children. Valero and colleagues (2000) studied the orthologous region on mouse chromosome 5G and showed that the human WBS deletion region is inverted in mice, with breakpoints at the sites where the human 7q11.23 low-copy repeats are located—

an evolutionary inversion. Osborne et al. (2001) studied twelve families of children with WBS who had a demonstrable WBS deletion and identified an inversion of the WBS region of chromosome 7q11.23 in one parent in each of four families (33%) The deleted chromosome in the child with WBS was inherited from the parent with the inversion.

Management

Genetic counseling should be given to parents who have a child with WBS. The empiric recurrence risk is ~1%. Testing a parent for the inversion is not yet routine. Families at risk can have reliable prenatal testing for the deletion in the fetus by fluorescent in situ hybridization (FISH) of tissue from chorionic villous sampling or amniocentesis. There is no prenatal screening test for the general population.

Clinical Implications: Summary of Recommended Ongoing Evaluations and Tests

This summary is adapted from American Academy of Pediatrics, "Health Care Supervision for Children with Williams-Beuren Syndrome," *Pediatrics* 107(2001):1192–1204.

Evaluations

The majority of the recommended evaluations should be done annually, unless noted otherwise. Optimally, these tests should be performed in a multidisciplinary Williams-Beuren syndrome clinic.

1. Complete physical and neurologic examination
2. Growth parameters plotted on WBS and general population growth charts
3. Cardiology evaluation by a pediatric cardiologist (may be needed less frequently); exam should include
   (a) four-limb blood pressure measurements
   (b) echocardiography
4. Genitourinary system evaluation
5. Ophthalmologic evaluation
6. Dental evaluation
7. Multidisciplinary developmental evaluation: educational, physical therapy, occupational therapy, speech/feeding therapy
8. Gynecologic evaluation in late childhood–early adolescence

Anticipatory Guidance

1. Review of increased risk for otitis media
2. Continuing feeding and dietary assessment
3. Prevention/treatment of constipation
4. Appropriate therapy: physical, occupational (including sensory integration), feeding, speech and language, and music therapies
5. Monitoring of renal tract
   (a) evaluate for urinary tract infection if there is unexplained fever.
   (b) evaluate urinary frequency for dystocia-dyssynergy

6. Monitoring of growth (linear and weight) and puberty, using general and Williams-Beuren syndrome graphs
7. Discussion of developmental status, early intervention programs, and preschool programs
8. Psychosocial and vocational counseling for adolescents
9. Family support by other family members, friends, clergy, support groups

Laboratory and Radiologic Tests

1. FISH to confirm Williams-Beuren syndrome by demonstrating elastin gene (*ELN*) deletion
2. Annual urinalysis
3. Annual ionized (preferred) or total calcium measurement, if
   (a) the level was elevated at baseline
   (b) the child becomes symptomatic; if level was normal at baseline, measurements every two to three years until mid-childhood
4. Urinary calcium/creatinine ratio every two years
5. Serum creatinine level every two to four years
6. Renal ultrasonography
   (a) annually if patient has calcinosis and/or diverticula or if renal signs/symptoms develop
   (b) every two years until later childhood in the absence of calcinosis and/or diverticula
   (c) every five years in adolescence and adulthood in the absence of calcinosis and/or diverticula
7. Thyroid function test every four to five years if asymptomatic
8. Puberty (if early)
   Boys: testosterone
   Girls: TSH, LH, estradiol, pelvic ultrasound

Future Directions

In the past few decades, the management of dysfunction in multiple organs and systems has greatly improved the outcome for people with WBS. However, there are still many areas in which our understanding of pathophysiology, prevention, and treatment is not optimal. Future research in clinical and laboratory environments must focus on the medical problem areas: hypercalcemia, hyperactivity, anxiety, abnormal sleep patterns, arterial narrowing, hypertension, gastroesophageal reflux, and urinary tract dysfunction. To improve quality of life and adaptive behavior, research attention should be directed to the psychosocial problems related to the awareness of being "different" experienced by adolescents and adults with WBS.

REFERENCES

Ahearn, W. H., Kerwin, M. E., Eicher, P. S., and Lukens, C. T. 2001. An ABAC comparison of two intensive interventions for food refusal. *Behavior Modification* 25:385–405.
American Academy of Pediatrics Committee on Genetics. 2001. Health care supervision for children with Williams-Beuren syndrome. *Pediatrics* 107:1192–1204.

Ardinger, R. H., Jr., Goertz, K. K., and Mattioli, L. F. 1994. Cerebrovascular stenoses with cerebral infarction in a child with Williams-Beuren syndrome. *American Journal of Medical Genetics* 51:200–202.

Arens, R., Wright, B., Elliott, J., Zhao, H., Wang, P. P. P., Brown, L. W., Namey, T., and Kaplan, P. 1998. Periodic limb movement in sleep in children with Williams-Beuren syndrome. *Journal of Pediatrics* 133:670–674.

Bawden, H. N., MacDonald, G. W., and Shea, S. 1997. Treatment of children with Williams-Beuren Syndrome with methylphenidate. *Journal of Child Neurology* 12:248–252.

Bellugi, U., Mills, D., Jernigan, T., Hickok, G., and Galaburda, A. 1999. Linking cognition, brain structure and brain function in Williams-Beuren syndrome. In *Neurodevelopmental disorders: Contributions to a new framework from the cognitive neurosciences*, ed. H Tager-Flusberg, 111–136. Cambridge: MIT Press.

Biesecker, L. G., Laxova, R., and Friedman, A. 1987. Renal insufficiency in Williams-Beuren syndrome. *American Journal of Medical Genetics* 28:131–135.

Bini, R., and Pela, I. 2004. New case of thyroid dysgenesis and clinical signs of hypothyroidism in Williams syndrome. *American Journal of Medical Genetics A* 127:183–185.

Bird, L. M., Billman, G. F., Lacro, R. V., Spicer, R. L., Jariwala, L. K., Hoyme, E., Zamora-Salinas, R., Morris, C., Viskochil, D., Frikke, M. J., and Jones, M. C. 1996. Sudden death in Williams-Beuren syndrome: Report of ten cases. *Journal of Pediatrics* 129:926–931.

Bockoven, J. R., Kaplan, P., Namey, T., and Gleason, M. 1996. Williams-Beuren syndrome: The first decade is crucial for cardiovascular monitoring. Paper presented at the Eighth International Williams-Beuren Syndrome Professional Conference, Dearborn, MI.

Bonnet, D., Cormier, V., Villain, E., Bonhoeffer, P., and Kachaner, J. 1997. Progressive left main coronary artery obstruction leading to myocardial infarction in a child with Williams-Beuren syndrome. *European Journal of Pediatrics* 156:751–753.

Breault, D., Carpenter, T., and Pober, B. 2000. Prevalence of hypothyroidism and compensated hypothyroidism in Williams-Beuren syndrome. Paper presented at the Eighth International Williams-Beuren Syndrome Professional Conference, Dearborn, MI.

Broder, K., Reinhardt, E., Ahern, J., Lifton, R., Tamborlane, W., and Pober, B. 1999. Elevated ambulatory blood pressure in 20 subjects with Williams-Beuren syndrome. *American Journal of Medical Genetics* 83:356–360.

Cammareri, V., Vignati, G., Nocera, G., Beck-Peccoz, P., and Persani, L. 1999. Thyroid hemiagenesis and elevated thyrotropin levels in a child with Williams-Beuren syndrome. *American Journal of Medical Genetics* 85:491–494.

Chapman, C. A., du Plessis, A., and Pober, B. R. 1995. Neurologic findings in children and adults with Williams-Beuren syndrome. *Journal of Child Neurology* 10:63–65.

Cherniske, E. M., Sadler, L. S., Schwartz, D., Carpenter, T. O., and Pober, B. R. 1999. Early puberty in Williams-Beuren syndrome. *Clinical Dysmorphology* 8:117–121.

Cote, G., Jequier, S., and Kaplan, P. 1989. Increased renal medullary echogenicity in patients with Williams-Beuren syndrome. *Pediatric Radiology* 19:481–483.

Crawfurd, M. d'A., Kessel, I., Liberman, M., McKeown, J. A., Mandalia, P. Y., and Ridler, M. A. C. 1979. Partial monosomy 7 with interstitial deletions in two infants with differing congenital abnormalities. *Journal of Medical Genetics* 16:453–460.

Deering, R. P., Nicolson, S., and Kaplan, P. 2000. Safety of anesthesia in Williams-Beuren syndrome: evaluation of a large unselected cohort. Paper presented at the Eighth International Williams-Beuren Syndrome Professional Conference, Dearborn, MI.

Douchi, T., Maruta, K., Kuwahata, R., and Nagata, Y. 1999. Precocious puberty in a Williams-Beuren syndrome patient. *Obstetrics and Gynecology* 94:860.

Einfeld, S. L., Tonge, B. J., and Florio, T. 1997. Behavioral and emotional disturbance in individuals with Williams-Beuren syndrome. *American Journal of Mental Retardation* 102:45–53.

Giannotti, A., Tiberio, G., Castro, M., Virgilii, F., Colistro, F., Ferretti, F., Digilio, M. C., Gambarara, M., and Dallapiccola, B. 2001. Coeliac disease in Williams-Beuren syndrome. *Journal of Medical Genetics* 38:767–768.

Giordano, U., Turchetta, A., Giannotti, A., Digilio, M. C., Virgilii, F., and Calzolari, A. 2001. Exercise testing and 24-hour ambulatory blood pressure monitoring in children with Williams-Beuren syndrome. *Pediatric Cardiology* 22:509–511.

Greenberg, F., and Lewis, R. A. 1988. The Williams-Beuren syndrome: Spectrum and significance of ocular features. *Ophthalmology* 95:1608–1612.

Hertzberg, J., Nakisbendi, L. A., Needleman, H. L., and Pober, B. 1994. Williams-Beuren syndrome: Oral presentation of 45 cases. *Pediatric Dentistry* 16:262–267.

Ichinose, M., Tojo, K., Nakamura, K., Matsuda, H., Tokudome, G., Ohta, M., Sakai, S., and Sakai, O. 1996. Williams-Beuren syndrome associated with chronic renal failure and various endocrinological abnormalities. *Internal Medicine (Tokyo, Japan)* 35:482–488.

Ingelfinger, J. R., and Newburger, J. W. 1991. Spectrum of renal anomalies in patients with Williams-Beuren syndrome. *Journal of Pediatrics* 119:771–773.

Jernigan, T. L., and Bellugi, U. 1990. Anomalous brain morphology on magnetic resonance images in Williams syndrome and Down syndrome. *Archives of Neurology* 47:529–533.

Johnson, L. B., Comeau, M., and Clarke, K. D. 2001. Hyperacusis in Williams-Beuren syndrome. *Journal of Otolaryngology* 30:90–92.

Kahler, S. G., Adhvaryu, S. G., Helali, N., and Qumsiyeh, M. B. 1995. Microscopically visible deletion of chromosome 7 in a child with features of Williams-Beuren syndrome. *American Journal of Medical Genetics* 57:A117.

Kaplan, A., Stallings, V. A., Zemel, B., Green, K., and Kaplan, P. 1998. Body composition, energy expenditure and energy intake in Williams-Beuren syndrome. *Journal of Pediatrics* 132:223–227.

Kaplan, P., Kirschner, M., Watters, G., and Costa, M. T. 1989. Contractures in patients with Williams-Beuren syndrome. *Pediatrics* 84:895–899.

Kaplan, P., Levinson, M., and Kaplan, B. S. 1995. Cerebral artery stenoses in Williams-Beuren syndrome cause strokes in childhood. *Journal of Pediatrics* 126:943–945.

Kapp, M. E., von Noorden, G. K., and Jenkins, R. 1995. Strabismus in Williams-Beuren syndrome. *American Journal of Ophthalmology* 119:355–360.

Kara-Mostefa, A., Raoul, O., Lyonnet, S., Amiel, J., Minnich, A. A., Vekemans, M., Magnier, S., Ossareh, B., and Bonnefont, J. P. 1999. Recurrent Williams-Beuren syndrome in a sibship suggestive of maternal germ-line mosaicism. *American Journal of Human Genetics* 64:1475–1478.

Kawai, M., Nishikawa, T., Tanaka, M., Ando, A., Kasajima, T., Higa, T., Tanikawa, T., Kagawa, M., and Momma, K. 1993. An autopsied case of Williams-Beuren syndrome complicated by moyamoya disease. *Acta Paediatrica Japan* 35:63–67.

Klein, A. J., Armstrong, B. L., Greer, M. K., and Brown, F. R., 3rd. 1990. Hyperacusis and otitis media in individuals with Williams-Beuren syndrome. *Journal of Speech and Hearing Disorders* 55:339–344.

Lacro, R. V., Perry, S. B., Keane, J. F., Castaneda, A. R., and Lock, J. E. 1994. Combined transcatheter and surgical therapy for severe bilateral outflow obstruction in Williams-Beuren syndrome and familial supravalvar aortic stenosis. *Circulation* 90:I-587.

Lazar, L., Kauli, R., Pertzelan, A., and Phillip, M. 2002. Gonadotropin-suppressive therapy in girls with early and fast puberty affects the pace of puberty but not total pubertal growth or final height. *Journal of Clinical Endocrinology and Metabolism* 87:2090–2094.

Martin, N. D. T., Snodgrass, G. J. A. I., and Cohen, R. D. 1984. Idiopathic infantile hypercalcemia—a continuing enigma. *Archives of Disease in Childhood* 59:605–613.

Mathias, R. S. 2000. Rickets in an infant with Williams-Beuren syndrome. *Pediatric Nephrology* 14:489–492.

Mercuri, E., Atkinson, J., Braddick, O., Rutherford, M. A., Cowan, F. M., Counsell, S., Dubowitz, L. M., and Bydder, G. 1997. Chiari I malformation in asymptomatic young children with Williams-Beuren syndrome: Clinical and MRI study. *European Journal of Paediatric Neurology* 5:177–181.

Miani, C., Passon, P., Bracale, A. M., Barotti, A., and Panzolli, N. 2001. Treatment of hyperacusis in Williams-Beuren syndrome with bilateral conductive hearing loss. *European Archives of Otorhinolaryngology* 258:341–344.

Mizugishi, K., Yamanaka, K., Kuwajima, K., and Kondo, I. 1998. Interstitial deletion of chromosome 7q in a patient with Williams-Beuren syndrome. *Journal of Human Genetics* 43:178–181.

Morris, C. A., Thomas, I. T., and Greenberg, F. 1993. Williams-Beuren syndrome: Autosomal dominant inheritance. *American Journal of Medical Genetics* 47:478–481.

Olitsky, S. E., Sadler, L. S., and Reynolds, J. D. 1997. Subnormal binocular vision in the Williams syndrome. *Journal of Pediatric Ophthalmology and Strabismus* 34:58–60.

O'Reilly, M. F., and Lancioni, G. E. 2001. Treating food refusal in a child with Williams-Beuren syndrome using the parent as therapist in the home setting. *Journal of Intellectual Disability Research* 45:41–46.

Osborne, L. R., Li, M., Pober, B., Chitayat, D., Bodurtha, J., Mandel, A., Costa, T., Grebe, T., Cox, S., Tsui, L. C., and Scherer, S. W. 2001. A 1.5 million–base pair inversion polymorphism in families with Williams-Beuren syndrome. *Nature Genetics* 29:321–325.

Pagon, R. A., Bennett, F. C., La Veck, B., Stewart, K. B., and Johnson, J. 1987. Williams-Beuren syndrome: Features in late childhood and adolescence. *Pediatrics* 80:85–91.

Pankau, R., Partsch, C.-J., Gosch, A., Oppermann, H. C., and Wessel, A. 1992. Statural growth in Williams-Beuren syndrome. *European Journal of Pediatrics* 151:751–755.

Pankau, R., Partsch, C.-J., Winter, M., Gosch, A., and Wessel, A. 1996. Incidence and spectrum of renal abnormalities in Williams-Beuren syndrome. *American Journal of Medical Genetics* 63:301–304.

Partsch, C.-J., Dreyer, G., Gosch, A., Winter, M., Schneppenheim, R., Wessel, A., and Pankau, R. 1999. Longitudinal evaluation of growth, puberty, and bone maturation in children with Williams-Beuren syndrome. *Journal of Pediatrics* 134:82–89.

Patel, J., and Harrison, M. J. 1991. Williams-Beuren syndrome: Masseter spasm during anaesthesia. *Anaesthesia* 46:115–116.

Pérez Jurado, L. A., Peoples, R., Kaplan, P., Hamel, B. C. J., and Francke, U. 1996. Molecular definition of the chromosome 7 deletion in Williams syndrome and parent-of-origin effects on growth. *American Journal of Human Genetics* 59:781–792.

Picchietti, D. L., England, S. J., Walters, A. S., Willis, K., and Verrico, T. 1998. Periodic limb movement disorder and restless legs syndrome in children with attention-deficit hyperactivity disorder. *Journal of Child Neurology* 13:588–594.

Pober, B. R., and Filiano, J. J. 1995. Association of Chiari I malformation in Williams-Beuren syndrome. *Pediatric Neurology* 12:84–88.

Pober, B. R., Lacro, R. V., Rice, C., Mandell, V., and Teele, R. L. 1993. Renal findings in 40 patients with Williams-Beuren syndrome. *American Journal of Medical Genetics* 46:271–274.

Power, T. J., Blum, N. J., Jones, S. M., and Kaplan, P. 1997. Response to methylphenidate in 2 children with Williams-Beuren syndrome. *Journal of Autism and Developmental Disorders* 27:79–87.

Radford, D. J., and Pohlner, P. G. 2000. The middle aortic syndrome: An important feature of Williams-Beuren syndrome. *Cardiology in the Young* 10:597–602.

Rodd, C., and Goodyer, P. 1999. Hypercalcemia of the newborn: Etiology, evaluation, and management. *Pediatric Nephrology* 13:542–547.

Rose, C., Wessel, A., Pankau, R., Partsch, C. J., and Bursch, J. 2001. Anomalies of the abdominal aorta in Williams-Beuren syndrome—another cause of arterial hypertension. *European Journal of Pediatrics* 160:655–658.

Ruangdaraganon, N., Tocharoentanaphol, C., Kotchabhakdi, N., and Khowsathit, P. 1999. Williams-Beuren syndrome and the elastin gene in Thai patients. *Journal of the Medical Association of Thailand* 82 (suppl. 1): S174–S178.

Sadler, L. S., Olitsky, S. E., and Reynolds, J. D. 1996. Reduced stereoacuity in Williams-Beuren syndrome. *American Journal of Medical Genetics* 66:287–288.

Sadler, L. S., Gingell, R., and Martin, D. J. 1998. Carotid ultrasound examination in Williams-Beuren syndrome. *Journal of Pediatrics* 132:354–356.

Sargent, J. D., Stukel, T. A., Kresel, J., and Klein, R. Z. 1993. Normal values for random urinary calcium to creatinine ratios in infancy. *Journal of Pediatrics* 123:393–397.

Sarimski, K. 1996. Specific eating and sleeping problems in Prader-Willi and Williams-Beuren syndrome. *Child: Care, Health, and Development* 22:143–150.

Schulman, S. L., Zderic, S., and Kaplan, P. 1996. Increased prevalence of urinary symptoms and voiding dysfunction in Williams-Beuren syndrome. *Journal of Pediatrics* 129:466–469.

Scothorn, D. J., and Butler, M. G. 1997. How common is precocious puberty in patients with Williams-Beuren syndrome? *Clinical Dysmorphology* 6:91–93.

Sheih, C. P., Liu, M. B., Hung, C. S. Yang, K. H., Chen, W. Y., and Lin, C. Y. 1989. Renal abnormalities in Chinese schoolchildren. *Pediatrics* 84:1086–1090.

Soper, R., Chaloupka, J. C., Fayad, P. B., Greally, J. M., Shaywitz, B. A., Awad, I. A., and Pober, B. R. 1995. Ischemic stroke and intracranial multifocal cerebral arteriopathy in Williams-Beuren syndrome. *Journal of Pediatrics* 126:945–948.

Steiger, M. J., Rowe, P. A., Innes, A., and Burden, R. P. 1988. Williams-Beuren syndrome and renal failure. *Lancet* 2:804.

Tanner, J. M., Goldstein, H., and Whitehouse, R. H. 1970. Standards for children's height at ages 2–9 years allowing for heights of parents. *Archives of Disease in Childhood* 45:755–762.

Tsao, C. Y., and Westman, J. A. 1997. Infantile spasms in two children with Williams-Beuren syndrome. *American Journal of Medical Genetics* 71:54–56.

Tuvemo, T., Gustafsson, J., and Proos, L. A., Swedish Growth Hormone Group. 2002. Suppression of puberty in girls with short-acting intranasal versus subcutaneous depot GnRH agonist. *Hormone Research* 57:27–31.

Valero, M. C., de Luis, O., Cruces, J., and Perez Jurado, L. A. 2000. Fine-scale comparative mapping of the human 7q11.23 region and the orthologous region on mouse chromosome 5G: The low-copy repeats that flank the Williams-Beuren syndrome deletion arose at breakpoint sites of an evolutionary inversion(s). *Genomics* 69:1–13.

Van Borsel, J., Curfs, L. M., and Fryns, J. P. 1997. Hyperacusis in Williams-Beuren syndrome: A sample survey study. *Genetic Counseling* 8:121–126.

Wang, P. P. P., Hesselink, J. R., and Jernigan, T. L. 1992. Specific neurobehavioural profile of Williams-Beuren syndrome is associated with neocerebellar hemispheric preservation. *Neurology* 42:1999–2002.

Wilson, R. D., and Baird, P. A. 1985. Renal agenesis in British Columbia. *American Journal of Medical Genetics* 21:153–169.

Winter, M., Pankau, R., Amm, M., Gosch, A., and Wessel, A. 1996. The spectrum of ocular features in the Williams-Beuren syndrome. *Clinical Genetics* 49:28–31.

Wollack, J. B., Kaifer, M., LaMonte, M. P., and Rothman, M. 1996. Stroke in Williams-Beuren syndrome. *Stroke* 27:143–146.

Young, R. S., Weaver, D. D., Kubolich, M. K., Heerema, N. A., Palmer, C. G., Kawira, E. L., and Bender, H. A. 1984. Terminal and interstitial deletions of the long arm of chromosome 7: A review with five new cases. *American Journal of Medicine* 17:437–450.

Zackowski, J. L., Raffel, L. J., Blank, C. A., and Schwartz, S. 1990. Proximal interstitial deletion of 7q: A case report and review of the literature. *American Journal of Medical Genetics* 36:328–332.

Cardiovascular Disease in Williams-Beuren Syndrome

5

Ronald V. Lacro, M.D., and Leslie B. Smoot, M.D.

The spectrum of cardiovascular manifestations associated with Williams-Beuren syndrome (table 5.1) was of integral importance in the initial recognition and description of the disorder and in the elucidation of its underlying molecular genetic etiology. To put things into perspective, we present here a brief review of the investigations implicating the elastin gene in familial supravalvular aortic stenosis (SVAS) and Williams-Beuren syndrome (WBS). A more detailed account is given in chapter 1. We now know that SVAS is just one manifestation of a more diffuse arteriopathy associated with mutations or deletions involving the elastin gene at chromosome 7q11.23 (elastin arteriopathy).

Supravalvular aortic stenosis, characterized primarily by narrowing of the ascending aorta, occurs most commonly as an isolated autosomal dominant trait (familial SVAS) or as part of WBS. In 1961, J. C. P. Williams, a cardiologist in New Zealand, described four unrelated children with characteristic facies, developmental delay, and SVAS, a cardiovascular defect that is uncommon in the general population (Williams et al. 1961). Linkage to chromosome 7q11 was initially established in two kindreds with familial SVAS (Ewart et al. 1993b). A family in which SVAS cosegregates with a balanced reciprocal translocation, t(6;7)(p21.1;q11.23), which disrupts the elastin gene (*ELN*), provided further evidence that familial SVAS is the result of a mutation of elastin at 7q11.23 (Curran et al. 1993; Morris et al. 1993). A variety of mutations involving *ELN* have since been reported in additional families with SVAS (Ewart et al. 1994; Li et al. 1997; Tassabehji et al. 1997). Finally, hemizygosity at the elastin locus was shown in WBS, which is usually caused by de novo heterozygous microdeletions of a 1.5 to 2.0 Mb genomic DNA segment in chromosomal region 7q11.23 (Ewart et al. 1993a). To summarize, mutations in *ELN* cause familial SVAS, whereas de novo heterozygous microdeletions involving chromosomal region 7q11.23 cause most cases of

Table 5.1.
Review of the Most Important Publications Dealing with Cardiovascular Malformations in Williams-Beuren Syndrome

Reference	No. of patients	No. of heart cath.	SVAS (%)	PPS (%)	SVPS (%)	PS (%)	AS (%)	CoA (%)	AoHy (%)	ASD (%)	VSD (%)	PDA (%)	Other, no. of patients
Williams et al. 1961	4	3	100										
Beuren et al. 1962	4	3	100						25				
Beuren et al. 1964	10	10	100	60									
Ecklof et al. 1964	2		50	50		50							
Beuren et al. 1966	23	23	100	100					30				
Jones and Smith 1975	19	7	37	16		26	5		16	10	10		
Wesselhoft et al. 1980	79	79	100	82	2.5	5		5	70	1.3	2.5	2.5	
Martin et al. 1984	41	21	39	27		2.4		2.4					
Pernot et al. 1984	1											100	TOF, 1
Maisuls et al. 1987	8		62	50		12.5		25					MR, 2
Hallidie-Smith and Karas 1988	61	7	34						1.6	1.6	1.6		
Ino et al. 1988	2	2	100	100				50					
Morris et al. 1988	59	11	68	39	10/17	10		5					
Zalzstein et al. 1991	49	16	57	10				4					
Lopez-Rangel et al. 1992	10	1	40				20						MVP, 3
Pankau et al., unpubl.	124	78	77	48	0.8	0.8	1.6	6	29	1.6	2.4		IAA, 1; TOF, 1

Source: Adapted from Wessel et al. 1994.

Abbreviations: Cath,, catherization; SVAS, supravalvular aortic stenosis; PPS, peripheral pulmonary artery stenosis; SVPS, supravalvular pulmonary stenosis; PS, valvular pulmonary stenosis; AS, vavular aortic stenosis; CoA, coarctation; AoHy, aortic hypoplasia; ASD, atrial septal defect; VSD, ventricular septal defect; PDA, patent ductus arteriosus; TOF, tetralogy of Fallot; MR, mitral regurgitation; MVP, mitral valve prolapse; IAA, interrupted aortic arch.

WBS. These microdeletions include *ELN*, which accounts for the cardiovascular disease, as well as twenty other genes, which account for the nonvascular manifestations of WBS. Consistent with their common molecular etiology involving abnormalities in elastin, the vascular defects in familial SVAS and WBS are clinically and pathologically indistinguishable (O'Connor et al. 1985).

SVAS and other vascular abnormalities associated with the elastin arteriopathy continue to be an important part of the clinical management of individuals with WBS. The characteristic vascular narrowing, especially SVAS, often contributes to an earlier diagnosis of WBS, particularly in male patients (Sadler et al. 2001). Pediatric cardiologists have grown accustomed to suspecting and confirming the diagnosis of WBS based on the association with vascular stenoses, particularly SVAS and peripheral pulmonary artery stenosis (PPS). The clinical significance of the elastin arteriopathy depends on the location and severity of the vascular involvement. For example, in SVAS, typically there is thickening of the sinotubular junction of the aorta with narrowing of the lumen, leading to left ventricular outflow tract obstruction and left ventricular hypertrophy. Narrowing of the branch pulmonary arteries leads to right ventricular (RV) hypertension and RV hypertrophy. Renal artery stenosis can lead to renovascular hypertension. Rarely, coronary artery stenosis can result in myocardial ischemia, myocardial infarction, and sudden death; and stenosis of the cerebral arteries can cause stroke.

Supravalvular Aortic Stenosis and the Elastin Arteriopathy

Supravalvular aortic stenosis is a narrowing of the aortic lumen most typically associated with thickening of the sinotubular ridge of the ascending aorta, just above the origin of the coronary arteries. The narrowing can be discrete, diffuse—involving the entire ascending aorta—or diaphragmatic. Although SVAS is the most common cardiovascular abnormality associated with WBS, virtually all muscular arteries, both systemic and pulmonary, can be affected (fig. 5.1). The cardiovascular pathology of WBS consists of medial hypertrophy, which results in lumen narrowing. Although some individuals with WBS do not manifest any clinically important vascular obstructions, virtually all have some degree of thickening and/or narrowing of the arterial tree. Sadler and colleagues (1998) performed carotid ultrasound examination in a group of twenty individuals with WBS and twenty-five control subjects and found increased carotid arterial wall thickness in a wide range of individuals with WBS, demonstrating the pervasive nature of the arteriopathy of this disorder. The increased arterial wall thickness was observed in all WBS patients studied; thickness did not vary significantly with gender, patient age, the presence or absence of stenotic cardiac disease, or the

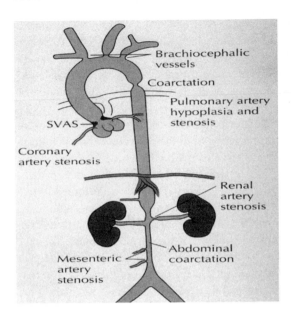

Fig. 5.1. Supravalvular stenosis is the most common cardiovascular abnormality associated with WBS, but virtually all muscular arteries, both systemic and pulmonary, can be affected.

presence or absence of hypertension. Using intravascular ultrasound imaging (performed with catheter-directed transducers from within the vessels), Rein and colleagues (1993) documented the cardiovascular pathology in three patients with WBS. The two most striking findings disclosed by the imaging were the basic pathologic features of medial hypertrophy in both systemic and pulmonary arteries, with secondary lumen narrowing, and the diffuse nature of the condition, involving all systemic and pulmonary arteries examined (fig 5.2).

The clinical importance of the vascular disease depends on the location and severity of the stenoses, which can vary greatly from individual to individual. The determinants of penetrance, distribution, and severity of the elastin arteriopathy in individuals with WBS and familial SVAS are not clearly understood. In a retrospective review of 127 individuals with WBS, Sadler et al. (2001) found that the severity of both SVAS and total cardiovascular disease was significantly greater in male patients than female patients. This difference was not accounted for by differences in height, weight, body mass index, or head circumference. The clinical diagnosis of WBS was made at a significantly younger age in male patients, partly because of the increased incidence and severity of cardiovascular disease in males. The authors hypothesized that the differences in arterial stenosis by gender may be related to prenatal hormonal effects.

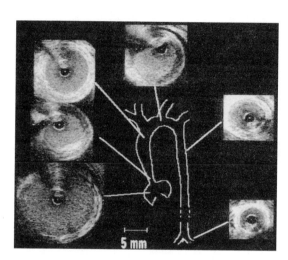

Fig. 5.2. Intravascular ultrasound imaging shows medial hypertrophy with secondary lumen narrowing in both systemic and pulmonary arteries and the diffuse nature of the condition. These images were obtained with an ultrasound transducer in the aorta. Note the thickness of the aortic wall at various levels (normal wall thickness, 0.25–0.35 mm) and narrowing of the aortic lumen at the level of the sinotubular junction. *Source:* Rein et al. 1993. Generalized Arteriopathy in Williams Syndrome, *Journal of the American College of Cardiology* 21(7):1727–1730. Reprinted with permission from the American College of Cardiology Foundation.

Elastin Arteriopathy: Clinical Implications
Supravalvular Aortic Stenosis

As noted above, SVAS is the most common vascular obstructive abnormality associated with WBS (fig. 5.3). The affected individual usually presents with an asymptomatic murmur. The anatomy and degree of obstruction can be confirmed by two-dimensional and Doppler echocardiography, particularly in younger individuals. Echocardiography is also useful for assessing the degree of left ventricular hypertrophy. Magnetic resonance imaging (MRI), cardiac catheterization, and angiography are also useful for further imaging and hemodynamic assessment. In most centers, including our own, cardiac catheterization is performed before surgical repair. SVAS is not generally amenable to balloon dilation.

Stamm and colleagues (1997) retrospectively reviewed the anatomic findings of SVAS by echocardiography and angiography of thirty-seven patients and correlated their findings with the pathologic findings in eight anatomic specimens. Echocardiography and angiography demonstrated discrete hourglass stenosis at the sinotubular junction in 77% of cases and diffuse tubular narrowing of the entire ascending aorta in 23% of cases. No cases of the so-called diaphragmatic lesion were encountered. Morphologic studies of

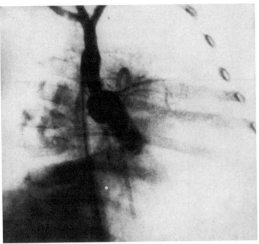 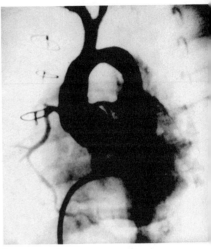

a   b

Fig. 5.3. Supravalvular aortic stenosis in an infant with WBS (*a*) before and (*b*) after surgical repair.

the aortic root revealed that the entire valvular apparatus is always affected by the so-called supravalvular stenosis. Partial adhesion of the leaflets to the stenosing supravalvular ridge was observed in 54% of cases, and the leaflets were thickened and less mobile in 30%. In all anatomic specimens, a marked redundancy of the leaflets was observed. Forty-five percent of the angiograms showed evidence of coronary ostial stenosis. Marked dilation and tortuosity of one or both coronary arteries was observed angiographically in 23% (5/22) of cases. The sinuses of Valsalva were significantly enlarged in 75% of the cases. Changes in dimensions of the aortic root were demonstrated more clearly by angiography than by echocardiography.

Several studies have documented the potential for progression in the severity of the left ventricular outflow tract obstruction associated with SVAS (Giddins et al. 1989; Wessel et al. 1994; Kim et al. 1999). Wessel and colleagues (1994) reported on three decades of follow-up of aortic and pulmonary vascular lesions in WBS, describing fifty-nine patients who were seen at least twice in their institution. Follow-up periods ranged from 2.1 to 28.2 years. Among forty-five individuals with SVAS and a mean follow-up period of 12.9 years, pressure gradients of less than 20 mm Hg in infancy generally remained unchanged during the first two decades of life. Pressure gradients exceeding 20 mm Hg increased from an average of 35.5 mm Hg to 52.7 mm Hg in thirteen patients. Of these, eight required surgical relief of the narrowing. The risk for restenosis after repair of SVAS was higher when diffuse aortic hypoplasia was present preoperatively. Kim and colleagues (1999) also found a tendency for SVAS to progress. They suggested that failure of growth of the sinotubular junction might be responsible for the progression of the aortic lesion. Patients with coronary arterial abnormalities (dilation and stenosis) had significantly smaller sinotubular junction dimensions (corrected for body surface area) and higher gradients from left ventricle to aorta, compared with those with normal coronary arteries.

Stamm et al. (1997) emphasized the pathologic involvement of the entire aortic root in SVAS, including the valvular apparatus, sinuses of Valsalva, and sinotubular junction, and suggested that anatomic restoration of the aortic root should ideally take into account all the deformed components by enlarging all three sinuses of Valsalva at the sinotubular junction. Reviewing forty-one years of surgical experience with congenital SVAS at our institution, including WBS and familial SVAS cases, Stamm and colleagues (1999) noted that postoperative results improved greatly after the introduction of more symmetric reconstructions of the aortic root (fig. 5.3). Multiple-sinus reconstructions, including inverted bifurcated patch plasty and three-sinus reconstruction, resulted in superior hemodynamics (lower residual gradients and less aortic valvular insufficiency) and were associated with reductions in both mortality rate and the need for reoperation. Diffuse stenosis of the ascending aorta was a risk factor for both mortality and reoperation.

Supravalvular Pulmonary Stenosis and Peripheral Pulmonary Artery Stenosis

Vascular obstruction in the pulmonary arterial tree can involve the main pulmonary artery (SVPS) and the branch or peripheral pulmonary arteries (PPS) (fig. 5.4). The distribution and severity of the stenoses are extremely variable. Most individuals have no significant symptoms. Although SVAS has the potential to progress in elastin arteriopathy, pulmonary artery stenosis often becomes less severe during childhood, particularly when the obstruction is mild. There is a strong likelihood that mild to moderate pulmonary artery stenosis will improve spontaneously over time. Severe pulmonary artery obstruction presenting in infancy may not undergo similar improvement (especially when combined with diffuse aortic disease). Long-standing pulmonary artery obstruction can result in asymmetric pulmonary blood flow and/or RV hypertension. Fortunately, the long-term prognosis for the vast majority of individuals is generally good, and older individuals with WBS usually have normal RV systolic pressures (Giddins et al. 1989; Wessel et al. 1994; Kim et al. 1999). Two-dimensional and Doppler echocardiography can detect stenosis of the main pulmonary artery and proximal branch pulmonary arteries and is useful for assessment of RV pressure and RV hypertrophy. MRI, cardiac catheterization, and angiography are also useful for

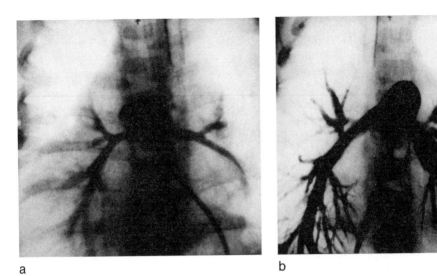

a   b

Fig. 5.4. Peripheral pulmonary artery stenosis in an infant with WBS (*a*) before and (*b*) after balloon dilations and surgical repair of the proximal branch pulmonary arteries. Note the diffuse pulmonary artery hypoplasia before treatment.

further hemodynamic assessment and anatomic imaging, particularly of the distal pulmonary arteries.

For the relatively small subset of patients with elastin arteriopathy who have more significant pulmonary artery stenosis that does not regress, significant RV hypertension and RV hypertrophy can develop. These patients may respond to a combination of balloon dilation in the cardiac catheterization laboratory and surgical repair. Obstruction of the distal branch pulmonary arteries is not accessible to the surgeon and requires cardiac catheterization and balloon dilation, whereas obstruction of the main pulmonary artery and proximal branch pulmonary arteries is amenable to surgical repair. In some cases, multiple balloon dilation procedures are necessary. Geggel and colleagues (2001) reviewed fifteen years of experience in our institution with balloon dilation of PPS in cases of WBS. Criteria for successful dilation included an increase of more than 50% in predilation diameter and a decrease of more than 20% in the ratio of RV to aortic systolic pressure. Median age and weight were 1.5 years and 9.5 kg. There were 134 dilations during thirty-nine procedures in twenty-five patients. The success rate for initial dilations was 51%. In multivariate analysis, successful dilation was more likely (1) in distal than in central pulmonary arteries, (2) if the balloon waist resolved with inflation, and (3) with larger balloon/stenosis ratio. RV pressure was unchanged after dilation, primarily because of failure to enlarge central pulmonary arteries. The aortic pressure increased and the RV/aortic pressure ratio decreased. Aneurysms developed after 24 dilations (18%) and were not related to balloon/stenosis ratio. Balloon rupture in 12 dilations produced an aneurysm in all seven cases in which the rupture was in a hypoplastic segment. Three patients died, none from pulmonary artery trauma, and all the deaths occurred before 1994. Despite successful dilation of distal pulmonary arteries, there was only modest initial hemodynamic improvement, mainly because of persistent central pulmonary artery obstruction. The authors suggest that a serial approach of distal dilations followed by surgical repair of proximal obstruction may be a rational and successful therapy (fig. 5.4).

Biventricular Outflow Tract Obstruction

Patients with a combination of SVAS and PPS, so-called biventricular outflow tract obstruction, are at an increased risk for cardiac complications including sudden death, particularly during diagnostic and surgical procedures requiring sedation or anesthesia. In the presence of bilateral outflow tract obstruction, there is biventricular hypertrophy and biventricular hypertension, increasing the risk for decreased cardiac output, myocardial ischemia, and dysrhythmias. These patients may respond to a combination of transcatheter and surgical therapy (Lacro et al. 1994; Stamm et al. 2000; Geggel et al. 2001).

Coarctation of the Aorta Including Middle Aortic Syndrome

In addition to obstruction in the ascending aorta, individuals with WBS less frequently present with obstruction of the aortic arch, its branches (innominate, left common carotid, and left subclavian arteries), the descending thoracic aorta, and/or the abdominal aorta. Infants and children with coarctation (narrowing) of the thoracic aorta can present with ductal dependent circulation at birth, congestive heart failure, decreased femoral pulses, and/ or systemic hypertension of the upper extremities. Some individuals are asymptomatic. Coarctation of the aorta is usually suspected clinically in patients with decreased lower extremity pulses and a blood pressure gradient between the upper and lower extremities; it is confirmed by echocardiography. MRI, cardiac catheterization, and angiography are useful diagnostic modalities. Native, or unrepaired, coarctation is usually managed surgically, most commonly with resection of the narrowed segment and direct reanastomosis of the proximal and distal segments of the aorta. Balloon dilation, with or without stenting, is usually reserved for recurrent coarctation.

Long-segment aortic hypoplasia or obstruction may require more complex repairs including aortic arch augmentation, subclavian artery flap repair, or conduits. Severe aortic hypoplasia is often associated with hypoplasia of more peripheral arterial branches including those to the head and neck, the renal arteries, and the mesenteric arteries (celiac, superior mesenteric, and inferior mesenteric arteries).

Abdominal coarctation or middle aortic syndrome generally presents in older children and can be associated with symptoms and signs of coarctation (decreased pulses, blood pressure gradient between upper and lower extremities), systemic hypertension, or abdominal pain (rarely), or without symptoms. Abdominal aortic obstruction is best diagnosed by angiography, although computed tomography (CT) and MRI are also useful imaging modalities. Surgical repair of diffuse abdominal aortic coarctation can be quite difficult. Individuals with systemic hypertension should consult with a nephrologist for diagnostic evaluation and management.

Narrowing of the thoracic and abdominal aorta is a frequent morphologic manifestation of the elastin arteriopathy associated with WBS. Rose and colleagues (2001) reported on the pattern of stenotic lesions of the abdominal aorta and the incidence of systemic hypertension. Of their 112 patients with WBS, 25 had undergone abdominal aortic angiography. The diameter of the thoracic aorta and the change in diameter to the iliac bifurcation were compared with normal data. Of the 25 patients, 20 had vascular stenosis; 19 patients were affected by segmental narrowing of either the thoracic aorta (n = 9) or the abdominal aorta (n = 7) or both (n = 3). Only one patient had a solitary stenosis of the renal artery.

Hypoplasia of the abdominal aorta was characterized by the smallest diameters at the renal artery level and an increased diameter of the infrarenal abdominal aorta. Renal artery stenosis was suspected when the proximal vessel diameter was less than 50% of the distal diameter. Isolated renal artery stenosis was rare; it was more frequently combined with a narrowed aorta. Eleven patients had renal artery stenosis, associated with narrowing of other aortic segments in ten cases. Systemic hypertension was a common symptom in the affected group and must be regarded as a manifestation of generalized arteriopathy rather than renal hypoperfusion. Hypertension was diagnosed in seventeen patients, two of them with no vascular lesions; in the remaining fifteen patients stenosis was present in more than one segment (aorta in six, renal artery in one, both in eight) (Rose et al. 2001).

Coronary Artery Stenosis and Myocardial Infarction

The true incidence of coronary artery disease, both symptomatic and asymptomatic, is unclear. Major complications involving the coronary arteries are rare. Mild stenosis of the coronary arteries, usually at the ostia, is often asymptomatic and often noted incidentally during cardiac catheterization and angiography for SVAS or coarctation of the aorta. However, there are reports of acute and chronic myocardial ischemia, myocardial infarction, and sudden death (Bird et al. 1996; Suares-Mier and Morentin 1999; Imashuku et al. 2000). Sudden death is rare. Some instances of sudden death occurred before confirmation of a diagnosis of WBS. Although not completely understood, risk factors for sudden death include coronary artery narrowing with acute and chronic myocardial ischemia and infarction, as well as biventricular outflow tract obstruction (combined SVAS and PPS) (Bird et al. 1996).

Coronary artery abnormalities include dilation, stenosis, and occlusion of the ostium by the aortic valve leaflets. The coronary artery origins are usually below the level of supravalvular obstruction, so the coronary arteries, subject to the increased pressure proximal to the obstruction, are often dilated. Coronary ischemia can result from coronary artery narrowing due to the elastin arteriopathy. In other cases, ischemia can result from occlusion of the coronary artery ostium by the aortic valve leaflets adhering to the thickened supravalvular ridge (Stamm et al. 1997).

Although echocardiography may show dilation of the coronary arteries and abnormally high origins of the coronary arteries, the best imaging modality for coronary artery stenosis or ostial occlusion is selective coronary artery angiography. The diagnostic evaluation for suspected or proven coronary artery disease in WBS includes electrocardiography, ambulatory electrocardiograph monitoring (Holter monitor), exercise test with and without radionuclides (e.g., stress MIBI [radiolabeled protein]), and stress echocardiography. There is no standard evaluation protocol, and the degree of testing should be directed by the clinical history of individual cases.

Information about medical and surgical treatment for coronary artery disease in WBS is limited. Family history and lipid profiles should be reviewed to rule out additional risk factors for coronary artery disease. Aspirin has been used empirically, but there are no data about its efficacy in preventing coronary complications specifically in WBS.

Cerebral Artery Stenosis and Cerebrovascular Accident (Stroke)

Fortunately the incidence of stroke or cerebrovascular accident associated with stenosis of the cerebral arteries is rare in WBS (Ardinger et al. 1994; Soper et al. 1995; Putnam et al. 1995; Wollack et al. 1996). Prospective screening for cerebral artery narrowing is generally not recommended, though a heightened awareness of symptoms related to potential vascular events is warranted. Any symptoms suggestive of a stroke or transient ischemia should prompt a consultation with a neurologist and appropriate diagnostic evaluation (brain CT or MRI, angiography). Treatment of stroke may initially be the same as for other causes, with long-term management dependent on details of vascular anatomy and available therapeutic options. Empiric treatment with aspirin has been suggested, but there are no data to support routine use in WBS.

Mesenteric Artery Stenosis

Mesenteric artery stenosis (narrowing of the celiac trunk, superior mesenteric artery, and inferior mesenteric artery) is most often identified in the course of abdominal vascular imaging, usually MRI or abdominal angiography. Mesenteric artery narrowing may be an incidental finding during evaluation of other sites of vascular disease or, less commonly, may be found during investigation of specific abdominal symptoms. Despite findings of mesenteric artery narrowing, it may be difficult to connect these findings to specific symptoms. Abdominal pain, cramping, gastroesophageal reflux, constipation, diverticulosis, and diverticulitis are common in WBS but are most often associated with nonvascular causes. Because of the extensive redundancy in blood flow to the intestinal tract associated with abundant collateral circulation, it is extremely rare for discrete vascular obstruction to cause bowel ischemia or require specific intervention. However, the potential for vascular compromise should be considered in any patient with abdominal symptoms without a clear cause.

Renal Artery Stenosis and Hypertension

Hypertension is common, particularly in older teenagers and adults with WBS. Most individuals are asymptomatic or present with nonspecific signs and symptoms. Routine screening for hypertension is extremely important for all individuals with WBS. The differential diagnosis for hypertension in WBS includes renovascular hypertension (Daniels et al. 1985); generalized arteriopathy related to elastin deficiency and/or atherosclerosis in adulthood; anxiety; and pseudohypertension (Narasimhan et al. 1993). Renovascular hypertension can be due to coarctation of the thoracic aorta, coarctation of the abdominal aorta (middle aortic syndrome), renal artery stenosis, and/or renal parenchymal disease (e.g., nephrocalcinosis) (Daniels et al. 1985; Broder et al. 1999; Giordano et al. 2001; Pober et al. 1993; Pankau et al. 1996).

In pseudohypertension, often reported in elderly subjects but unusual in children, the blood pressure measured by cuff sphygmomanometry is inappropriately high when compared with true intraarterial pressure. This condition is believed to be due to thickening of the vessel wall requiring a higher pressure in the cuff to occlude the stiff artery. In the elderly, pseudohypertension reflects a higher prevalence of arteriosclerosis, while in WBS it reflects arterial wall thickening due to the elastin arteriopathy. Normal blood pressure detected by direct measurement of the arterial pressure confirms the diagnosis of pseudohypertension. Although pseudohypertension has been reported in a child with WBS, it seems to be a rare phenomenon (Narasimhan et al. 1993). True hypertension is more prevalent in WBS.

Two studies have used twenty-four-hour ambulatory blood pressure monitoring to evaluate systemic hypertension in WBS. Broder and colleagues (1999) studied twenty subjects with WBS evaluated through a multidisciplinary WBS clinic and thirty-five age- and gender-matched controls. They found that subjects with WBS had significantly higher ambulatory blood pressures than controls. After controlling for age, gender, and weight, the diagnosis of WBS added approximately 10 mm Hg to mean daytime and nighttime blood pressures. Hypertension, as defined by elevated mean daytime blood pressure, was present in 40% of WBS subjects versus 14% of controls ($P < 0.05$). Among the children studied, this difference was even more dramatic, with 46% of WBS children versus 6% of control children classified as hypertensive ($P = 0.01$). The study demonstrated normal diurnal blood pressure variation but no evidence of a "white coat" effect or increased blood pressure variability. Interestingly, parental reporting of a history of infantile hypercalcemia was strongly associated with the presence of hypertension ($P = 0.008$). Giordano and colleagues (2001) also noted that ambulatory blood pressure measurement values showed higher systolic blood pressures both during the day and at night. Maximum heart rate and maximum systolic blood pressure during exercise were higher than in normal children.

The diagnostic evaluation for systemic hypertension consists first of documenting blood pressure (including the time, setting, and state of the individual), method of measurement (automated or manual cuff, direct arterial, etc.), and site and, if necessary, ambulatory twenty-four-hour blood pressure monitoring. Many individuals with WBS, especially young children, will not tolerate blood pressure monitoring, especially with an automated cuff. Four extremity blood pressures are useful for the diagnosis of coarctation of the thoracic or abdominal aorta. Additional studies include renal ultrasound with Doppler, cardiac evaluation and echocardiogram (with attention to thoracic and/or abdominal coarctation of the aorta), and angiography with renal vein renin sampling if indicated. Consultation with a nephrologist who has experience with WBS is recommended.

Nonvascular Congenital Heart Defects

Nonvascular intracardiac abnormalities, such as mitral valve prolapse, septal defects, and bicuspid aortic valve, are much less common than SVAS and other vascular stenoses in WBS (table 5.1). Hallidie-Smith and Karas (1988) reported a 15% clinical and echocardiographic incidence of mitral valve prolapse and an 11.6% incidence of bicuspid aortic valve. Conotruncal malformations, including tetralogy of Fallot and interrupted aortic arch, have been reported but are rare. There has been speculation that mitral valve prolapse is a cardiac manifestation of an elastin-related connective tissue disorder. Abnormalities of the aortic and pulmonary valves, including bicuspid aortic valve, are part of the SVAS spectrum. The relationship of other nonvascular congenital heart defects to elastin is unclear. Although some cardiovascular defects might be related to deletion of other genes in the WBS critical region, there is no direct evidence to support this hypothesis.

Elastin Arteriopathy: Pathophysiology

With the discovery of the association between familial supravalvular aortic stenosis, Williams-Beuren syndrome, and elastin, genetic evidence pointed to functional haploinsufficiency of elastin as the primary cause of this arteriopathy. Subsequent investigation confirmed that, in virtually all cases of elastin arteriopathy examined, mutations in *ELN* resulted in premature truncation of the elastin message. Thus, familial SVAS and WBS are functionally identical with respect to elastin haploinsufficiency. What was not known was how a reduction in elastin transcription contributed to the progressive arterial disease observed clinically in WBS.

Elastin fibers form the scaffolding for many tissues, providing tensile strength and resilience in skin, connective tissue, and blood vessels. Elastic fibers consist primarily of covalently cross-linked elastin molecules in extracellular matrix. Elastin is secreted as a precursor protein, tropoelastin, by a variety of cell types including fibroblasts, smooth muscle cells, and endothelial cells (Arteaga-Solis et al. 2000; Milewicz et al. 2000). Large elastic arteries normally contain highly organized elastic lamella, which can be seen with selective histologic staining. In the elastic arteries of individuals with WBS, there is disruption of these organized lamellar structures amid more normal-appearing vessel. Initial hypotheses assumed that reduced elastin deposition in the arterial wall led to reduced vessel compliance. It was largely assumed that *mechanical stress* in the vasculature led to secondary smooth muscle proliferation, which led to vascular obstruction. This hypothesis seemed to account for the predominant location of vascular obstruction.

In 1998, Li and colleagues demonstrated obstructive arterial disease in mice with targeted disruption of one *ELN* allele. These elastin-deficient mice showed subendothelial and smooth muscle proliferation even in isolated arteries grown in cell culture, devoid of hemodynamic stress. The authors proposed that elastin played a significant role in the *regulation* of smooth muscle proliferation. Other researchers have also suggested a regulatory role of elastin in other conditions that disrupt elastin (transplant vasculopathy, coronary angioplasty) (Urban et al. 2002; Rabinovitch 1999). In these models, disruption of vascular integrity is associated with a breakdown of insoluble elastin and generation of elastin breakdown products. Accumulation of these elastin-derived peptides has been associated with a proliferative and less differentiated response of vascular smooth muscle. These findings offer insight into additional molecular pathways leading to the smooth muscle proliferation and de-differentiation observed clinically in elastin arteriopathy and may offer new opportunities for intervention.

Clinical Implications of Cardiovascular Disease

The clinical implications of vascular disease in WBS are both significant and well recognized in their most severe forms. The effect of elastin haploinsufficiency in asymptomatic individuals with WBS is less well defined. Diffuse arteriopathy is assumed but may not be clinically relevant in early childhood or adolescence. As the population of older individuals with WBS increases, we hope to become more knowledgeable about the subtle changes that may affect vascular health throughout the life span. With a better understanding of the underlying pathophysiology, we should be able to implement preventive measures, as is done in the general population for diabetes mellitus and hyperlipidemia.

Future Directions

Since the initial recognition of the role of elastin in Williams-Beuren syndrome and familial vasculopathy, major advances have been made in understanding the mechanisms by which this protein interacts with multiple components of the vasculature and circulation. Although effects of the elastin deficiency were initially thought to represent a defect in the structural architecture of blood vessels, more recent and exciting research implicates elastin as a signaling molecule in pathways that influence smooth muscle proliferation and de-differentiation, which lead to vascular stenosis. These findings offer increasing possibilities for gene- and protein-specific therapeutic intervention for WBS, familial SVAS, and other vasculopathies. In the future, new therapies will be aimed at preventing the body's secondary abnormal proliferative response that accounts for most obstructive vascular disease.

REFERENCES

Ardinger, R. H., Jr., Goertz, K. K., and Mattioli, L. F. 1994. Cerebrovascular stenoses with cerebral infarction in a child with William syndrome. *American Journal of Medical Genetics* 51:200–202.
Arteaga-Solis, E., Gayraud, B., and Ramirez, F. 2000. Elastic and collagenous networks in vascular diseases. *Cell Structure and Function* 25:69–72.
Beuren, A. J., Apitz, J., and Harmjanz, D. 1962. Supravalvular aortic stenosis in association with mental retardation and a certain facial appearance. *Circulation* 26:1235–1240.
Beuren, A. J., Schulze, C., Eberle, P., Harmjanz, D., and Apitz, J. 1964. The syndrome of supravalvular aortic stenosis, peripheral pulmonary stenosis, mental re-

tardation and similar facial appearance. *American Journal of Cardiology* 13:471–482.

Beuren, A. J., Apitz, J., Stoermer, J., Kaiser, B., Schlange, H., von Berg, W., and Jorgensen, G. 1966. Vitamin D-hypercalcamische Herz- und Gefasserkrankung. Monatsschrift fur Kinderheilkunde 114:457–470.

Bird, L. M., Billman, G. F., Lacro, R. V., Spicer, R. L., Jarwala, L. K., Hoyme, E., Zamora-Salinas, R., Morris, C., Viskochil, D., Frikke, M. J., and Jones, M. C. 1996. Sudden death in Williams syndrome: Report of ten cases. *Journal of Pediatrics* 129:926–931.

Broder, K., Reinhardt, E., Ahern, J., Lifton, R., Tamborlane, W., and Pober, B. 1999. Elevated ambulatory blood pressure in 20 subjects with Williams syndrome. *American Journal of Medical Genetics* 83:356–360.

Curran, M. E., Atkinson, D. L., Ewart, A. K., Morris, C. A., Leppert, M. F., and Keating, M. F. 1993. The elastin gene is disrupted by a translocation causing supravalvular aortic stenosis. *Cell* 73:159–168.

Daniels, S. R., Loggie, J. M. H., Schwartz, D. C., Strife, J. L., and Kaplan, S. 1985. Systemic hypertension secondary to peripheral vascular anomalies in Williams syndrome. *Journal of Pediatrics* 106:249–251.

Ecklof, O., Ilha, D. O., and Zetterqvist, P. 1964. Aortic hypoplasia. *Acta Paediatrica Supplementum* 53:377–387.

Ewart, A. K., Morris, C. A., Atkinson, D., Jin, W., Sternes, K., Spallone, P., Stock, A. D., Leppert, M., and Keating, M. T. 1993a. Hemizygosity at the elastin locus in a developmental disorder, Williams syndrome. *Nature Genetics* 5:11–16.

Ewart, A. K., Morris, C. A., Ensing, G. K., Loker, J., Moore, C. A., Leppert, M., and Keating, M. 1993b. A human vascular disorder, supravalvular aortic stenosis, maps to chromosome 7. *Proceedings of the National Academy of Sciences USA* 90:3226–3230.

Ewart, A. K., Jin, W., Atkinson, D., Morris, C. A., and Keating, M. T. 1994. Supravalvar aortic stenosis associated with a deletion disrupting the elastin gene. *Journal of Clinical Investigation* 93:1071–1077.

Geggel, R. L., Gauvreau, K., and Lock, J. E. 2001. Balloon dilation angioplasty of peripheral pulmonary stenosis associated with Williams syndrome. *Circulation* 103:2165–2170.

Giddins, N. G., Finley, J. P., Nanton, M. A., and Roy, D. L. 1989. The natural course of supravalvular aortic stenosis and peripheral pulmonary artery stenosis in Williams syndrome. *British Heart Journal* 62:315–319.

Giordano, U., Turchetta, A., Giannotti, A., Digilio, M. C., Virgilii, F., and Calzolari, A. 2001. Exercise testing and 24-hour ambulatory blood pressure monitoring in children with Williams syndrome. *Pediatric Cardiology* 22:509–511.

Hallidie-Smith, K. A., and Karas, S. 1988. Cardiac anomalies in Williams-Beuren syndrome. *Archives of Disease of Childhood* 63:809–813.

Imashuku, S., Hayshi, S., Kuriyama, K., Hibi, S., Tabta, Y., and Todo, S. 2000. Sudden death of a 21-year-old female with Williams syndrome showing rare complications. *Pediatrics International* 42:322–324.

Ino, T., Nishimoto, K., Iwahara, M., Akimoto, K., Boku, H., Kaneko, K., Tokita, A., Yabuta, K., and Tanaka, J. 1988. Progressive vascular lesions in Williams-Beuren syndrome. *Pediatric Cardiology* 9:55–58.

Jones, K. L., and Smith, D. W. 1975. The Williams elfin facies syndrome. *Journal of Pediatrics* 86:718–723.

Kim, Y. M., Yoo, S.-Y., Choi, J. Y., Kim, S. H., Bae, E. J., and Lee, Y. T. 1999. Natural course of supravalvar aortic stenosis and peripheral pulmonary arterial stenosis in Williams' syndrome. *Cardiology in the Young* 9:37–41.

Lacro, R. V., Perry, S. B., Keane, J. F., Castaneda, A. R., and Lock, J. E. 1994. Combined transcatheter and surgical therapy for severe bilateral outflow tract obstruction in Williams syndrome and familial supravalvar aortic stenosis. *Circulation* 90:I-587.

Li, D. Y., Toland, A. E., Boak, B. B., Atkinson, D. L., Ensing, G. J., Morris, C. A., and Keating, M. T. 1997. Elastin point mutations cause an obstructive vascular disease, supravalvular aortic stenosis. *Human Molecular Genetics* 6:1021–1028.

Li, D. Y., Brooke, B., Davis, E. C., Mecham, R. P., Sorensen, L. K., Boak, B. B., Eichwald, E., and Keating, M. T. 1998. Elastin is an essential determinant of arterial morphogenesis. *Nature* 393:276–280.

Lopez-Rangel, E., Maurice, M., McGillivray, B., and Friedman, J. M. 1992. Williams syndrome in adults. *American Journal of Medical Genetics* 44:720–729.

Maisuls, H., Alday, L. E., and Thuer, O., 1987. Cardiovascular findings in Williams-Beuren syndrome. *American Heart Journal* 114:897–899.

Martin, N. D. T., Snodgrass, G. J. A. I., and Cohen, R. D. 1984. Idiopathic infantile hypercalcemia—a continuing enigma. *Archives of Disease in Childhood* 59:605–613.

Milewicz, D. M., Urban, Z., and Boyd, C. 2000. Genetic disorders of the elastic fiber system. *Matrix Biology* 19:471–480.

Morris, C. A., Demsey, S. A., Leonard, C. O., Dilts, C., and Blackburn, B. L. 1988. Natural history of Williams syndrome: Physical characteristics. *Journal of Pediatrics* 113:318–326.

Morris, C. A., James, L., Ensing, G., and Stock, A. D. 1993. Supravalvular aortic stenosis cosegregates with a familial 6;7 translocation which disrupts the elastin gene. *American Journal of Medical Genetics* 46:737–744.

Narasimhan, C., Alexander, T., and Krishnaswami, S. 1993. Pseudohypertension in a child with Williams syndrome. *Pediatric Cardiology* 14:124–126.

O'Connor, W. N., Davis, J. B., Geissler, R., Cottrill, C. M., Noonan, J. A., and Todd, E. P. 1985. Supravalvular aortic stenosis: Clinical and pathologic observations in six patients. *Archives of Pathology and Laboratory Medicine* 109:179–185.

Pankau, R., Partsch, C.-J., Winter, M., Gosch, A., and Wessel, A. 1996. Incidence and spectrum of renal abnormalities in Williams-Beuren syndrome. *American Journal of Medical Genetics* 63:301–304.

Pernot, C., Woums, A. M., Macom, F., and Admant, P. 1984. Facies de Williams-Beruen avec retard mental et tetralogie de Fallot. *Pediatrie* 39:53–58.

Pober, B. R., Lacro, R. V., Rice, C., Mandell, V., and Teele, R. 1993. Renal findings in individuals with Williams syndrome. *American Journal of Medical Genetics* 46:271–274.

Putnam, C. M., Chaloupka, J. C., Eklund, J. E., and Fulbright, R. K. 1995. Multifocal intracranial occlusive vasculopathy resulting in stroke: An unusual manifestation of Williams syndrome. *American Journal of Neuroradiology* 16:1536–1538.

Rabinovitch, M. 1999. EVE and beyond, retro and prospective insights. *American Journal of Physiology* 277 (1, pt. 1): L5–L12.

Rein, A. J. J. T., Preminger, T. J., Perry, S. B., Lock, S. E., and Sanders, S. P. 1993. Generalized arteriopathy in Williams syndrome: An intravascular ultrasound study. *Journal of the American College of Cardiology* 21:1727–1930.

Rose, C., Wessel, A., Pankau, R., Partsch, C. J., and Bursch, J. 2001. Anomalies of the abdominal aorta in Williams-Beuren syndrome—another cause of arterial hypertension. *European Journal of Pediatrics* 160:655–658.

Sadler, L. S., Gingell, R., and Martin, D. J. 1998. Carotid ultrasound examination in Williams syndrome. *Journal of Pediatrics* 132:354–356.

Sadler, L. S., Pober, B. R., Grandinetti, A., Scheiber, D., Fekete, G., Sharma, A. N., and Urban, Z. 2001. Differences by sex in cardiovascular disease in Williams syndrome. *Journal of Pediatrics* 139:849–852.

Soper, R., Chaloupka, J. C., Fayad, P. B., Greally, J. M., Shaywitz, B. A., Awad, I. A., and Pober, B. R. 1995. Ischemic stroke and intracranial multifocal cerebral arteriopathy in William syndrome. *Journal of Pediatrics* 126:945–948.

Stamm, C., Li, J., Ho, S. Y., Redington, A. N., and Anderson, R. H. 1997. The aortic root in supravalvular aortic stenosis: The potential surgical relevance of morphologic findings. *Journal of Thoracic and Cardiovascular Surgery* 114:16–24.

Stamm, C., Kruetzer, C., Zurakowski, D., Nollert, G., Friehs, I., Mayer, J. E., Jonas, R. A., and del Nido, P. J. 1999. Forty-one years of surgical experience with congenital supravalvular aortic stenosis. *Journal of Thoracic and Cardiovascular Surgery* 118:874–885.

Stamm, C., Friehs, I., Moran, A. M., Zurakowski, D., Bacha, E., Mayer, J. E., Jonas, R. A., and del Nido, P. J. 2000. Surgery for bilateral outflow tract obstruction in elastin arteriopathy. *Journal of Thoracic and Cardiovascular Surgery* 120:755–763.

Suares-Mier, M.-P., and Morentin, B. 1999. Supravalvular aortic stenosis, Williams syndrome and sudden death: A case report. *Forensic Science International* 106:45–53.

Tassabehji, M., Metcalfe, K., Donnai, D., Hurst, J., Reardon, W., Burch, M., and Read, A. P. 1997. Elastin: Genomic structure and point mutations in patients with supravalvular aortic stenosis. *Human Molecular Genetics* 6:1029–1036.

Urban, Z., Riazi, S., Seidl, T. L., Katahira, J., Smoot, L. B., Chitayat, D., Boyd, C. D., and Hinek, A. 2002. Connection between elastin haploinsufficiency and increased cell proliferation in patients with supravalvular aortic stenosis and Williams-Beuren syndrome. *American Journal of Human Genetics* 71:30–44.

Wessel, A., Pankau, R., Kececioglu, D., Ruschewski, W., and Bursch, J. H. 1994. Three decades of follow-up of aortic and pulmonary vascular lesions in the Williams-Beuren syndrome. *American Journal of Medical Genetics* 52:297–301.

Wesselhoft, H., Salomon, F., and Grimm, T. 1980. Spektrum der supravalvularen Aortenstenose: Untersuchungsergebisse bei 150 Patienten mit Williams-Beuren-Syndrom und der isolierten Form der supravalvularen Aortenstenose. *Zeitschrift für Kardiologie* 69:131–140.

Williams, J. C. P., Barratt-Boyes, B. G., and Lowe, J. B. 1961. Supravalvular aortic stenosis. *Circulation* 24:1311–1318.

Wollack, J. B., Kaifer, M., LaMonte, M. P., and Rothman, M. 1996. Stroke in Williams syndrome. *Stroke* 27:143–146.

Zalstein, E., Moes, C. A. F., Musewe, N. N., and Freedom, R. M. 1991. Spectrum of cardiovascular anomalies in Williams-Beuren syndrome. *Pediatric Cardiology* 12:219–213.

Evidence-Based Medical Management of Adults with Williams-Beuren Syndrome   6

Barbara R. Pober, M.D.

Since the initial recognition of Williams-Beuren syndrome (WBS) as a distinct clinical entity approximately forty years ago, most of the medical literature has focused on problems found in children with this disorder. The recent availability of objective diagnostic testing, heightened awareness of WBS in the lay press and the general population, and increasing self-advocacy by adults with WBS have raised awareness about issues specifically affecting adults. Many of the medical problems of WBS that complicate the early years of life continue into adulthood, but additional problems seemingly unique to adults also develop. Furthermore, varying degrees of emotional and psychiatric problems are extremely common among adults with WBS and often have a greater effect on their quality of life than do the concomitant medical problems.

No study on life expectancy in WBS has been published. However, elderly patients with WBS are reported in the medical literature and are also seen in our clinic, indicating that longevity is possible. Quality of life and life expectancy among adults with WBS are likely to be optimized with proper medical management. The recommendations for management in this chapter are based on findings in the published literature complemented by findings from our own research and clinical experience. Although several of the published medical series on adults with WBS are more than a decade old, they comprise an important source of information for medical management and are therefore cited in this chapter.

General Overview of Adults with Williams-Beuren Syndrome

Several series profiling adults with WBS have been published (Morris et al. 1988, 1990; Nicholson and Hockey 1993; Plissart et al. 1994; Udwin 1990; Lopez-Rangel et al. 1992). Data from these reports and our own series collectively demonstrate that most adults with WBS continue to experience significant medical problems and require a higher level of support than similarly aged adults in the general population. Case reports on older persons with WBS have been published but are potentially biased toward the more severe end of the disease spectrum and may not portray the typical picture of WBS adulthood. Some of the more common medical problems described in multiple reports are vascular stenosis, hypertension, gastrointestinal problems such as constipation and diverticular disease, musculoskeletal problems such as contractures or spinal curvature, dental malocclusion, urinary frequency, neurologic abnormalities, and premature graying of the hair. Our own work confirms that these problems are common and, in addition, highlights the presence of endocrine abnormalities and hearing loss. Several investigators have reported a very high frequency of behavioral problems such as social isolation, somaticization, and excess worry (Udwin 1990; Davies et al. 1998). Our data, which include direct interviews of adults with WBS by an expert psychiatrist, confirm a heightened level of anxiety in most adults with WBS and a variety of other psychiatric disturbances (Pober et al. 1998).

This chapter focuses on medical problems that can complicate the lives of adults with WBS. It is important to point out that no person with WBS will have all the potential medical problems discussed here and that, although intensive medical monitoring is often needed, with proper medical care most adults with WBS can enjoy relatively good health.

In 1988, Morris et al. reported on seventeen adults with WBS with an average age of 23.5 years (range 17–34 years). In a 1990 paper, Morris and colleagues presented details on sixteen adults (average age 28.5 years) with WBS; some patients seem to be tabulated in both series, so here I cite data primarily from the 1990 paper. Plissart et al. (1994) reported on eleven adults (average age 36.4 years), and Lopez-Rangel et al. reported on ten adults (average age 26.4 years). Nicholson and Hockey (1993) published data on a series of eighteen patients with WBS (average age 17.5 years); the age range of this series was very broad (4–35 years) and the manner in which the data were presented precludes identification of the adults, so these data are not cited in this review.

Ophthalmologic Problems

A history of strabismus and/or persistence of strabismus was present in the majority of WBS adults in two published series—in seven of thirteen cases (Morris et al. 1990) and seven of ten cases (Lopez-Rangel et al. 1992)—though it was present in only two of eleven cases reported by Plissart et al. (1994). Problems with visual acuity were also commonly reported, hyperopia more frequently than myopia. Two groups, primarily looking at children, performed detailed ophthalmologic examinations (Greenberg and Lewis 1988; Winter et al. 1996). One woman of forty-six years had "initial cataract in both eyes," but no other findings specific to adults were described. An autopsy of a forty-two-year-old man with WBS demonstrated calcium deposition in the cornea and sclera of the eye, though clinical ophthalmologic examination had shown only astigmatism and right exotropia (Jensen et al. 1976). Clinical evidence of calcium deposition in the eyes was not observed in either detailed ophthalmologic study (Greenberg and Lewis 1988; Winter et al. 1996).

In our series of adult WBS patients, we found a similarly high frequency of strabismus and several patients with cataracts (B. Pober et al., unpublished data). Several older adults required reading glasses for presbyopia.

A high frequency of problems dating from childhood (strabismus, abnormal visual acuity, and possible hypercalcemia) can combine with age-related visual problems such as presbyopia and cataracts to create a high potential for visual dysfunction. Thus, adults with WBS should undergo ophthalmologic monitoring at least annually and perhaps more frequently, depending on the clinical findings. Fortunately, serious visual disability does not seem to be common among adults with WBS, but regular ophthalmologic monitoring is essential.

Ear, Nose, and Throat/Audiologic problems

The previously published series of adults with WBS mention only two adults with hearing loss-type unspecified (Plissart et al. 1994) and left-sided congenital sensorineural hearing loss (Lopez-Rangel et al. 1992). However, several recent publications draw attention to the finding that hearing problems can develop in adulthood. Moderate to severe bilateral conductive hearing loss was found in a twenty-seven-year-old woman with hyperacusis and tinnitus (Miani et al. 2001). Her hearing loss was thought to be caused by otosclerosis; her hyperacusis was treated with auditory training.

In another study, nine patients with WBS, ages ranging from nine to twenty-five years, underwent a complete audiologic workup (Johnson et al. 2001). Among the four patients older than eighteen, three had moderate high-frequency sensorineural hearing loss in at least one ear. This loss was accompanied by absent transient evoked otoacoustic emissions, leading the authors to suggest that cochlear dysfunction may underlie the hearing loss.

Hyperacusis and recurrent otitis media are frequent problems during childhood. Hyperacusis persists throughout adulthood but seems to be clinically less bothersome for most adults (Van Borsel et al. 1987). Otitis media is an uncommon problem of adulthood. However, we have observed recurrent buildup of ear wax in the majority of adult patients with WBS seen at our clinic. Furthermore, we confirm the finding of mild to moderate hearing loss, primarily of the high-frequency sensorineural type, on standard audiologic evaluation (Pober et al. 2002).

Based on these findings, recommendations for monitoring include prompt audiologic or ear, nose, and throat valuation when a patient experiences difficulty "hearing" (to screen for hearing loss and wax buildup); baseline audiologic evaluation at thirty years of age, even for asymptomatic patients; and repeat evaluations every two to three years until there is no evidence of hearing loss or a stable audiogram pattern is documented. If persistent snoring develops, this should be evaluated with a sleep study because we have seen obstructive sleep apnea in a few of our adult patients.

Dental Problems

Dental problems in WBS, either structural or functional, have received little attention in the published literature. In her 1990 series, Morris listed twelve of thirteen patients as having "dental problems," most commonly dental malocclusion and enamel hypoplasia. One adult was described as having poor dentition and another as having "malimplantation" (Plissart et al. 1994). In another series, three of ten adults had malformations of the teeth or malocclusion; all were described as having micrognathia, and one underwent jaw reconstruction (Lopez-Rangel et al. 1992). Combining data from all these series, we find that a minority of adults received orthodontic treatment. In one study, patients with WBS underwent systematic oral evaluation by a dentist/orthodontist; thirteen of these forty-five patients had their permanent teeth (Hertzberg et al. 1994). Many had abnormal incisor morphology (peg-shaped incisors), smaller than normal incisor dimensions, and a significantly increased frequency of occlusal abnormalities. Generalized and localized enamel hypoplasia were uncommon. Oral examinations performed as part of the routine physical examination of WBS patients at our clinic revealed poor dental hygiene leading to caries and gum disease in most adults (B. Pober et al., unpublished data). We suspect that the poor visuospatial motor skills that are common in WBS contribute to the inability to perform proper tooth brushing and flossing.

Given the high frequency of morphologic and occlusal abnormalities, difficulty in performing proper dental hygiene, and a high frequency of cardiovascular disease, adults with WBS need consistent dental monitoring and care. Adults may require assistance with daily brushing, or at least should undergo weekly "oral" checks at home. They should be seen by a dentist for thorough cleanings every three to four months, rather than at six-month intervals. The pros and cons of orthodontics or reconstructive jaw surgery are complex, encompassing medical, ethical, and financial decisions. These matters should be discussed among the appropriate professionals, family members, and the adult with WBS to allow informed decisions about the risks and benefits of these treatments.

Cardiovascular Disease

A detailed discussion of the spectrum and management of cardiovascular disease in WBS is the focus of chapter 5. A few specific points relating to cardiovascular disease in adults are presented here.

Hypertension is common in both children and adults with WBS, with several but not all studies suggesting increased frequency with advancing age (Broder et al. 1999; Wessel et al. 1997; Morris et al. 1990; Lopez-Rangel et al. 1992). The hypertension is often "idiopathic"—that is, not secondary to an identifiable vascular stenosis in the descending aorta or renal arteries. However, imaging studies must be undertaken to rule out such causes, as they have been reported in adults with WBS (Radford and Pohlner 2000, Rose et al. 2001; Pankau et al. 2000). The frequency of descending aorta hypoplasia, mesenteric artery stenosis, and renal artery stenosis in adults is currently unknown. Intrinsic vascular anomalies caused by elastin gene (*ELN*) hemizygosity presumably underlie the hypertension in the many cases where discrete vascular stenosis cannot be documented (Sadler et al. 1998). Stroke is relatively uncommon but has been reported in adults with WBS (Wollack et al. 1996; Kawai et al. 1993). We have identified a few adult patients who experienced asymptomatic stroke, noted incidentally on magnetic resonance imaging (MRI) performed for another indication. There are no data to support recommendations for prophylactic treatment with low-dose daily aspirin to minimize the risk of stroke in adults with WBS.

Gastrointestinal Problems

Gastrointestinal problems are common throughout the life span of patients with WBS. During adulthood, frequently mentioned problems in the published literature are constipation, abdominal pain, and diverticulitis. In the series providing the most detailed information on gastrointestinal problems during adulthood (Morris et al. 1990), constipation was present in seven of thirteen adults and diverticulitis in three of thirteen. A few patients with gallstones have been reported (Morris et al. 1990). Problems associated with chronic constipation that require ongoing medical management or surgery include hemorrhoids, rectal prolapse, and diverticular disease (Lopez-Rangel et al. 1992; Davies et al. 1997).

Potential causes of recurrent or chronic abdominal pain include gastroesophageal reflux, diverticular disease, anxiety, and celiac disease. One study found antibody evidence of celiac disease in ~10% of sixty-three children with WBS (Gianotti et al. 2001), but the presence of celiac disease has not been documented in adults.

Physicians should perform a complete history, physical examination, and laboratory workup, as appropriate, to investigate medical causes of abdominal pain in adults with WBS. Although anxiety can cause abdominal pain (B. Pober, personal observation), this is a diagnosis of exclusion. Symptoms of gastroesophageal reflux merit documentation of reflux through endoscopy or imaging; if reflux is confirmed, a proper course of medical treatment is necessary. Signs of weight loss or abdominal pain that are associated with fever require prompt evaluation for diverticulitis. This should be done with great urgency, as some patients have suffered bowel perforation caused by diverticulitis (Giannotti et al. 2001). Celiac disease should be considered in the differential diagnosis of chronic abdominal pain, weight loss, and diarrhea.

A very important aspect of gastrointestinal medical management is prevention of chronic constipation. Constipation seems to increase the risk of rectal prolapse, hemorrhoids, diverticulosis, and diverticulitis. Aggressive treatment with dietary additives such as fiber or roughage should be incorporated into the diet of patients with chronic constipation. If constipation persists, then prescription medications are required and management should be under the care of a physician.

Endocrine Abnormalities
Calcium Metabolism

The most frequently described endocrine abnormality complicating WBS is hypercalcemia. Despite many studies, the incidence and etiology of hypercalcemia remain unknown. Elevated blood calcium levels have been documented in adults, as has ectopic vascular calcification and calcification of the basal ganglia and the anterior faux, detected by computed tomography (CT) scan (Morris et al. 1988, 1990). Although the risk of developing hypercalcemia is lower in adults than in young children, the magnitude of this risk remains unknown. Isolated hypercalciuria without hypercalcemia or nephrocalcinosis occurs in a small percentage of adults (Morris et al. 1988; B. Pober, personal observations). The etiology of this is unclear, even after routine diagnostic tests such as vitamin D levels, parathyroid hormone levels, and bone densitometry scans.

Long-term management of eucalcemic adults with no prior documented hypercalcemia consists of maintenance of the normal recommended daily allowance of calcium and vitamin D intake for age, and periodic determination of blood and urine calcium levels (American Academy of Pediatrics Committee on Genetics 2001). If a patient has a history of hypercalcemia during adolescence or adulthood, more frequent monitoring of calcium status is indicated. No published data on osteopenia or osteoporosis in WBS are available. Accordingly, bone density studies should be performed in asymptomatic WBS adults according to general population guidelines, and they certainly should be included as part of the workup of patients with hypercalcemia or hypercalciuria.

Thyroid Function

Hypothyroidism has been reported in children with WBS, but no reports confirm its presence in adults. In our series of adults with WBS, compensated or "subclinical" hypothyroidism occurs more commonly than true or actual hypothyroidism (Pober et al. 2000). Subclinical hypothyroidism may require hormone supplementation if the level of thyroid stimulating hormone (TSH) is sufficiently high or if, over time, there is progression to actual hypothyroidism. Periodic monitoring of thyroid function, including TSH level, is indicated in adults with WBS.

Diabetes

Diabetes mellitus has been reported in adults with WBS, with age of onset as early as twenty-one years (Imashuku et al. 2000; Nakaji et al. 2001; Plissart et al. 1994; Morris et al. 1988; Lopez-Rangel et al. 1992). We have observed clinical diabetes in several adults with WBS. Additionally, we have found an increased frequency of elevated glucose levels on standard oral glucose tolerance tests (Pober et al. 2001). It is not known whether the diabetes in individuals with WBS is best classified as type I or type II. However, we suspect that being overweight confers additional risk of developing abnormal glucose tolerance. Medical treatment guidelines specific for Williams-Beuren syndrome are under development. We recommend that all adults over thirty years of age undergo standard oral glucose tolerance testing. Additionally, efforts should be made to prevent weight gain and to maintain an activity level as high as is approved by the patient's primary physician or cardiologist. Individuals with abnormal glucose tolerance should be considered candidates for treatment with agents that improve glucose control.

Growth

Published growth curves document that children and adults with WBS are shorter than comparably aged controls (Morris et al. 1988; Pankau et al. 1992). In one study, average height for females eighteen years of age or older was ~155 cm (61 inches) and for males was ~168 cm (66 inches) (Pankau et al. 1992). There are several reports of adults with WBS who have become overweight or obese (Morris et al. 1990; Lopez-Rangel et al. 1992; Davies et al. 1997). Our observations indicate that adults with WBS can gain excess weight most often in a central or pear-shaped distribution; a small minority develop nonpitting edema or thickness in the legs (B. Pober, unpublished data). It is unclear whether the major determinants of this weight gain are the genetics of WBS, lifestyle, or some contribution from medications used to treat psychiatric disturbances. Ideally, excess weight gain should be prevented through education about healthy food choices and exercise; some adults with WBS have successfully lost weight by adhering to diets and increasing their activity level.

Genitourinary Abnormalities

A variety of renal abnormalities, including solitary kidney, duplicated kidney, hypoplastic kidneys, and renal scarring, have been identified on ultrasonography in ~15% to 20% of patients with WBS (Pober et al. 1993; Pankau et al. 1996). Nephrocalcinosis has also been documented, presumably secondary to hypercalcemia. There are reports of adults with recurrent urinary tract infections, often resulting from structural anomalies of the kidneys or ureters (Morris et al. 1990; Lopez-Rangel et al. 1992), but culture-proven urinary tract infections have been uncommon in the adults evaluated in our clinic (B. Pober, personal observations). Renal failure has been reported in a few cases, possibly caused by nephrocalcinosis, renal dysplasia, recurrent infections, or renal artery stenosis (Steiger et al. 1988; Biesecker et al. 1987; Ichinose et al. 1996; Davies et al. 1997).

Bladder diverticula have been detected on ultrasound examination in adults with WBS (Morris et al. 1990; Schulman et al. 1996). Bladder diverticula and abnormal detrusor contractions may contribute to the most common genitourinary problem in WBS: voiding frequency and incontinence (Schulman et al. 1996).

Given the potential for a variety of genitourinary problems, regular monitoring of renal status in adults with WBS is essential. An ultrasound examination of the kidney and bladder should be obtained on diagnosis of WBS; if the initial results are normal, scans should be repeated every five years in asymptomatic adults and more frequently in the event of recurrent infections, a change in voiding patterns, or loss of continence. Urine cultures should be obtained if symptoms are suggestive of a urinary tract infection. Blood and urine assessments of renal function should follow the published guidelines (American Academy of Pediatrics 2001). Persistent increased voiding frequency or enuresis merit a urologic referral for a more detailed evaluation of the genitourinary system and for possible consideration of bladder training or medication.

Musculoskeletal Abnormalities

Musculoskeletal abnormalities are a common complication of Williams-Beuren syndrome and, based on parental reports, seem to worsen over time. Five adults over the age of eighteen years were carefully studied by Kaplan et al. (1989). All five had contractures of the fingers; most had additional contractures involving the larger joints of the extremities, and one had scoliosis.

Contractures involving the lower extremities and a variety of spinal abnormalities (kyphosis, scoliosis, and/or lordosis) were observed in most of the adults previously reported (Morris et al. 1990; Lopez-Rangel et al. 1992). Severe kyphoscoliosis requiring spinal fusion and rod insertion is uncommon but has been reported (Osebold and King 1994). Radioulnar synostosis is found in 5% to 25% of persons with WBS (Bzduch 1994).

Our experience concurs with the published findings of decreased joint range of motion typically affecting the heel cords, hamstrings, and fingers in most adults with WBS. Almost paradoxically, a few adults have ligamentous laxity leading to problems such as recurrent dislocation of the patella (Davies et al. 1997). The most common spinal abnormality in our patient population is kyphosis, followed by lordosis and then scoliosis. Based on clinical examination, decreased range of motion at the elbow limiting either extension or pronation is present in ~20% of adults. The etiology of the joint contractures is unclear and could possibly result from intrinsic joint problems or neurologic abnormalities, such as hypertonia.

Ideally, contractures should be prevented or minimized by physical therapy to improve the strength of the upper body and the abdominal musculature. Direct stretching exercises should also be done to improve range of motion in the lower extremity joints. Most adults with WBS received physical therapy services during their school years, which were discontinued by adolescence. We recommend an individual physical therapy consultation for each adult, with the goal of developing a small set of exercises, to be performed at home, that target the involved areas. The degree of curvature of scoliosis is not likely to progress during adulthood, but kyphosis and lordosis can worsen over time.

Integument Problems

Patients with WBS are often described as having "soft" skin; concern has also been raised about premature aging of the skin (Ewart et al. 1993). Microscopic analysis of the skin in WBS demonstrates abnormal elastin fibers with reduced amounts of amorphous elastin and decreased elastic fiber volume and diameter (Urban et al. 2000; Ghomrasseni et al. 2001).

Presumably, the ultrastructural changes in elastin are responsible for the mild skin phenotype found in patients with WBS. Anecdotally, we often observe generalized dry skin and an increased frequency of psoriatic/scaling-type lesions on the face and scalp in a small number of adults with WBS. Standard skin care, with the use of moisturizers and sun protection, is recommended.

Most adults with WBS have premature graying of the hair (Morris et al. 1988). Our own observations confirm this, with graying starting as early as sixteen years of age (B. Pober, personal observation). The cause of the premature graying is unknown. It is often treated with readily available hair coloring products.

Neurologic Problems

Increased deep tendon reflexes were present in most of the adults with WBS who were examined by Morris (1990), with one patient noted to have fine tremor and dysdiadochokinesia. Another adult, who concomitantly was shown to have a de novo apparently balanced chromosome 12;15 translocation, was reported to have "tremor, hyperreflexia and spastic paraparesis" (Plissart et al. 1994). Only a few systematic neurologic examinations of adults by a neurologist have been published. Among seven WBS patients with an average age of 21.8 years, the majority were noted to have hypertonia, hyperreflexia, and gait and fine motor abnormalities (Chapman and Pober 1996). In a larger series of patients, the following abnormalities were found in a high proportion of adults: hyperreflexia, impairment of oculomotor control, dysmetria, dysdiadochokinesia, and limb and gait ataxia (Pober and Szekely 1999). Collectively, these findings suggest that cerebellar dysfunction is one of the characteristic neurologic features in adults with WBS. In addition, some older adults displayed slowing in movement execution, postural instability, intention and resting tremor, and frontal release signs.

Symptomatic Chiari malformation type I has been reported in adults with WBS (Pober and Filiano 1995; Wang et al. 1992). In our larger series, this malformation was diagnosed at a relatively young age in approximately one-tenth of the subjects (Pober and Szekely 1999). Nevertheless, the presence of Chiari malformation type I is sufficiently rare that it cannot provide a common mechanism to explain the characteristic spectrum of "abnormal" neurologic findings consistently seen in adults with WBS.

The precise cellular and molecular basis underlying the spectrum of abnormal neurologic features in WBS is unclear. In a single case, neuropathologic examination of a thirty-five-year-old man clinically diagnosed with WBS demonstrated the presence of Alzheimer-type changes (Golden et al. 1995). Neuropathologic examination in three other adults with WBS did not have these findings, but the histologic staining methodologies were not entirely comparable (Gallaburda and Bellugi 2001).

It is important for physicians caring for adults with WBS to perform a detailed neurologic examination and to be aware that the baseline examination generally shows disturbances in motor control, increased muscle tone and reflexes, and cerebellar abnormalities. We do not routinely recommend an MRI scan, but we have a low threshold for obtaining a scan and consulting with a neurologist. Furthermore, any acute changes merit further investigation to rule out stroke or symptomatic Chiari malformation, among other possibilities. In some older patients, tremor, both resting and intention, becomes quite marked and can interfere with daily living skills. This seems to be part of the natural history of WBS in some patients, potentially exacerbated by anxiety and medications. Symptomatic treatment may be attempted, though it is challenging because many of these drugs have significant central nervous system and/or cardiovascular side effects.

Miscellaneous Medical Concerns
Reproductive Issues

Most adolescents with WBS undergo early pubertal development (Cherniske et al. 1999; Partsch et al. 1999). Adults seem to have normal reproductive capabilities and several have had children (Ewart et al. 1993; Ounap et al. 1998). No information about the timing of menopause is yet available. Adult women with WBS need to have routine gynecologic care. Both men and women need to be taught about appropriate sexual relations, inappropriate sexual behavior, contraception, and their 50% risk of having a child with WBS. Approximately one-third of the adult women seen at our clinic have undergone sterilization procedures; rigorous steps must be taken to ensure that appropriate informed consent is obtained.

Cancer Screening

There are rare case reports of malignancy in adults with WBS (Marles et al. 1993; Felice et al. 1994). Among sixteen WBS patients in the Danish Cytogenetic Registry, none were recorded as having cancer in the Danish Cancer Registry (Hasle et al. 1998). One of the women evaluated at our center has been diagnosed with endometrial cancer. The available information indicates that WBS is not a "cancer-predisposition" syndrome, but too few adults have been studied to exclude a small increase in risk for developing malignancy compared with the general population. Recommendations at this time are to follow general population screening guidelines, superceded, as necessary, by guidelines based on specific family history.

Life Expectancy and Sudden Death

No studies have focused on life expectancy in WBS, though case reports and personal observations confirm the presence of elderly adults with WBS (Fryns et al. 1991). However, there seems to be increased morbidity and mortality, most often secondary to cardiovascular and gastrointestinal complications. Two reports describe sudden death in adults with WBS, one due to severe vascular stenosis and one due to less clear causes, possibly portal hypertension (Imashuku et al. 2000; Paz Suarez-Mier and Morentin 1999). In two other studies, the recurring risk factors for sudden death, primarily in children, were severe supravalvular aortic stenosis and/or biventricular outflow obstruction, coronary artery stenosis, or renal insufficiency (Kececioglu et al. 1993; Bird et al. 1996). For patients with these problems, the very low risk of sudden death may be slightly exacerbated following exposure to anesthesia. Identification of coronary artery stenosis by standard stress testing is difficult in adults with WBS because most cannot exercise sufficiently to reach the requisite heart rates (Kececioglu et al. 1993). The incidence of coronary artery stenosis and the risk for myocardial ischemia in adults with WBS remain unknown.

Possible Premature Aging

The question has been raised, by both parents and professionals, whether WBS represents a premature aging syndrome. In support of this possibility are the premature graying of the hair and earlier-than-expected onset of puberty, cataracts, diabetes, high-frequency sensorineural hearing loss, and tremor, among other findings. Additionally, parents often report decreased "energy level with easy fatigability" and subtle cognitive decline among adults with WBS in their thirties and forties, although these latter findings have yet to be substantiated in any scientific study. More data will need to be collected longitudinally on a cohort of patients to determine whether physical decline, cognitive decline, or both, occur at an earlier-than-expected age among adults with WBS.

Behavior and Mental Health

Findings from psychiatric studies of individuals with WBS are reviewed in chapter 12, but this discussion would not be complete without mention of behavioral and emotional problems, given their effects on quality of life for most adults with WBS.

Many studies on children with WBS report an increased frequency of a variety of behavior problems. Among adults, Udwin (1990) found that more than 50% were described by their caregivers as solitary, restless, irritable, worried, miserable, fearful, complaining of aches and pains, overfriendly with strangers, engaging in incessant chatter, and having preoccupations/obsessions. Despite the high frequency of such problems, only a minority of these adults were receiving therapy or counseling. Another questionnaire study confirmed the presence of most problems noted by Udwin; anxiety, social disinhibition, and preoccupations/obsessions were particularly common or disruptive or both (Davies et al. 1998). Again, despite the high frequency of these problems, only a minority of these individuals had been under the care of a mental health professional, though most who had received such care felt it was not effective. A study of older adolescents and adults with several different diagnoses reported that persons with WBS were rated as "having many fears" but were also described as "social" but having difficulty "maintaining friendships" (Dykens and Rosner 1999).

In our work, an experienced psychiatrist directly interviewed adults with WBS, in addition to asking parents or caregivers to complete standard questionnaires (Pober et al. 1998). Based on information from these multiple sources, all fifteen patients studied met either threshold or subthreshold DSM-IV criteria for a generalized anxiety disorder, and twelve of the fifteen met the criteria for a phobic disorder. A lower frequency of other diagnoses, such as depression or separation anxiety, was noted. Importantly, internalizing disorders such as anxiety were underdiagnosed when information from only parents or caregivers was considered.

The constellation of behavioral and emotional problems seen in adults with WBS is characteristic and can cause considerable distress both to the individuals with WBS and to their families. Caregivers should be aware of the high risk for psychopathology and must not be deceived by the superficial friendliness and "everything is fine" response most adults provide on initial questioning. Among the adults we have seen, the majority received or continue to receive counseling or therapy services; many have been prescribed antianxiety medication. The response to medication is variable, and no scientific studies exist to guide recommendations for treatment. Our anecdotal experience to date is that persons with WBS are very sensitive to medications of the serotonin selective reuptake inhibitor (SSRI) class and seem to require lower-than-standard doses.

A few adults with WBS have been treated for the diagnosis of a "psychotic" disorder (Bradley and Udwin 1989). Our center has been involved in the care of several adults who experienced significant deterioration in affect, function, and thought following a major life stress. These patients have generally been hospitalized and treated with antipsychotic medications, with varying degrees of success. As Bradley and Udwin also found, caution must be exercised before concluding whether these episodes truly represent psychosis or result from significant environmental triggers superimposed on the baseline WBS personality profile. Most of our patients have returned to baseline or close to baseline following intense therapy, antianxiety medication, and/or modifications in the vocational/living environment.

Future Directions

There are many unanswered questions about the natural history of Williams-Beuren syndrome, especially among older adults. Studies are needed to evaluate the frequency of potentially serious medical problems such as coronary artery stenosis, stroke (and possible therapeutic strategies to minimize the risk of stroke), diverticular disease, and celiac disease. Further studies to characterize the mechanism underlying abnormal glucose tolerance and to develop treatment options are essential. Well-controlled clinical trials to assess the efficacy and risks of pharmacologic and nonpharmacologic interventions for anxiety and other emotional/behavioral problems are urgently needed. Some of these studies may best be done as multicenter collaborative projects so that an adequate number of patients can be evaluated in a reasonable time. Finally, longitudinal follow-up of a cohort of adults with WBS is the best way to collect information that will substantiate or refute concerns about accelerated physical and cognitive aging among older adults.

ADDENDUM

Results from the author's original work on adults with Williams-Beuren syndrome have recently been published (Cherniske et al. 2004) and confirm many of the literature observations reviewed in this chapter. This work extends findings to older adults and demonstrates a high prevalence of diverticular disease, abnormal glucose metabolism, excess weight gain, high-frequency sensorineural hearing loss, and anxiety. Based on their findings, in conjunction with observations from the literature, we have developed medical management guidelines (table 6.1).

Table 6.1.
Recommendations for Medical Monitoring of Adults with Williams Syndrome

The recommendations listed below are intended to assist in the ongoing management of adults with WS. Recommendations for the initial medical assessment of the newly diagnosed patient with WS have been recently published elsewhere [2001]. We have expanded on these recommendations, especially those specific to adults over the age of 30 years.
General
   Comprehensive annual medical evaluation, preferably by a physician with expertise in WS
General well-being and nutrition
   Nutrition education focused on preventing excess weight gain
   Calcium & Vitamin D intake not to exceed RDA
   ADA diet if needed (see endocrine section below)
   Encourage active lifesyle & focused exercise regimen assuming there are no cardiovascular contraindications
Ophthalmologic
   Annual vision evaluation to monitor for strabismus, refractive errors, & cataracts
ENT/Audiologic
   Baseline audiologic evaluation @ 30 years of age to rule out sensorineural hearing loss
   Audiologic evaluation every 5 years or more frequently until existing hearing loss stabilizes
   Prevent ear wax build-up with softening drops & cleanouts as needed
Dental
   Supervision of brushing & flossing
   Consider use of an electric toothbrush
   Comprehensive dental cleaning every 3–4 months
   Consider use of a short acting oral anxiolytic prior to dental cleanings and procedures
Cardiovascular
   Cardiology evaluation every 3–5 years, even in the presence of stable cardiovascular disease
   Annual auscultation of abdomen to screen for bruit
   Evaluation of bruit by Doppler ultrasound and/or non-invasive imaging
   Blood pressure monitoring
     a. If normotensive—biannual blood pressure determination
     b. If hypertensive—evaluate for stenoses, renal disease, & hypercalcimia. No preferred pharmacologic treatment
       for "idiopathic" hypertension yet identified
   Evaluate for stroke only if symptomatic

(continued)

Table 6.1.
(*Continued*)

Gastrointestinal
  Medically treat documented reflux
  Monitor for constipation, rectal prolapse, and/or hemorrhoids
  Prevent constipation with dietary manipulation or medical management if needed
  Prompt evaluation of severe or recurrent abdominal pain (to rule out divericular disease)
Genitourinary
  Annual BUN, creatinine & urinalysis
  Renal & bladder ultrasound for symptomatology, or every decade for ongoing monitoring
  Increased vigilance for urinary tract infections
  Routine gynecologic care and prostate screening
Endocrine
  Blood calcium determination every 1–2 years (but more frequently if abnormal)
  Spot urine calcium to creatinine ratio annually
  For documented hypercalcemia and/or persistent hypercalciuria
    a. Three day diet history to calculate calcium & vitamin D intake; if intake exceeds RDA then decrease to 80% of the RDA and retest
    b. Twenty-four hour urine for calcium to creatinine ratio (normal adult ratio ≤0.22; normal adult calcium excretion <0.4 mg/kg/24 hr)
    c. Renal ultrasound to assess for nephrocalcinosis
    d. Fasting determinations of biointact PTH, 1,25 (OH)$_2$ and 25-OH vitamin D
    e. DEXA scan to assess bone mass
    f. Referral to endocrinologist if hypercalcemia and/or hypercaciuria persist, or if regulatory hormone levels are abnormal
  Baseline DEXA scan
    a. If normal repeat in 5 years; repeat sooner if fractures occur
    b. For mild ostopenia (bone mineral density T-score between −1.5 and −1.8 SD below the mean) **and** no other risk factors for a bone fracture
      i. Check urinary markers of bone turnover
      ii. Check 24 hr urine calcium, creatinine, and sodium excretion
      iii. Check 25-OH vitamin D level
      iv. If these studies are normal, repeat DEXA in 1 year
      v. Do **not** begin calcium supplementation
    c. For more severe bone loss (bone mineral density T-score −1.8 or −2.0 SD below the mean)
      i. Evaluate for secondary causes of bone loss such as hyperparathyroidism, hyper- or hypo-thyroidism, hypogonadism, Cushings disease, etc.
      ii. Consider treatment with a bisphosphonate
        • Monitor carefully for gastroesophageal reflux if using a biophosphonate
  Thyroid function tests and thyroid stimulating hormone (TSH) level every 3 years
    a. If abnormal obtain anti-thyroid antibodies
    b. For compensated hypothyroidism, check TFTs, & TSH annually and consider thyroid hormone replacement if TSH >10
  Baseline 2 hr oral glucose tolerance test (OGTT) at 30 years
    a. Repeat OGTT every 5 years or sooner if rapid weight gain
    b. Hemoglobin A1C is not a good screening tool in WS adults
    c. Control impaired glucose tolerance with exercise and diet
    d. Manage silent diabetes with exercise, diet, & consider medication
    e. Patients with clinical diabetes should be managed like adults in the general population with diabetes
  Routine gynecologic care & mammography
    a. Consider use of a short acting oral anxiolytic prior to pelvic examination
    b. Use pediatric speculum
Musculoskeletal/integument
  Physical therapy consultation to assess for contractures and/or scoliosis
  Limited exercise regimen to maintain joint range of motion & posture
  Seek specialist assessment for lower extremity lipedema; consider treatment with compressive stockings and wraps
Neurologic
  Acute neurological symptoms, asymmetry on neurological exam, and/or worsening of chronic low grade neurological problems require prompt evaluation by a neurologist as well as neuroimaging
  Baseline neuroimaging, without any clinical indication, is not recommended
Cancer screening
  Routine cancer surveillance, including mammography, prostate, testicular, and colon cancer screening should be performed as dictated by age and family history

(*continued*)

Table 6.1.
(*Continued*)

Psychiatry
    Low threshold for psychiatric intervention given prevalence of anxiety disorders as well as increased frequency of other psychopathology including depression
        Begin with low doses of medication as patients seem to have an increased sensitivity to standard adult doses
        Caution against diagnosis of psychotic disorder without careful and longitudinal mental status assessment
Social & Vocational
    Tailor residential placement to maximize independence while taking into consideration the strengths and weaknesses of WS cognitive functioning
        Encourage vocational opportunities, even volunteer positions
        Foster social outings and networking

Source: E. M. Cherniske et al., "Multisystem study of 20 older adults with Williams syndrome," *American Journal of Medical Genetics* 131A (2004): 255–264.
Abbreviations: WS, Williams syndrome; RDA, recommended daily allowance; ADA, American Dietetic Association; ENT, ear, nose, and throat; BUN, blood urea nitrogen; PTH, parathyroid hormone; TFTs, thyroid function tests.

ACKNOWLEDGMENTS

Funding for research evaluations of adults with WBS came from several sources: grant NICHD5-P01-HD03008-35 from the National Institute of Child Health and Human Development; a Yale Pepper Center Pilot Project; and a Williams Syndrome Association Pilot Project. I thank Elizabeth Cherniske for her many valuable insights and comments on this chapter and Dr. Anna Szekely for her input on the neurology section. Finally, I thank all the people with WBS and their families who participated in our research projects so that we could learn more about their disorder.

REFERENCES

American Academy of Pediatrics Committee on Genetics. 2001. Health care supervision for children with Williams syndrome. *Pediatrics* 107:1192–1204.
Biesecker, L., Laxova, R., and Friedman, A. 1987. Renal insufficiency in Williams syndrome. *American Journal of Medical Genetics* 28:131–135.
Bird, L., Billman, G., Lacro, R., Spicer, R., Jariwala, L., Hoyme, E., Zamora-Salinas, R., Morris, C., Viskochil, D., Frikke, M., and Jones, M. 1996. Sudden death in Williams syndrome: Report of ten cases. *Journal of Pediatrics* 129:926–931.
Bradley, E. A., and Udwin, O. 1989. Williams syndrome in adulthood: A case study focusing on psychological and psychiatric aspects. *Journal of Mental Deficiency Research* 33:175–184.
Broder, K., Reinhardt, E., Ahern, J., Lifton, R., Tamborlane, W., and Pober, B. 1999. Elevated ambulatory blood pressure in 20 subjects with Williams syndrome. *American Journal of Medical Genetics* 83:356–360.
Bzduch, V. 1994. Radioulnar synostosis in Williams syndrome: A historical overview. *American Journal of Medical Genetics* 50:386.
Chapman, C., and Pober, B. 1996. Neurologic findings in children and adults with Williams syndrome. *Journal of Child Neurology* 11:63–65.
Cherniske, E. M., Carpenter, T. O., Klaiman, C., Young, E., Bregman, J., Insogna, I., Schultz, R. T., and Pober, B. R. 2004. Multisystem study of 20 older adults with Williams syndrome. *American Journal of Medical Genetics* 131A:255–264.

Cherniske, E. M., Sadler, L. S., Schwartz, D., Carpenter, T. O., and Pober, B. 1999. Early puberty in Williams syndrome. *Clinical Dysmorphology* 8:117–121.

Davies, M., Howlin, P., and Udwin, O. 1997. Independence and adaptive behavior in adults with Williams syndrome. *American Journal of Medical Genetics* 70:188–195.

Davies, M., Udwin, O., and Howlin, P. 1998. Adults with Williams syndrome: Preliminary study of social, emotional and behavioral difficulties. *British Journal of Psychiatry* 172:273–276.

Dykens, E., and Rosner, B. 1999. Refining behavioral phenotypes: Personality-motivation in Williams and Prader-Willi syndromes. *American Journal of Mental Retardation* 104:158–169.

Ewart, A., Morris, C., Atkinson, D., Jin, W., Sternes, K., Spallone, P., Stock, A. D., Leppert, M., and Keating, M. 1993. Hemizygosity at the elastin locus in a developmental disorder, Williams syndrome. *Nature Genetics* 5:11–16.

Felice, P. V., Ritter, S. D., and Anto, J. 1994. Occurrence of non-Hodgkin's lymphoma in Williams syndrome—case report. *Angiology* 45:167–170.

Fryns, J. P., Borghgraef, M., Volke, P., and Van den Berghe, H. 1991. Adults with Williams syndrome. *American Journal of Medical Genetics* 40:253.

Gallaburda, A., and Bellugi, U. 2001. Cellular and molecular cortical neuroanatomy in Williams syndrome. In *Journey from cognition to brain to gene: Perspectives from Williams syndrome,* ed. U. Bellugi and M. St. George, 123–146. Cambridge: MIT Press.

Ghomrasseni, S., Dridi, M., Bonnefoix, M., Septier, D., Gogly, G., Pellat, B., and Godeau, G. 2001. Morphometric analysis of elastic skin fibres from patients with: Cutis laxa, anetoderma, pseudoxanthoma elasticum, and Buschke-Ollendorff and Williams-Beuren syndromes. *Journal of the European Academy of Dermatology and Venereology* 15:305–311.

Giannotti, A., Tiberio, G., Castro, M., Virgilii, F., Colistro, F., Ferretti, F., Digilio, M. C., Gambarara, M., and Dallapiccola, B. 2001. Coeliac disease in Williams syndrome. *Journal of Medical Genetics* 38:767–768.

Golden, J. A., Gunnlauger, P., Pober, B., and Hyman, B. 1995. The neuropathology of Williams syndrome. *Archives of Neurology* 52:209–212.

Greenberg, F., and Lewis, R. 1988. The Williams syndrome: Spectrum and significance of ocular features. *Ophthalmology* 95:1608–1612.

Hasle, H., Olsen, J. H., Hansen, J., Friedrich, U., and Tommerup, N. 1998. Occurrence of cancer in a cohort of 183 persons with constitutional chromosome 7 abnormalities. *Cancer Genetics and Cytogenetics* 105:39–42.

Hertzberg, J., Nakisbendi, L., Needleman, H., and Pober, B. 1994. Williams syndrome—oral presentation of 45 cases. *Pediatric Dentistry* 16:262–267.

Ichinose, M., Tojo, K., Nakamura, K., Matsuda, H., Tokudome, G., Ohta, M., Sakai, S., and Sakai, O. 1996. Williams syndrome associated with chronic renal failure and various endocrinological abnormalities. *Internal Medicine (Tokyo, Japan)* 35:482–488.

Imashuku, S., Hayashi, S., Kuriyama, K., Hibi, S., Tabata, Y., and Todo, S. 2000. Sudden death of a 21-year-old female with Williams syndrome showing rare complications. *Pediatrics International* 42:322–324.

Jensen, O. A., Warburg, M., and DuPont, A. 1976. Ocular pathology in the elfin face syndrome. *Ophthalmologica Basel* 172:343–444.

Johnson, L., Comeau, M., and Clarke, K. 2001. Hyperacusis in Williams syndrome. *Journal of Otolaryngology* 30:90–92.

Kaplan, P., Kirschner, M., Watters, G., and Costa, M. T. 1989. Contractures in patients with Williams syndrome. *Journal of Pediatrics* 84:895–899.

Kawai, M., Nishikawa, T., Tanaka, M., Ando, A., Kasajima, T., Higa, T., Tanikawa, T., Kagawa, M., and Momma, K. 1993. An autopsied case of Williams syndrome complicated by moyamoya disease. *Acta Paediatrica Japan* 35:63–67.

Kececioglu, D., Kotthoff, S., and Vogt, J. 1993. Williams-Beuren syndrome: A 30 year follow-up of natural and postoperative course. *European Heart Journal* 14:1458–1464.

Lopez-Rangel, E., Maurice, M., McGillivray, B., and Friedman, J. 1992. Williams syndrome in adults. *American Journal of Medical Genetics* 44:720–729.

Marles, S., Goldber, N., and Chudley, A. 1993. Mucinous cystadenoma of ovary in a patients with Williams syndrome. *American Journal of Medical Genetics* 46:349.

Miani, C., Passon, P., Bracale, A. M., Barotti, A., and Panzolli, N. 2001. Treatment of hyperacusis in Williams syndrome with bilateral conductive hearing loss. *European Archives of Otorhinolaryngology* 258:341–344.

Morris, C., Demsey, S., Leonard, C., Dilts, C., and Blackburn, B. 1988. Natural history of Williams syndrome. *Journal of Pediatrics* 113:318–326.

Morris, C., Leonard, C., Dilts, C., and Demsey, S. 1990. Adults with Williams syndrome. *American Journal of Medical Genetics* 6:102–107.

Nakaji, A., Kawame, Y., Nagai, C., and Iwata, M. 2001. Clinical features of a senior patient with Williams syndrome. *Rinsho Shinkeigaku* 41:592–598.

Nicholson, W. R., and Hockey, K. A. 1993. Williams syndrome: A clinical study of children and adults. *Journal of Paediatrics and Child Health* 29:468–472.

Osebold, W., and King, H. 1994. Kyphoscoliosis in Williams syndrome. *Spine* 19:367–371.

Ounap, K., Laidre, P., Bartsch, O., Rein, R., and Lipping-Sitska, M. 1998. Familial Williams-Beuren syndrome. *American Journal of Medical Genetics* 80:491–493.

Pankau, R., Partsch, C. J., Gosch, A., Oppermann, H., and Wessel, A. 1992. Statural growth in Williams-Beuren syndrome. *European Journal of Pediatrics* 151:751–755.

Pankau, R., Partsch, C., Winter, M., Gosch, A., and Wessel, A. 1996. Incidence and spectrum of renal anomalies in Williams-Beuren syndrome. *American Journal of Medical Genetics* 63:301–304.

Pankau, R., Partsch, C. J., Gosch, A., Siebert, R., Schneider, M., Schneppenheim, R., Winter, M., and Wessel, A. 2000. Williams Beuren syndrome 35 years after the diagnosis of one of the first Beuren patients. *American Journal of Medical Genetics* 91:322–324.

Panzolli, N. 2001. Treatment of hyperacusis in Williams syndrome with bilateral conductive hearing loss. *European Archives of Otorhinolaryngology* 258:341–344.

Partsch, C. J., Dreyer, G., Gosch, A., Winter, M., Schneppenheim, R., Wessel, A., and Pankau, R. 1999. Longitudinal evaluation of growth, puberty, and bone maturation in children with Williams syndrome. *Journal of Pediatrics* 134:82–89.

Paz Suarez-Mier, M., and Morentin, B. 1999. Supravalvar aortic stenosis, Williams syndrome and sudden death: A case report. *Forensic Science International* 106:45–53.

Plissart, L., Borghgraef, M., Volcke, P., Van den Berghe, H., and Fryns, J. P. 1994. Adults with Williams-Beuren syndrome: Evaluation of the medical, psychological and behavioral aspects. *Clinical Genetics* 46:161–167.

Pober, B. R., and Filiano, J. J. 1995. Association of Chiari I malformation and Williams syndrome. *Pediatric Neurology* 12:84–88.

Pober, B., and Szekely, A. 1999. Distinct neurological profile in Williams syndrome. *American Journal of Human Genetics* 65:367A.

Pober, B., Lacro, R., Rice, C., Mandell, V., and Teele, R. 1993. Renal findings in 40 individuals with Williams syndrome. *American Journal of Medical Genetics* 46:271–274.

Pober, B., Schultz, R., Teague, B., Bronen, R., and Bregman, J. 1998. Psychiatric assessment and neuroimaging in subjects with Williams syndrome. Paper presented at the 19th David W. Smith Workshop on Malformations and Morphogenesis, Whistler, Canada.

Pober, B., Carpenter, T., and Breault, D. 2000. Prevalence of hypothyroidism and compensated hypothyroidism in Williams syndrome. Paper presented at the 21st David W. Smith Workshop on Malformations and Morphogenesis, La Jolla, CA.

Pober, B., Wang, E., Petersen, K., Osborne, L., and Caprio, S. 2001. Impaired glucose tolerance in Williams syndrome. *American Journal of Human Genetics* 69:302A.

Pober, B., Wang, E., Morgan, T., Cherniske, E., Young, E., Petersen, K., Osborne, L., and Caprio, S. 2002. Abnormal glucose tolerance and sensorineural hearing loss in adults with Williams syndrome. Paper presented at the 9th International Professional Conference on Williams syndrome, Long Beach, CA.

Radford, D. J., and Pohlner, P. G. 2000. The middle aortic syndrome: An important feature of Williams syndrome. *Cardiology of the Young* 10:597–602.

Rose, C., Wessel, A., Pankau, R., Partsch, C. J., and Bursch, J. 2001. Anomalies of the abdominal aorta in Williams-Beuren syndrome—another cause of arterial hypertension. *European Journal of Pediatrics* 160:655–658.

Sadler, L. S., Gingell, R., and Martin, D. J. 1998. Carotid ultrasound examination in Williams syndrome. *Journal of Pediatrics* 132:354–356.

Schulman, S., Zderic, S., and Kaplan, P. 1996. Increased prevalence of urinary symptoms and voiding dysfunction in Williams syndrome. *Journal of Pediatrics* 129:466–469.

Steiger, M. J., Rowe, P. A., Innes, A., and Burden, R. P. 1988. Williams syndrome and renal failure. *Lancet* 2:804.

Udwin, O. 1990. A survey of adults with Williams syndrome and idiopathic hypercalcemia. *Developmental Medicine and Child Neurology* 32:129–141.

Urban, Z., Peyrol, S., Plauchu, H., Zabot, M. T., Lebwohl, M., Schilling, K., Green, M., Boyd, C. D., and Csiszar, K. 2000. Elastin gene deletions in Williams syndrome patients result in altered deposition of elastic fibers in skin and a subclinical dermal phenotype. *Pediatric Dermatology* 17:12–20.

Van Borsel, J., Curfs, L. M. G., and Fryns, J. P. 1987. Hyperacusis in Williams syndrome: A sample survey study. *Genetic Counseling* 8:121–126.

Wang, P. P., Hesselink, J. R., Jernigan, T. L., Doherty, S., and Bellugi, U. 1992. Specific neurobehavioral profile of Williams' syndrome is associated with neocerebellar hemispheric preservation. *Neurology* 42:1999–2002.

Wessel, A., Motz, R., Pankau, R., and Bursch, J. H. 1997. Arterial hypertension and blood pressure profile in patients with Williams-Beuren syndrome. *Zeitschrift fur Kardiologie* 86:251–257.

Winter, M., Pankau, R., Amm, M., Gosch, A., and Wessel, A. 1996. The spectrum of ocular features in the Williams-Beuren syndrome. *Clinical Genetics* 49:28–31.

Wollack, J. B., Kaifer, M., LaMonte, M. P., and Rothman, M. 1996. Stroke in Williams syndrome. *Stroke* 27:143–146.

II. Behavioral Neuroscience Research

The Behavioral Neuroscience of Williams-Beuren Syndrome

An Overview

Paul P. Wang, M.D.

7

The neurobehavioral characterization of Williams-Beuren syndrome (WBS) dates from the earliest reports on the syndrome. The physician scientists who first wrote about WBS provided only a "broad-brush" description of its associated cognition and behavior, but their observations set the stage for decades of progressively more sophisticated neurobehavioral studies. During the late 1990s, neurobehavioral research on WBS evolved quickly, reflecting the increasingly interdisciplinary nature of neurobehavioral research and its increasingly sophisticated techniques. Indeed, the literature on WBS illustrates the development of the field of cognitive neuroscience as it advanced from psychological and neuroanatomic phenomenology to the study of the interactions among genetic, neurobiological, and environmental factors during development. Methodologic advances in the psychological and the biological sciences also are evident in the WBS literature, with many of the early studies being superceded by later studies of greater technical merit and theoretical rigor.

Psychologists' and neuroscientists' interests in WBS stem from the syndrome's striking profile of general cognitive, visuospatial, linguistic, and social-emotional traits. This profile is evident to the most casual of observers, though its explication requires rigorous investigation. Champions of various theoretical perspectives have hoped to find fodder for their arguments in WBS, and biomedical investigators have sought to find in WBS a biological basis for complex cognitive functions. One result of these pursuits is that the quantity of research on WBS is itself remarkable, given the limited number of individuals who are diagnosed with WBS. In this chapter, I provide some theoretical and historical context (through the mid-1990s) for the discussions of the behavioral neuroscience of WBS in the following chapters, as well as providing sources, especially historical references and those not cited elsewhere.

Early Observations

The first twenty-five years of research on WBS focused predominantly on its biological etiology and its medical complications. Despite this emphasis and despite the lack of neurobehavioral expertise on the part of the early WBS investigators, important elements of the behavioral profile of WBS began to be appreciated. To begin with, the triad of defining criteria described by Williams and coworkers (1961) included mental retardation, supravalvular aortic stenosis, and the distinctive facial appearance of the syndrome. Beuren and colleagues (1962) also recognized mental retardation as a cardinal feature of the syndrome. Von Arnim and Engel's more detailed observations of six cases were published only shortly after recognition of the syndrome, but their behavioral description of WBS touched on almost all the facets that continue to be topics of active investigation today: "Mentally, the children also show great similarities. Their IQ is about 40–50 but they show outstanding loquacity and a great ability to establish interpersonal contacts. This stands against a background of insecurity and anxiety" (von Arnim and Engel 1964, 376). The authors observed further that their patients with WBS had poor motor coordination and typically had an "amicable attitude" but that "their friendliness is not returned by others as expected" (375). Later findings on language, visuospatial skills, sociability, and psychopathology in WBS all are consistent with von Arnim and Engel's observations. About fifteen years later, Bennett et al. (1978) initiated the systematic neuropsychological study of WBS when they administered standardized psychometric tests to experimental cohorts of children and adults with WBS. With the publication of their results, the objective definition of the WBS neurobehavioral profile began.

A Diagnostic Caveat. A seminal point in the history of research on WBS was the identification by Ewart and colleagues (1993) of the 7q11.23 microdeletion as the genetic basis of the syndrome. The diagnostic fluorescent in situ hybridization (FISH) test for WBS became widely available over the next few years. Studies conducted before that time and other studies that do not establish the WBS diagnosis by FISH may be confounded by the inclusion of subjects who do not have WBS.

General Cognitive Abilities

Estimates of the average intelligence level of individuals with WBS have gained accuracy as a result of the intertwining of advances in genetic and neurobehavioral research. Before the development of a genetic test for WBS, medical authorities generally asserted that mental retardation was a cardinal and therefore mandatory feature of WBS. As a consequence, the diagnosis of WBS was unlikely to be made for any patient who did not have such levels of cognitive impairment. In some cases, diagnosed individuals had profound retardation and were nonverbal, presenting a very low and flat profile of cognitive skills. The appreciation that WBS is associated with a broader range of cognitive skills emerged gradually, and the advent of molecular diagnostic methods cemented the understanding that WBS can be associated, in some cases, with very mild cognitive impairments.

No rigorous epidemiologic study of intelligence quotient has been conducted for WBS, but it is now believed that average intelligence among individuals with WBS is in the range of mild mental retardation, with mean IQ scores of 55 to 60 (Morris et al. 1988; Udwin et al. 1996). The extant studies suggest that the variability of IQ in WBS is similar to that among nonsyndromic individuals (i.e., a standard deviation of about fifteen points). Thus, a large majority of persons with WBS are mildly or moderately retarded, with small numbers either more or less severely impaired. There seem to be a handful of persons with WBS who have IQ scores in the normal range (K. Levine, personal communication). The day-to-day "adaptive function" of individuals with WBS is typically commensurate with IQ scores, though the data on adaptive skills are few (Mervis et al. 2001). The data on age-related change in IQ are also limited. Only a handful of studies report longitudinal data on IQ, and the data for these studies date from before the advent of molecular diagnosis (Udwin et al. 1996; Gosch and Pankau 1996). These studies do not support the presence of significant changes in IQ with age. They suggest that slow but steady gains are evident for many individuals with WBS through the adolescent years (Howlin et al. 1998). Cognitive decline has been reported anecdotally in some adult patients in their fifth or sixth decades (B. Pober, personal communication).

Language

Even casual interactions with individuals who have WBS give the impression that their profile of cognitive skills is highly uneven. Specifically, linguistic skills may seem to be well preserved. These individuals speak with a fluency, grammatical accuracy, and pragmatic facility that casual observers often regard as surprisingly high for the general cognitive abilities typically associated with WBS. Neurobehavioral scientists' interest in WBS was initially based on these impressions and continues to be driven by the contrast between the linguistic behavior of individuals with WBS and that of individuals with other neurodevelopmental disabilities.

Over the first quarter-century of investigation on WBS, a handful of studies attempted to illuminate the language skills of people with this disorder. The interpretation of these studies, however, was limited by their use of measures that confounded linguistic skills with other cognitive skills. As an example, some investigators posited that the putative linguistic strengths of persons with WBS could be documented by comparing their verbal IQ scores with their performance IQ scores. Such analyses neglected the critical demands placed by the verbal IQ tests on nonlinguistic skills. For example, in the Wechsler intelligence tests, arithmetic is one of the subtests that contribute to the verbal IQ score. Consequently, the comparisons of "verbal" and "nonverbal" skills in the early literature on WBS often failed to demonstrate significant contrasts between language and other domains of cognitive ability (e.g., MacDonald and Roy 1988; Greer et al. 1997).

Studies by Bellugi and her colleagues were the first to employ tasks that focused on linguistic skills rather than drawing on a panoply of unspecified other cognitive abilities. In their early investigations, Bellugi et al. (1988) demonstrated that the grammatical skills of adults with WBS were clearly superior to those of individuals with Down syndrome who were matched for age and general cognitive abilities. The WBS advantage extended from grammatical comprehension to sentence production and metacognitive tasks that require the subjects to repair nongrammatical sentences. Later studies by Bellugi's group (Reilly et al. 1991; Bellugi et al. 2000) showed that the superiority of persons with WBS (vs. Down syndrome) also was evident in their spontaneous productions, which contain fewer grammatical errors, use more complex grammatical forms, and more frequently employ prosody to convey emotional affect.

Bellugi's findings established WBS as a fascinating paradigm for cognitive neuroscience. For cognitive psychologists, her findings seemed to make WBS an illustration of the modularity of language in the human mind. For developmental psychology, WBS became an intriguing condition in which language seemed to develop normally despite the impairment of general cognitive abilities. For biological scientists, WBS was an opportunity to fathom the genetic and neurobiological foundations of language. An abundance of more recent research on language in WBS demonstrates that the scientific community's early interpretations of Bellugi's seminal data were sometimes hyperbolic. The recent data, derived from studies performed in many different countries, across many different languages, show consistently that language skills in WBS are not fully preserved in the face of mental retardation. Indeed, the overall level of language abilities in WBS is similar to the level of general cognitive abilities. Initial claims of atypical semantic organization in WBS also have been revisited. (These recent studies are reviewed by Mervis in chapter 8.)

Recent linguistic research on WBS reflects the more nuanced character of current theories of psycholinguistics. In the domain of word morphology, for example, some contend that there are distinct brain systems for processing regular versus irregular verbs (e.g., walk/walked vs. run/ran, respectively) and that this distinction is mirrored in the linguistic profile of WBS. The relationship of language-processing skills to working-memory capacity is another topic of recent investigation (as further discussed below). New research also examines language development in children with WBS, with multiple research teams following the trajectory of language development in WBS and its relationship to the acquisition of general cognitive skills in childhood. Of important clinical relevance is the finding that young children with WBS are typically quite delayed in early language development. Mervis (chapter 8) and Karmiloff-Smith and coauthors (chapter 11) detail these and other recent topics in language research on WBS.

Visuospatial Cognition

Bellugi and her associates also pioneered the systematic study of visuospatial skills in Williams-Beuren syndrome, starting in the late 1980s (Bellugi et al. 1988). Their widely published illustration contrasting a young adult's verbal description of an elephant and her line drawing of an elephant from memory is a dramatic demonstration of the contrast between linguistic and visuospatial performance in WBS. Data from Bellugi's laboratory, confirmed by many other labs, show that visual-motor skills in WBS constitute a clear weakness in the neuropsychological profile of the syndrome. Although linguistic skills in WBS almost always exceed those in Down syndrome, the reverse is typically true for visuospatial tasks requiring motor performance (Wang et al. 1995). The weakness in visual-motor skills is so characteristic of WBS that Mervis and colleagues (2000) were able to operationalize a definition of the "Williams Syndrome cognitive profile" that is heavily based on deficits on a block construction task. As a marker for WBS, this profile shows a sensitivity of more than 95% and a fairly high specificity, although individuals with other genetic syndromes may sometimes show a similar profile (Bearden et al. 2002).

Bellugi and colleagues also illuminated a peculiar pattern in the visual-motor performances of individuals with WBS (Bihrle et al. 1989). When asked to copy drawings that have an organization that can be dichotomized into "global" and "local" levels, individuals with WBS tend to produce figures that contain the correct local details but lack correct global organization. The same pattern can be seen in the block constructions of individuals with WBS. This pattern of local versus global preference and the larger profile of linguistic versus visuospatial abilities led to the interpretation that the neuropsychological profile of WBS resembled that of patients with right-hemisphere brain damage.

Here again, recent research suggests that the cognitive profile of WBS is more complicated than the early data reflect. In further examining the global-local dichotomy in WBS, Pani et al. (1999) found no local preference in visual perception, despite the documented visual-motor preference for the local level of detail. Other studies of visual-perceptual abilities show a WBS strength in some skills, such as in facial recognition and in the identification of objects that are presented in a noncanonical view (e.g., a chair depicted from a bird's-eye view) (Wang et al. 1995; see also Landau et al.'s discussion in chapter 9). Subjects with WBS may have a weakness in the perception of motion, however, although this point is not resolved (Atkinson et al. 1997). The profile of visual-perceptual skills in WBS has been noted to map onto the dichotomy between the functions of the ventral and dorsal cortical pathways for visuospatial processing (the "what" vs. "where" pathways, respectively) (Wang et al. 1995).

Research on the development of visuospatial skills in WBS also has begun, and the results suggest that the poor global organization of drawings by children with WBS may represent a normal stage of visuospatial skill development, rather than an altogether deviant pattern. Landau and coauthors (chapter 9) and Karmiloff-Smith and coauthors (chapter 11) explore these issues in greater detail. In particular, Landau et al. describe recent studies that delve into the fundamental cognitive processes that underlie the visuospatial performance of persons with WBS.

Social Cognition and Social Behavior

Von Arnim and Engel's observations (1964) on the sociability of individuals with WBS and other early investigators' reports on the strong social orientation of individuals with WBS provided the foundation for a third important and growing domain of investigation on WBS: social cognition. Subsequent studies have taken two tracks, one attempting to document the sociability associated with WBS and the other examining the social cognitive skills of individuals with WBS.

In pursuit of the first objective, several investigators have studied the temperamental and personality traits of persons with WBS. Unfortunately, many of their studies were limited by the use of norms or control groups that were less than ideal. Recent work by Klein-Tasman and Mervis (2003), however, shows convincingly that there is a distinct personality profile in WBS and that a very low rating for shyness is among its prime features. In analogy to the "Williams Syndrome cognitive profile," Klein-Tasman and Mervis proposed a "Williams Syndrome personality profile," which also has high statistical sensitivity for the diagnosis of WBS. Consistent with these findings are other data on temperament in WBS, collected for about fifty individuals under the age of nine and for matching cohorts of children with velocardiofacial syndrome (another contiguous gene deletion syndrome) and children with mental retardation of unknown etiology, all assessed with the Revised Colorado Children's Temperament Inventory (Buss and Plomin 1984). These temperament data also show very low ratings for shyness in WBS and high ratings for emotionality (P. Wang, unpublished observations). Detailed behavioral observations of infants with WBS also show exceptionally intense "looking" behaviors directed toward other people rather than toward alternative stimuli (Mervis et al. 2003). Jones et al. (2000) also have documented, in experimental settings, "hypersocial" behaviors in individuals with WBS across a wide age range.

In chapter 10, Plesa-Skwerer and Tager-Flusberg describe research on the social cognitive abilities of individuals with WBS. These studies demonstrate that the ability to perceive and correctly label the facial emotions displayed by other persons is well preserved but the ability to reason about social motivations and social problems is significantly impaired. The gap between these skills is perhaps not surprising to parents and other keen observers of WBS, who have seen that children and adults with WBS often are frustrated in their desires to engage socially with their peers. Thus, the social cognitive profile of WBS appears to hold clear clinical implications.

An additional aspect of the social profile of WBS remains poorly investigated despite the intrigue it has generated in many observers. After an infantile period of fussy, colicky behavior, most individuals with WBS appear to be biased toward an unusually happy and agreeable disposition (Levine and Wharton 2000). Although children with WBS can be oppositional toward their parents, and adults with WBS may develop anxiety and depression (see below), the disposition that teachers, social acquaintances, and nonfamily authority figures most often observe is a cheerful and accommodating one. Experiments by Bellugi's group (1999) suggest that individuals with WBS also are unusually predisposed to attribute positive characteristics to pictures of unfamiliar people. No other research groups have yet studied these WBS traits, and as yet there is no clear theoretical context in which these traits should be interpreted. One possibility is that they are related to the high sociability that typifies the syndrome.

Memory and Music

Over the past decade, several research groups have reported on the memory skills of individuals with WBS. At least two theoretical points are of particular interest in this area of investigation. First, WBS is associated with significantly stronger short-term memory for phonological or verbal stimuli than for visuospatial stimuli (Wang and Bellugi 1994; Vicari et al. 1996; Jarrold et al. 1999). While a similar distinction can be found in some other disorders, in WBS it suggests the possibility of a distinct genetic basis for these cognitive skills. The relationships of both phonological or verbal working memory and of spatial memory to language are the second focus of investigation on memory. Mervis reviews this literature in chapter 8 and posits that language development and language processing may be even more strongly dependent on memory capacity in individuals with WBS than in others.

Two reports on the procedural or implicit learning abilities of individuals with WBS have been published (Vicari et al. 2001; Don et al. 2003). These studies seem to indicate that implicit learning, a heterogeneous set of skills, may be somewhat impaired in WBS. Despite this impairment, individuals with WBS demonstrate some ability to implicitly acquire an artificial grammar. Further study of memory skills in WBS will be necessary to further elucidate the role of working memory and implicit learning in the development of other cognitive skills.

Anecdotal reports of outstanding musical abilities in WBS are plentiful, but scientific study of musical abilities began only with Don and colleagues in 1999. In chapter 16, Levitin and Bellugi review and discuss this emerging literature, and in chapter 15 Lenhoff focuses specifically on absolute pitch in WBS. Though data are still scant, there is a suggestion that memory for musical stimuli also is relatively well preserved, consistent with the hypothesis that phonological and tonal memory skills are closely related and that musical memory skills may underlie other musical performance abilities (Peretz and Coltheart 2003). The analogy to the relationship between memory and language skills is apparent (Patel 2003) and will likely be a focus of future study.

Clinical Psychology and Behavioral Medicine

Clinical psychologists and behaviorally oriented physicians from the United States, Western Europe, and Australia have produced a helpful literature on the psychopathology that is sometimes associated with Williams-Beuren syndrome. The highly sociable temperament associated with WBS, for example, can be reframed from the clinical perspective as "social disinhibition," which connotes the often inappropriate socially forward behaviors of persons with WBS. Other behavioral difficulties frequently seen in WBS include attention deficits, mood disorders, sleep disturbances, and especially anxiety disorders and specific phobias. Dykens and Rosner summarize this literature in chapter 12, and in chapter 13 Mason and Arens provide a review of sleep research in WBS. Of potential relevance to the psychopathology associated with WBS is the recent finding that syntaxin (the gene for which is deleted in WBS) may be involved in the pathophysiology of psychiatric disorders (Honer et al. 2002).

Research on therapeutic or prophylactic interventions for these behavioral problems and on educational interventions is regrettably rare. Save for two reports on the use of methylphenidate for attention deficit disorders (Power et al. 1997; Bawden et al. 1997), there is no published research on the treatment of neurobehavioral problems in WBS. I hope future reviews of research on WBS will include much more of such content.

Neurobiology and Genetics

Enormous technical advances in neuroimaging have paralleled the increases in neuroscientific interest in WBS over the past decade. As a corollary, the recent in vivo morphometric studies of the brain in individuals with WBS are technically far superior to their earlier counterparts (Wang et al. 1992a, 1992b; Jernigan and Bellugi 1990; Jernigan et al. 1993). In chapter 14, Feinstein and Reiss summarize the recent morphometric studies as well as the few neuropathologic studies and the single neurochemical study (magnetic resonance spectroscopy) that have been published.

Despite the growing sophistication of these studies, the relationship between the neuroanatomic and cognitive profiles of WBS can only be conjectured. The conjectures that have been made, however, accord fairly well with standard neuropsychological models. The WBS weakness in visual-motor skills is accompanied by relative curtailment of parietal brain regions, and the behavioral strengths in auditory and phonological skills are accompanied by relative preservation of temporal lobe regions. Jernigan's early study of brain morphology in WBS also showed preservation of a mesial temporal brain area that included much of the limbic portions of the temporal lobe (Jernigan et al. 1993). These regions may well be related to the temperamental characteristic of high emotionality and to the affectively charged language that individuals with WBS so readily produce. Functional neuroimaging studies of WBS are just beginning and will surely contribute to a more secure understanding of brain-behavior relationships. The electrophysiologic studies reviewed by Feinstein and Reiss (chapter 14) indicate some of the promise that future neurofunctional studies hope to fulfill.

The study of gene-behavior relationships in WBS also promises much for the future. To date, it has proven difficult to definitely link any feature of the cognitive or behavioral profile of WBS to specific genes (see Morris's discussion in chapter 3 and Karmiloff-Smith and coauthors' discussion in chapter 11). As many writers have recently explained, genes are not linked directly to behavior. Rather, the complexities of development intervene between gene and mature behavioral profile, and the developmental process is richly and interactively affected by multiple converging factors, both biological and experiential.

Future Directions

Neurobehavioral and cognitive research on WBS has advanced tremendously over the past decade. It nonetheless remains fertile ground for continued research motivated by both theoretical and clinical concerns. Strong linguistic and other psychological claims have been made about the mature cognitive profile of WBS, but Karmiloff-Smith, Mervis, and others argue compellingly that these profiles must be reexamined in greater depth and with greater specificity. Recent research demonstrates that the WBS profile is more nuanced than originally appreciated and that the strong cognitive performance of individuals with WBS on certain cognitive tasks often depends on atypical underlying strategies. Thus, theoretical arguments on the modularity of language or other cognitive processes in WBS must be reconsidered. Arguments on the innateness or genetic specificity of the mature behavioral profile in WBS also must take into consideration the developmental processes that culminate in that profile. Genetics may provide a seed from which the later profile grows, but many other factors contribute to the final form of the WBS profile. Karmiloff-Smith's research suggests that, in some cases, the cognitive profile of WBS at very young ages differs markedly from the profile at later ages. In sum, the complex and richly interacting relationships among genetics, neurodevelopment, and behavior remain far removed from our current understanding.

As fascinating as these relationships are as subjects of academic study, the fervent hope of researchers, clinicians, and WBS families alike is that an understanding of some of these relationships will lead to the discovery of therapeutic interventions that can ameliorate some of the neurobehavioral impairments faced by persons with WBS. Clinicians, meanwhile, should attempt to advance on an empirical basis, drawing from their accumulated experience in the treatment of other populations with developmental disorders.

REFERENCES

Atkinson, J., King, J., Braddick, O., Nokes, L., Anker, S., and Braddick, F. 1997. A specific deficit of dorsal stream function in Williams' syndrome. *NeuroReport* 8:1919–1922.
Bawden, H. N., MacDonald, G. W., and Shea, S. 1997. Treatment of children with Williams syndrome with methylphenidate. *Journal of Child Neurology* 12:248–252.
Bearden, C. E., Wang, P. P., and Simon, T. J. 2002. Williams syndrome cognitive profile also characterizes velocardiofacial/DiGeorge syndrome. *American Journal of Medical Genetics (Neuropsychiatric Genetics)* 114:689–692.
Bellugi, U., Marks, S., Bihrle, A., and Sabo, H. 1988. Dissociation between language and cognitive functions in Williams syndrome. In *Language development in exceptional circumstances,* ed. D. Bishop and K. Mogford, 177–189. London: Churchill-Livingstone.
Bellugi, U., Adolphs, R., Cassady, C., and Chiles, M. 1999. Towards the neural basis for hypersociability in a genetic syndrome. *NeuroReport* 10:1653–1657.
Bellugi, U., Lichtenberger, L., Jones, W., Lai, Z., and St. George, M. 2000. The neurocognitive profile of Williams syndrome: A complex pattern of strengths and weaknesses. *Journal of Cognitive Neuroscience* 12 (suppl. 1): 7–29.
Bennett, F. C., LaVeck, B., and Sells, C. J. 1978. The Williams elfin facies syndrome:

The psychological profile as an aid in syndrome identification. *Pediatrics* 61:303–306.

Beuren, A. J., Apitz, J., and Harmjanz, D. 1962. Supravalvular aortic stenosis in association with mental retardation and a certain facial appearance. *Circulation* 26:1235–1240.

Bihrle, A. M., Bellugi, U., Delis, D., and Marks, S. 1989. Seeing either the forest or the trees: Dissociation in visuospatial processing. *Brain and Cognition* 11:37–49.

Buss, A. H., and Plomin, R. 1984. *Temperament: Early developing personality traits.* Hillsdale, NJ: Erlbaum.

Don, A., Schellenberg, E. G., and Rourke, B. P. 1999. Music and language skills of children with Williams syndrome. *Child Neuropsychology* 5:154–170.

Don, A. J., Schellenberg, E. G., Reber, A. S., DiGirolamo, K. M., and Wang, P. P. 2003. Implicit learning in children and adults with Williams syndrome. *Developmental Neuropsychology* 23:201–226.

Ewart, A. K., Morris, C. A., Atkinson, D., Jin, W., Sternes, K., Spallone, P., Stock, A. D., Leppert, M., and Keating, M. T. 1993. Hemizygosity at the elastin locus in a developmental disorder, Williams syndrome. *Nature Genetics* 5:11–16.

Gosch, A., and Pankau, R. 1996. Longitudinal study of the cognitive development in children with Williams-Beuren syndrome. *American Journal of Medical Genetics* 61:26–29.

Greer, M. K., Brown, F. R., Pai, G. S., Choudry, S. H., and Klein, A. J. 1997. Cognitive, adaptive, and behavioral characteristics of Williams syndrome. *American Journal of Medical Genetics (Neuropsychiatric Genetics)* 74:521–525.

Honer, W. G., Falkai, P., Bayer, T. A., Xie, J., Hu, L., Li, H. Y., Arango, V., Mann, J. J., Dwork, A. J., and Trimble, W. S. 2002. Abnormalities of SNARE mechanism proteins in anterior frontal cortex in severe mental illness. *Cerebral Cortex* 12:349–356.

Howlin, P., Davies, M., and Udwin, O. 1998. Cognitive functioning in adults with Williams syndrome. *Journal of Child Psychology and Psychiatry* 39:183–189.

Jarrold, C., Baddeley, A. D., and Hewes, A. K. 1999. Genetically dissociated components of working memory: Evidence from Down's and Williams syndrome. *Neuropsychologia* 37:637–651.

Jernigan, T. L., and Bellugi, U. 1990. Anomalous brain morphology on magnetic resonance images in Williams syndrome and Down syndrome. *Archives of Neurology* 47:529–533.

Jernigan, T. L., Bellugi, U., Sowell, E., Doherty, S., and Hesselink, J. R. 1993. Cerebral morphological distinctions between Williams and Down syndromes. *Archives of Neurology* 50:186–191.

Jones, K. L., and Smith, D. W. 1975. The Williams elfin facies syndrome: A new perspective. *Journal of Pediatrics* 86:718–723.

Jones, W., Bellugi, U., Lai, Z., Chiles, M., Reilly, J., Lincoln, A., and Adolphs, R. 2000. Hypersociability in Williams syndrome. *Journal of Cognitive Neuroscience* 12 (suppl. 1): 30–46.

Klein-Tasman, B. P., and Mervis, C. B. 2003. Distinctive personality characteristics of 8-, 9-, and 10-year olds with Williams syndrome. *Developmental Neuropsychology* 23:269–290.

Levine, K., and Wharton, R. 2000. Williams syndrome and happiness. *American Journal of Mental Retardation* 105:363–371.

MacDonald, G. W., and Roy, D. L. 1988. Williams syndrome: A neuropsychological profile. *Journal of Clinical and Experimental Neuropsychology* 10:125–131.

Mervis, C. B., Robinson, B. F., Bertrand, J., Morris, C. A., Klein-Tasman, B. P., and

Armstrong, S. C. 2000. The Williams syndrome cognitive profile. *Brain and Cognition* 44:604–628.

Mervis, C. B., Klein-Tasman, B. P., and Mastin, M. E. 2001. Adaptive behavior of 4-through 8-year-old children with Williams syndrome. *American Journal of Mental Retardation* 106:82–93.

Mervis, C. B., Morris, C. A., Klein-Tasman, B. P., Bertrand, J., Kwitny, S., Appelbaum, L. G., and Rice, C. E. 2003. Attentional characteristics of infants and toddlers with Williams syndrome during triadic interactions. *Developmental Neuropsychology* 23:243–268.

Morris, C. A., Demsey, S. A., Leonard, C. O., Dilts, C., and Blackburn, B. L. 1988. Natural history of Williams syndrome: Physical characteristics. *Journal of Pediatrics* 113:318–326.

Pani, J. R., Mervis, C. B., and Robinson, B. F. 1999. Global spatial organization by individuals with Williams syndrome. *Psychological Science* 10:453–458.

Patel, A. D. 2003. Language, music, syntax, and the brain. *Nature Neuroscience* 6:674–681.

Peretz, I., and Coltheart, M. 2003. Modularity of music processing. *Nature Neuroscience* 6:688–691.

Power, T. J., Blum, N. J., Jones, S. M., and Kaplan, P. E. 1997. Brief report: Response to methylphenidate in two children with Williams syndrome. *Journal of Autism and Developmental Disorders* 27:79–87.

Reilly, J. S., Klima, E. S., and Bellugi, U. 1991. Once more with feeling: Affect and language in atypical populations. *Developmental Psychopathology* 2:367–391.

Udwin, O., Davies, M., and Howlin, P. 1996. A longitudinal study of cognitive abilities and educational attainment in Williams syndrome. *Developmental Medicine and Child Neurology* 38:1020–1029.

Vicari, S., Brizzolara, D., Carlesimo, G. A., Pezzini, G., and Voltera V. 1996. Memory abilities in children with Williams syndrome. *Cortex* 32:503–514.

Vicari, S., Bellucci, S., and Carlesimo, G. A. 2001. Procedural learning deficit in children with Williams syndrome. *Neuropsychologia* 39:665–677.

von Arnim, G., and Engel, P. 1964. Mental retardation related to hypercalcemia. *Developmental Medicine and Child Neurology* 6:366–377.

Wang, P. P., and Bellugi, U. 1994. Evidence from two genetic syndromes for a dissociation between verbal and visual-spatial short-term memory. *Journal of Clinical and Experimental Neuropsychology* 16:317–322.

Wang, P. P., Doherty, S., Hesselink, J. R., and Bellugi, U. 1992a. Callosal morphology concurs with neurobehavioral and neuropathological findings in two neurodevelopmental syndromes. *Archives of Neurology* 49:407–411.

Wang, P. P., Hesselink, J. R., Jernigan, T. L., Doherty S., and Bellugi, U. 1992b. Specific neurobehavioral profile of Williams syndrome is associated with neocerebellar hemispheric preservation. *Neurology* 42:1999–2002.

Wang, P. P., Doherty, S., Rourke, S. B., and Bellugi, U. 1995. Unique profile of visuoperceptual skills in a genetic syndrome. *Brain and Cognition* 29:54–65.

Williams, J. C., Barrett-Boyes, B. G., and Lowe, J. B. 1961. Supravalvular aortic stenosis. *Circulation* 24:1311–1318.

Language Abilities in Williams-Beuren Syndrome 8

Carolyn B. Mervis, Ph.D.

In the study of Williams-Beuren syndrome (WBS), the topic that has generated the most controversy is language ability, especially relative to nonlinguistic cognitive ability. Based on data from her pioneering studies of adolescents with WBS, Bellugi and her colleagues claimed that WBS represents a clear dissociation between intact language abilities and severe cognitive deficits (e.g., Bellugi et al. 1988). In particular, individuals with WBS correctly use complex syntactic constructions such as passives, conditionals, relative clauses, and tag questions. They also have an unusual command of vocabulary. At the same time, they have severe or profound mental retardation. Bellugi and colleagues argued that this pattern of abilities and disabilities provided a strong demonstration of the independence of language (or a language module) from cognition (or a cognitive module). Bellugi's position, which was based on right-hemisphere (parietal) damage as the best model for WBS, catapulted WBS into the center of the modularity debate, with the result that researchers who previously had not even heard of WBS began to devote significant resources to its study. The outcome has been highly beneficial for individuals with WBS, their families, and the professionals who provide support to them. Much more is known today about the cognitive and language abilities of individuals with WBS than would have been learned had Bellugi not succeeded so well in focusing attention on this syndrome.

At the same time, most researchers now believe that both aspects of Bellugi's initial position are incorrect. Although language may be a relative strength, it is by no means "intact." Furthermore, with the exception of visuospatial construction, most nonlinguistic cognitive abilities are only mildly impaired. Although some researchers still approach WBS from a modularity perspective, most recent research has started from the premise that WBS is a developmental disorder and, as such, the most appropriate models are developmental ones. Furthermore, given that WBS is a genetic disorder present from conception, the brains of individuals with WBS may develop in atypical ways. As a result, even when individuals with WBS are matched to typically developing individuals for level of performance, these similar levels of performance may have developed through differential emphasis on particular processes (Karmiloff-Smith et al. 2003; Mervis 2003).

In this chapter, I review recent research on the language abilities of individuals with WBS from both perspectives. Recent research on nonlinguistic cognitive abilities is also reviewed briefly in the context of linguistic abilities.

Performance on Standardized Assessments

Standardized assessments provide important information about individuals' abilities relative to abilities of peers of the same chronological age (CA). Findings from more naturalistic settings also are important, and these data are considered later in the chapter in the discussion of lexical and grammatical development. Data from experiments designed to measure particular aspects of language provide a third source of information about language strengths and weaknesses and potential processing differences; these data are also considered in later sections.

When studying a rare syndrome, it is tempting to conduct one's research on small, relatively easily obtained samples of individuals varying widely in CA. My colleagues and I have taken a different approach. The data reported in this section (from Mervis et al. 2003) are based on large samples that include individuals from forty-two of the fifty states of the United States. Descriptive statistics for performance on a wide range of standardized assessments are presented in table 8.1.

Differential Ability Scales

The Differential Ability Scales (DAS; Elliott 1990) is a full-scale measure of intellectual functioning. The six core subtests included in the School Age version of the DAS are divided into three clusters. The Verbal cluster measures the ability to define words and to perform verbal reasoning tasks. The Nonverbal Reasoning cluster measures inductive and sequential reasoning abilities. The Spatial cluster measures visuospatial constructive abilities, spatial memory, and spatial reasoning. Visuospatial construction is known to be the area of greatest weakness for individuals with WBS (Bellugi et al. 1994; Mervis et al. 1999). Mean GCA (General Conceptual Ability; similar to IQ) is 58.14 (in the range of mild mental retardation). As illustrated in figure 8.1, however, the mean GCA is misleading. Mean standard scores on both the Verbal cluster and the Nonverbal Reasoning cluster are considerably higher than the GCA. In contrast, 50% of the individuals tested performed

Table 8.1.
Descriptive Statistics for Standardized Assessments of Persons with Williams-Beuren Syndrome

Measure	N	CA Range	Mean Standard Score	SD	Range
DAS (School Age): GCA	50	7;0–16;11	58.14	11.44	32–88
Verbal cluster	50	7;0–16;11	70.02	13.21	51–100
Nonverbal Reasoning cluster	50	7;0–16;11	67.56	12.09	52–98
Spatial cluster	50	7;0–16;11	54.74	6.07	50–79
Pattern construction T	210	5;0–51;6	23.25	5.52	20–53
Recall of Digits T	234	5;0–51;6	32.97	9.72	20–60
K-BIT: Composite IQ	250	4;0–51;6	67.38	15.39	40–108
Verbal IQ	250	4;0–51;6	71.77	15.45	40–108
Nonverbal IQ	250	4;0–51;6	68.52	17.12	40–108
Mullen Scales: Composite	34	2;9–5;5	62.32	11.64	49–88
Visual Reception T	34	2;9–5;5	30.12	10.12	20–46
Fine Motor T	34	2;9–5;5	21.65	3.45	20–31
Receptive Language T	34	2;9–5;5	30.47	9.82	20–55
Expressive Language T	34	2;9–5;5	33.21	9.59	20–48
PPVT-III	146	4;0–51;6	77.91	15.38	40–120
EVT	119	4;0–49;5	64.14	19.18	40–106
TRC	40	5;0–7;11	58.45	18.14	40–105
TROG	209	5;0–51;8	73.67	12.54	55–112

Source: Mervis et al. 2003. Reprinted with permission.
Note: For the general population, mean = 100 and SD = 15 for all measures not labeled "T." For all measures labeled "T," mean = 50 and SD = 10.
Abbreviations: CA, chronological age; DAS, Differential Ability Scales; GCA, General Conceptual Ability; K-BIT, Kaufman Brief Intelligence Test; PPVT-III, Peabody Picture Vocabulary Test (3rd ed.); EVT, Expressive Vocabulary Test; TRC, Test of Relational Concepts; TROG, Test for Reception of Grammar.

at floor on the Spatial cluster. Performance was best on the Recall of Digits subtest (a diagnostic subtest not included in the GCA) and worst on the Pattern Construction and Recall of Designs subtests (the subtests in the Spatial cluster).

Our research group used the pattern of performance of individuals with WBS on the DAS to quantify and test the Williams Syndrome Cognitive Profile (WSCP; Frangiskakis et al. 1996; Mervis et al. 2000). Four specific criteria were proposed, focusing on the extreme weakness in visuospatial construction, relative strength in verbal short-term memory, and uneven nature of verbal memory and language abilities relative to visuospatial construction abilities, even for individuals with very low IQ. Based on a sample of eighty-four individuals with WBS and fifty-six individuals with other forms of mental retardation or learning disabilities, the WSCP was found to have a sensitivity of 0.88 and specificity of 0.92 (Mervis et al. 2000). In a particularly important comparison, we considered the performance of eighteen individuals who had been clinically diagnosed with WBS but were later found to have a negative fluorescent in situ hybridization (FISH) test (and thus no deletion in the WBS region). Only two of the eighteen individuals fit the WSCP, yielding a specificity of 0.89 and providing further support for the argument that WBS is a genetic disorder involving a single etiology.

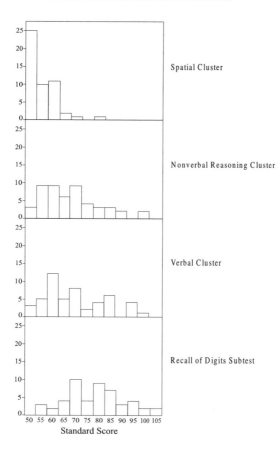

Fig. 8.1. Distribution of standard scores for DAS Spatial cluster, Nonverbal Reasoning cluster, Verbal cluster, and Recall of Digits subtest for fifty seven- to seventeen-year-olds with Williams-Beuren syndrome. Recall of Digits T score has been converted to the same scale as the cluster standard scores (mean, 100; SD = 15). *Source:* Mervis et al. 2003. Reprinted with permission.

Kaufman Brief Intelligence Test

The negative effect of the extreme weakness in visuospatial construction on IQ is well demonstrated by a comparison of the performance of individuals with WBS on the DAS and on the Kaufman Brief Intelligence Test (K-BIT; Kaufman and Kaufman 1990), an IQ test that measures only verbal ability and nonverbal reasoning ability (visuospatial construction ability is not tested on the K-BIT). The mean verbal standard scores on the DAS and K-BIT are within two points of each other; similarly, the mean nonverbal reasoning standard scores are only one point apart. In contrast, mean K-BIT IQ is nine points higher than mean DAS GCA.

Mullen Scales of Early Learning

The Mullen Scales provide a full-scale measure of intelligence for toddlers and preschoolers (Mullen 1995). The Mullen findings reported in table 8.1 indicate that the pattern of performance evident for school-aged children with WBS is present by age two years. Performance was weakest on the Fine Motor subtest (measuring primarily visuospatial construction); 79% of the participants scored at floor. Performance was considerably better for the two language subtests (averaging about the same as for the DAS and K-BIT verbal standard scores) and for the Visual Reception subtest, which measures many of the same types of abilities as the nonverbal reasoning sections of the DAS and K-BIT.

Thus, across the three measures of intelligence, a consistent pattern emerges, with standard scores for language abilities the highest. At one level, this pattern is consistent with prior assertions that language is a particular strength for individuals with WBS. However, level of performance is not consistent with the claim that language abilities are "excellent"; standard score means for language are in the borderline normal to mildly deficient range. Nonverbal reasoning standard scores are only slightly lower. Furthermore, mean IQ is considerably higher than the severe to profound mental retardation range. With this pattern in mind, I turn to standardized assessments that measure specific language abilities.

Peabody Picture Vocabulary Test (Third Edition)
and Expressive Vocabulary Test

The Peabody Picture Vocabulary Test (third edition) (PPVT-III; Dunn and Dunn 1997) measures receptive single-word vocabulary knowledge. Most words are names for objects, actions, or attributes, although some label more abstract concepts. On average, individuals with WBS earn their highest standard score on this measure. Mean performance was in the borderline normal range; 9% scored at least 100 (the mean for the general population).

The Expressive Vocabulary Test (EVT; Williams 1997) measures expressive single-word vocabulary. The participant is asked either to name a picture or an attribute of a picture or to provide a synonym for a name provided by the researcher. As in the PPVT-III, most target words are labels for objects, actions, or attributes. The EVT was co-normed with the PPVT-III, making standard scores on these measures easy to compare. Individuals with WBS typically have considerably more difficulty on the EVT, most likely because of the conceptual requirement of providing a synonym rather than simply naming a picture.

Test of Relational Concepts

The Test of Relational Concepts (TRC; Edmonston and Litchfield Thane 1988) measures comprehension of abstract relational concepts. Five types of concepts are included: temporal (e.g., before/after), quantitative (e.g., most/least), dimensional (e.g., tall/short), spatial (e.g., under/over, beginning/end), and other (same/different). We administered the TRC to forty five- to seven-year-olds with WBS who had a mean score of 87.03 on the PPVT-III (Mervis et al. 2003). In contrast, their mean score on the TRC was 58.45. (Standard scores on the TRC usually are expressed as T scores. To make it easier to compare performance on the PPVT-III and the TRC, I have converted the TRC standard scores to the same scale as the PPVT-III [mean, 100; SD = 15] and set the minimum standard score on the TRC at 40, the same as on the PPVT-III.) Percentage correct for each type of relational concept was similar to that for a group of typically developing children matched for TRC raw score. Performance on the TRC was the weakest of any language measure. This difficulty is likely related to the abstract/relational nature of the concepts being tested. The difficulty that children with WBS have with relational concepts as measured by the TRC is further considered later in the chapter (see "Semantics").

Test for Reception of Grammar

The Test for Reception of Grammar (TROG; Bishop 1989) measures receptive understanding of grammar. Constructions range in difficulty from single words to simple sentences, comparatives, passives, and sentences with relative or embedded clauses. Mean performance on this measure was in the borderline normal range, similar to that on the PPVT-III. The pattern of performance on the different grammatical constructions was similar to that found by Karmiloff-Smith et al. (1997) in their study of a considerably smaller British sample. In that study, particular difficulty was identified for embedded clauses. Zukowski (2001, 2004) reported the same difficulty in an elicited production task when individuals with WBS were prompted to describe a picture by using embedded clause constructions.

In summary, across all the language measures administered, average performance is consistently in the mildly deficient to borderline normal range in persons with WBS. This level of performance is considerably below that expected for CA, indicating that both lexical and grammatical abilities typically are well below the level expected for "excellent" language ability. It is important to note the great variability in language ability across the WBS population, which is strongly linked to both verbal short-term memory ability and verbal working-memory ability (Mervis 1999; Mervis et al. 2004), as discussed below (see "Relations between Verbal Memory Ability and Grammatical Ability").

Early Language Acquisition

Although people with WBS eventually develop relatively good language abilities, onset of language almost always is significantly delayed. We reported longitudinal data for a sample of thirteen children with WBS who were as-

Table 8.2.
Mean Chronological Age (CA, in months) and CA Range for Age of Acquisition of 10-, 50-, and 100-Word Expressive Vocabularies for 13 Children with Williams-Beuren Syndrome, Compared with MacArthur Communicative Development Inventory (CDI) Norms

Expressive Vocabulary Size	WBS		CA for CDI	
	Mean CA	CA Range	50th Percentile	5th Percentile
10 words	28.19	18.84–53.95	12–13	16–17
50 words	36.59	23.80–61.25	16–17	23–24
100 words	40.90	26.24–68.05	18–20	26–28

Source: Mervis et al. 2003. Reprinted with permission.

sessed monthly from the time of their first words (Mervis et al. 2003). Expressive vocabulary size was measured based on the 680-word vocabulary checklist included in the Words and Sentences form of the MacArthur Communicative Development Inventory (CDI; Fenson et al. 1993), a parental report measure of language acquisition that has very high reliability and validity (Fenson et al. 1993, 1994). Age of acquisition of a 10-word expressive vocabulary was below the fifth percentile (the lowest percentile provided) for the CDI norms for all thirteen children. Twelve children scored below the fifth percentile for age of acquisition of 50-word and 100-word expressive vocabularies. Mean chronological age and CA range for the WBS sample at acquisition of 10-, 50-, and 100-word expressive vocabulary sizes are indicated in table 8.2, along with the CAs corresponding to the fiftieth and fifth percentiles for the CDI.

Studies of the early language acquisition of children with WBS have focused on three topics. The first involves cross-sectional comparisons of children with WBS and children with Down syndrome; the second, relations between early language acquisition and verbal and nonverbal intelligence at age four years; and the third, relations between specific aspects of language and cognition.

Cross-Sectional Comparisons: Williams-Beuren Syndrome and Down Syndrome

School-aged children with WBS repeatedly have been found to have larger expressive vocabularies than CA-matched children with Down syndrome (DS) (Bellugi et al. 1994; Wang and Bellugi 1993). Singer Harris and colleagues (1997), however, argued that, initially, young children with DS have an expressive vocabulary advantage over young children with WBS; the advantage does not shift to children with WBS until after the onset of grammar. This position is based on Singer Harris et al.'s finding that, for children with expressive vocabularies of fewer than fifty words, children with DS had significantly larger expressive vocabularies than children with WBS. This comparison is methodologically problematic, however, in that Singer Harris et al. used the same variable (expressive vocabulary size) first as the criterion for inclusion in the sample and then as the dependent variable in the analysis. Thus, the outcome variable is confounded with the criterion for inclusion in the study, making the results uninterpretable. (See Mervis and Robinson 2000 for a more detailed argument.)

A more methodologically sound approach to comparing the expressive vocabulary sizes of children with WBS and children with DS would be to match the two groups closely on chronological age and then compare their expressive vocabulary sizes. Mervis and Robinson (2000) followed this approach, tightly matching a group of twenty-four two-year-olds with WBS to a group of twenty-eight two-year-olds with DS (mean CA, 2.55 years, for both groups). Two additional boys with WBS (ages 2.00 and 2.09 years) were excluded from the analyses because their expressive vocabulary sizes were much larger than those of any of the other children their age; descriptive data for these two children are provided separately. Expressive vocabulary size was derived from the CDI 680-word checklist. Parents were told to indicate that their child "said" a word if the child produced the word spontaneously, either in verbal or in signed form. Mean expressive vocabulary size was significantly greater for the WBS group (132.50 words; range, 3–391) than the DS group (66.35 words; range, 0–324).

The parents of nine toddlers with DS and thirteen toddlers with WBS had filled out the CDI vocabulary checklist when their children were between twenty-four and twenty-seven months old. To provide a comparison for a time even closer to the onset of expressive vocabulary acquisition, a second analysis was conducted. Mean CA was 2.16 years for each group. Once again, mean expressive vocabulary size was significantly larger for the WBS group (55.08 words; range, 5–120) than the DS group (19.67; range, 0–70). These results indicate that toddlers with WBS have, on average, a clear and significant expressive vocabulary advantage over children with DS who are of the same chronological age. Nevertheless, most of the WBS group was substantially delayed in acquisition of expressive vocabulary. Other than the two boys who were excluded from the analyses (and who were at the seventy-fifth percentile for the CDI norms, with vocabulary sizes of 412 and 439 words), no one in the WBS group was at even the tenth percentile for the CDI norms; 67% were below the fifth percentile. The wide range in expressive vocabulary size among toddlers with WBS presages the variability previously described for older children and adults on standardized tests of vocabulary.

Vicari and colleagues (2002) compared the language abilities of twelve Italian toddlers and preschoolers with WBS with two contrast groups similar in mental age (MA): a slightly older Down syndrome group and a considerably younger typically developing (TD) group. Mean MA for the WBS group was 2.83 years; mean CA was 4.85 years. Expressive vocabulary size and grammatical complexity were measured with the Italian version of the CDI (Caselli and Casadio 1995). Mean length of utterance (MLU) in words was calculated based on a twenty-minute spontaneous language sample, and children completed a sentence repetition test.

Expressive vocabulary size was very similar for the three groups: 452 words for the WBS group, 457 for the DS group, and 488 for the TD group. This finding suggests that matching young children with WBS and young children with DS on overall cognitive ability eliminates the differences in expressive vocabulary found when the groups were CA matched without taking cognitive ability into account (Mervis and Robinson 2000). The two sets of findings together indicate that, on average, children with WBS have higher overall cognitive ability than children with DS of the same chronological age; this pattern has been confirmed in a comparison between older children with WBS and those with DS (Klein and Mervis 1999).

Although the three groups had similar expressive vocabulary sizes, the TD group scored substantially and significantly higher than the DS group on sentence complexity (means of 28.8 and 13.1, of 37 possible). The WBS group (mean, 21.9) did not differ significantly from the other groups. The WBS group had a significantly longer MLU (3.1 words) than the DS group (2.4 words); the TD group (MLU, 2.9 words) did not differ significantly from the other groups.

Substantial individual differences in each group were found for vocabulary size, grammatical complexity, and MLU. Correlational analyses indicated that, for each group, there were strong and significant correlations between expressive vocabulary size and sentence complexity score ($r = 0.92$ for the WBS group) and expressive vocabulary size and MLU ($r = 0.85$ for the WBS group). Vicari et al. (2002) argued that these correlations indicate that grammatical development is not independent of lexical development even in WBS.

Analyses of performance on the sentence repetition test indicated that the WBS group (mean, 54.01% correct) and the TD group (mean, 57.1% correct) performed significantly better than the DS group (mean, 23.6% correct). Further analyses focusing on the percentages of various types of words repeated correctly indicated that the DS group was less likely to repeat correctly each type of word than were either of the other groups. The WBS group was significantly less likely to repeat nouns, verbs, and modifiers correctly than the TD group; no differences were found for articles and prepositions (the types of words that were most difficult for the TD children). Volterra and colleagues (2001) have shown that auditory processing ability plays an important role in mastery of function words. On this basis, Vicari et al. (2002) argued that the lack of differences between groups on prepositions and articles may be due to the good auditory processing abilities of individuals with WBS. Expressive vocabulary size was significantly correlated with percentage of correctly repeated sentences for all three groups ($r = 0.84$ for the WBS group).

Volterra and colleagues (2003) have reported more detailed analyses for a subset of the participants in the Vicari et al. (2002) study. Results of a standardized test of expressive vocabulary confirmed that the WBS, DS, and TD groups were well matched. Qualitative analyses indicated that the labels produced by the three groups (whether correct or incorrect) were similar; in contrast to the findings of Bellugi et al. (e.g., 1994), the children with WBS did not produce rare or unusual words. The WBS group correctly repeated significantly more sentences on the phrase repetition test than did the DS group. Sentences were considered to be repeated correctly if they were repeated verbatim or if the original sentence was repeated correctly but extra words were included. The WBS group was more likely than the other groups to produce the latter type of response. A qualitative analysis of the errors produced for sentences that a child had attempted to imitate indicated that, for each group, the most frequent error was omission. For both the WBS and DS groups, a significant proportion of errors involved bound morphology (e.g., tense marking, case marking); the TD group produced almost no errors of this type. For the TD group, lexical substitutions involved only nouns. In contrast, for the WBS and DS groups, lexical substitutions involved not only nouns but also articles, prepositions, and verbs. Italian is a language with relatively free word order. A significant proportion of the errors produced by the TD group involved word order inversions, and all these inversions resulted in utterances that were still grammatical. In contrast, although the WBS and DS groups produced a smaller proportion of word order errors, many of these errors resulted in ungrammatical utterances. The authors concluded that the language ability of children with WBS is not more advanced than expected for their mental age. Furthermore, the WBS group produced types of errors that were rarely or never made by the TD group but were made by the DS group, suggesting that these error types are likely associated with mental retardation rather than being unique to WBS.

Longitudinal Relations among Vocabulary, Grammar, and Cognitive Ability

Typically developing children evidence a strong relation between productive vocabulary size and grammatical development. Bates and Goodman (1997) argued that the onset of word combinations requires the accumulation of a "critical" mass of words in the child's expressive vocabulary size. These researchers noted that one of the strongest developmental relations is that between number of words in a young child's expressive vocabulary and the complexity of the child's spontaneous utterances. Vicari et al. (2002) provided cross-sectional evidence that this relation holds not only for TD children but also for children with WBS or Down syndrome.

Our research group has considered the relation between vocabulary development and grammatical development in an ongoing longitudinal study of twenty-three children with WBS (Mervis et al. 2003). The children's parents complete the CDI vocabulary checklist monthly. Once their child begins to combine words, parents also complete the CDI Early Sentence Checklist monthly; this checklist consists of thirty-seven pairs of phrases or sentences. The child's Sentence Complexity score is the number of utterance pairs for which the parents have marked the more complex version. CDI data are available for an average of 40 months per child (range, 8–66 months). Mean CA of the children when the parents began to complete the CDI was 26 months (range, 11–40 months).

To address the question of whether the onset of grammar was delayed, we used the data from the Early Sentence Checklist. Four of the twenty-two children (18%) had a Sentence Complexity score of at least 1 by age thirty months. (Sentence complexity data were not available for one of the twenty-three children.) Performance at this level corresponds to the tenth percentile for the general population. (Data are not available for the fifth percentile for this measure.) Based on this criterion, the onset of grammatical development is delayed for most children with WBS. However, once grammatical development begins, rate of development is the same as for TD children. The relation between productive vocabulary size and grammatical ability also was the same for the children with WBS as for the general population. This relation fell between the fifth and ninety-fifth percentiles for twenty-one of the twenty-two children, with individual children's data spread fairly evenly across this percentile range, suggesting that the amount of variability in the WBS sample was similar to that for TD children. Volterra et al. (2003), in a cross-sectional study of six Italian-speaking children, also found that grammatical complexity (as measured by the Italian CDI) is at the level expected for expressive vocabulary size.

Vocabulary growth curves based on data from the CDI vocabulary checklist follow a logistic shape for TD children (Robinson and Mervis 1999). Initially, vocabulary growth follows a linear pattern with a small slope. Eventually, however, rate of growth increases rapidly for a sustained period. As the child approaches the ceiling on the CDI checklist, rate of growth seems to slow down, leading to a logistic shape. (This reduced rate of growth is primarily an artifact of using a checklist with a constrained number of words.) Analysis of the monthly expressive vocabulary growth data indicated that the growth curves for twenty of the twenty-three children with WBS were logistic in shape. Two children evidenced slow linear growth until at least five years of age. The final child evidenced a growth pattern that was best characterized as "double linear." Until age forty-nine months, this child showed very slow linear growth. He then began to add words to his expressive vocabulary at an extremely fast pace that was maintained for several months, again yielding linear growth, but this time with a very steep slope.

To determine whether growth curve type was related to cognitive ability, we compared standardized test performances of the three sets of children at age forty-eight months (Mervis et al. 2003; Mervis 2004). The logistic growth group scored significantly higher on the PPVT-III, the Preschool DAS Verbal cluster, and forward digit span (the number of digits in the longest string of digits the child is able to repeat after hearing the string once; in this study, the researcher presented the strings at a rate of two digits per second). Impressively, this group also scored significantly higher on the DAS Nonverbal cluster. The child with a double-linear growth curve scored intermediate to the other groups. There was almost no overlap in standard scores between the logistic growth and linear growth groups. This pattern of findings suggests that the shape of vocabulary growth is closely linked not only to grammatical development and to other measures of verbal development but also to verbal short-term memory and to nonverbal aspects of development, including visuospatial construction, the area of greatest weakness for individuals with WBS.

Specific Relations between Lexical Development
and Cognitive Development

Based on studies of typically developing children and children with Down syndrome, several specific relations between particular aspects of early lexical acquisition and hypothetically linked aspects of early nonverbal cognitive development have been identified (see review in Mervis and Bertrand 1997). To address the question of whether these same links also hold for children with WBS, I review the findings of three research groups (Laing et al. 2002; Masataka 2001; Mervis and Bertrand 1997; Mervis et al. 2003).

Canonical Babble and Rhythmic Banging. Cobo-Lewis and colleagues (1995) argued that rhythmic (canonical or reduplicated) babble and rhythmic hand banging should begin at about the same time, because they reflect parallel manifestations of rhythmic behaviors. Canonical or reduplicated babble involves repetition of the same consonant-vowel syllable two or more times (e.g., *dada* or *mamama* but not *ga*). Both canonical babble and rhythmic hand banging appear before the onset of lexical comprehension or production. Because the rhythm of canonical babble fits the syllable patterns of mature speech, this type of babble is considered a very important step in the language acquisition process. Parents typically change the way they talk to their infants once canonical babble begins, and these changes likely facilitate the child's acquisition of an initial vocabulary.

Masataka (2001) conducted a longitudinal study of eight Japanese children with WBS to examine the relation between linguistic and motor milestones, including rhythmic banging and canonical babble. Infants entered the study at age six months and were observed every two weeks until age thirty months. Eight milestones were studied: two linguistic (canonical babble and first words) and six motor (rolls, reaches, sits, bangs, stands, walks). The canonical babble milestone was considered to be achieved when the proportion of canonical syllables relative to total syllables was at least 0.2. The first words milestone was considered to be achieved when the child's cumulative expressive vocabulary included twenty-five words. Rhythmic hand banging was considered to be achieved at the first session at which it occurred in two of four consecutive sessions. Masataka found that chronological age at onset of milestone was significantly correlated for only three pairs of milestones: canonical babble and first words, hand banging and first words, and hand banging and canonical babble. Furthermore, there were significant differences in CA at onset for all pairs of milestones except the canonical babble and hand banging pair and first words and first steps pair. The average CA at onset was 1.43 years for rhythmic hand banging, 1.47 years for canonical babble, 1.89 years for first words, and 1.92 years for first steps. This pattern of findings confirms that the predicted specific relation between onset of rhythmic hand banging and onset of canonical babble holds for WBS. Masataka argued that rhythmic hand banging may be a rate-limiting control parameter for the emergence of canonical babble; if so, the delay in onset of rhythmic hand banging would play an important role in the delayed onset of language in children with WBS.

Pointing and the Onset of Referential Production of Object Names. The second potential universal link involves the acquisition of the ability to refer. The cognitive manifestation of this link (referential pointing) is expected to precede the lexical manifestation (referential productive language, e.g., object labels). This sequential ordering is one of the most robust findings on the transition to language. Infants express communicative intentions nonverbally, by pointing, before expressing them verbally, by labeling (Adamson 1995). This link presumably obtains because the cognitive manifestation of reference (pointing) provides the child with an especially useful way to determine the reference of the words he or she hears. Adults use pointing gestures to indicate reference. Until the child is able to follow these gestures, he or she is likely to have difficulty determining the reference of the adult's words. At the same time, children use pointing gestures to elicit labels from adults.

Our research group considered the relation between the onset of referential pointing and the onset of referential language in a longitudinal study of ten children with WBS who entered the study between the ages of four and twenty-six months (Mervis and Bertrand 1997; Mervis et al. 2003). Children participated in monthly play sessions, after which their parents completed the CDI. Results indicate that the relation between referential pointing and referential language is very different for children with WBS than for TD children or other groups of children with developmental delay. Nine of the ten children with WBS began to produce referential labels several months (mean, six months) before the onset of either comprehension or production of referential pointing gestures. Only the most delayed child began to comprehend and produce referential pointing gestures before the onset of referential language—and only about three weeks before. These data make it clear that referential pointing skills are not necessary for the onset of referential language.

Nevertheless, comprehension and production of referential object labels almost certainly require that the child and adult be engaged in joint attention to an object at the time that the adult labels it. In positing that referential pointing should precede the onset of referential productive language, researchers likely were centering on the attention-focusing function of pointing. Thus, pointing may have been intended as a proxy for participation in episodes of joint attention to an object. The data from the children with WBS serve as a reminder that there are other ways to establish joint attention to objects. We identified three alternative methods for establishing such joint attention that were used by parents of children with WBS (Mervis and Bertrand 1997). First, the adult followed the child's focus of attention and then labeled that object. This method has been shown to be especially effective even for TD children (Dunham et al. 1993; Tomasello and Farrar 1986). Second, the adult picked up the object to which he or she wanted the child to attend, put it in the place where the child already was looking, and then labeled it. Third, the adult directed the child's attention to an object by tapping it. Once the child was looking at the object, the adult labeled it. These methods were successful in inducing children with WBS to comprehend and produce object labels referentially.

Laing et al. (2002) conducted a cross-sectional study of the social communication abilities of thirteen children with WBS (mean CA, 2.58 years; range, 1.42–4.58 years) matched for mental age to a group of thirteen younger TD toddlers. Mean MA for the WBS group was 1.16 years, with a range of 0.5 to 1.92 years. Mean expressive vocabulary size was 56 words (SD = 83.3 words) for the WBS group and 31.5 words (SD = 53.2 words) for the TD group. Each child completed the Early Social Communication Scales (Mundy and Hogan 1996), which measures initiation of joint attention, response to bids for joint attention, requests, responses to requests, and social interaction. The WBS group was significantly less likely to initiate requesting. Furthermore, the WBS group was less likely to initiate joint attention (P = 0.07) and more likely to engage in dyadic social interaction (P = 0.07). In contrast, the WBS group was significantly less likely than the TD group to point referentially or instrumentally, to combine eye contact with reaching for a desired object that the child could not obtain without help, or to make eye contact to request that the experimenter manipulate a toy. Overall, the TD group was more than twice as likely to produce socially referential behavior (simultaneous attention to both the experimenter and an object) as the WBS group. More generally, whereas the behavior of the TD group was usually triadic, the behavior of the WBS group was predominantly dyadic. Rate of responding to joint attention was significantly and strongly correlated with both receptive and expressive vocabulary size for both groups of children. In a follow-up study of comprehension and production of referential pointing gestures, the children with WBS were significantly less likely than the TD children to produce pointing gestures or follow the experimenter's pointing gesture. The results of a third study demonstrated that the infrequency of pointing gestures by the children with WBS was not due to fine motor problems. Laing and colleagues argued that their findings make it obvious that the characterization of WBS (e.g., by Pinker 1999) as an excellent example of intact language and social skills despite significant cognitive impairment is incorrect.

Priority of Basic-Level Categories: Labels and Play Patterns. Objects can be categorized at a variety of hierarchical levels. For example, the same object can be a beach ball (subordinate level), a ball (basic level), or a toy (superordinate level). The basic level is more fundamental than the other levels (Rosch et al. 1976). This is the most general level at which category members have similar overall shapes and at which a person uses similar motor actions for interacting with category members. Because of the salience of basic-level categories, they should be acquired first. Thus, children's initial functional play patterns (cognitive manifestation of categorization) and initial extensions of the object labels that they comprehend and produce (linguistic manifestation of categorization) should converge at the (child-) basic level.

Note that, although young children are expected to use the same principles (e.g., form-function correlation) to form basic-level categories, membership in these categories would not be expected to be identical to that for adult-basic-level categories labeled by the same name. The actual categories formed on the basis of these principles will vary because different groups attend to different attributes of the same object, as a function of different experiences or different levels of expertise (Mervis 1987). Because very young children may not share adults' knowledge of culturally appropriate functions of particular objects and the form attributes correlated with those functions, these children may deemphasize attributes that are important from an adult perspective. At the same time, very young children may notice a function (and its correlated form attributes) for an object that adults ignore, leading the children to emphasize features that are unimportant to adults. In these situations, although there will be significant overlap in membership between the child-basic and adult-basic categories labeled by the same word, the child-basic category will differ systematically from the corresponding adult-basic category.

This relation between the cognitive and linguistic manifestations of categorization has been confirmed by longitudinal research on TD children and children with Down syndrome, for the two categories for which it has been addressed: *ball* and *car*. Although for many categories, nonverbal play patterns are difficult to observe, especially in the laboratory, extensive data are available on children's first words from diary studies of TD children. Results indicate that basic-level labels are consistently acquired before subordinate- or superordinate-level labels (Mervis and Bertrand 1997).

Data from our longitudinal study indicate that basic-level categories had the same priority for the children with WBS as for TD children and children with DS (Mervis and Bertrand 1997; Mervis et al. 2003). During the play sessions, the children with WBS played with all the spherical objects (e.g., balls, spherical candles, sleigh bells) in the same manner, by rolling them. In contrast, they did not try to roll the nonspherical objects. The children's lexical behavior also indicated that they had formed a child-basic *ball* category; *ball* was comprehended and produced in reference to a wide range of spherical objects, whether or not an adult would have considered them to be balls, but not in relation to objects of other shapes. A parallel set of findings was obtained for the *car* category.

Examination of the data from the CDI vocabulary checklist and a specially constructed subordinate-category vocabulary checklist indicated that, in 96% of the cases, the basic-level name for an object was comprehended before the subordinate-level name; in 3% of the cases, the order of acquisition was unclear (the basic-level label and the label for a subordinate category subsumed under that basic-level category were acquired in the same month). The subordinate-level name was comprehended before the basic-level name in only 1% of the cases, involving two subordinate categories (toothbrush, school bus) that are atypical of their basic-level categories. None of the children comprehended or produced any superordinate-level labels before comprehending at least one basic-level label for an object subsumed under that superordinate.

Spontaneous Exhaustive Sorting, the Vocabulary Spurt, and Fast Mapping. Gopnik and Meltzoff (1987, 1992) argued that spontaneous exhaustive sorting and the vocabulary spurt should occur at about the same time because they reflect parallel insights: all objects belong to some category (cognitive insight) and all objects have a name (linguistic insight). We have argued that a better linguistic manifestation of this insight is the ability to fast map— that is, the ability to use the Novel Name–Nameless Category (N3C) principle (Mervis and Bertrand 1993, 1994). According to this principle, the child should assume that novel words map to categories for which the child does not yet have a name. Before children have this principle, they must rely on other people to provide an explicit connection between a new word and its referent (e.g., by showing an object to a child and then labeling it, or by labeling an object to which the child is already attending). Once children acquire the N3C principle, however, they no longer need to depend on someone else to make an explicit connection between a label and its referent. The indirect connection provided by hearing a novel word in the presence of an object for which the child does not yet have a name is sufficient for mapping to take place. For both TD children and children with DS, the onsets of spontaneous exhaustive sorting, the vocabulary spurt, and fast mapping have been found to occur at about the same time.

Much of this pattern does not hold for children with WBS. In particular, none of the children with WBS in our study (Mervis et al. 2003) evidenced a temporal link between the onset of spontaneous exhaustive sorting and the vocabulary spurt or between the onset of the vocabulary spurt and fast mapping. One child showed spontaneous exhaustive sorting and the ability to fast map five months before she began her vocabulary spurt. The other nine children had a vocabulary spurt six to twelve or more months before the onset of spontaneous exhaustive sorting or fast mapping ability. Some of the children with WBS had more than five hundred words in their productive vocabularies before they were able to fast map. These data indicate the presence of a viable alternative path to rapid vocabulary acquisition. Although fast mapping is an excellent facilitator of rapid acquisition of new words, other ways must be possible. For individuals with WBS, an increase in verbal short-term memory provides a likely alternative path. This possibility is consistent with Bates and Carnevale's position (1993) that the onset of the vocabulary spurt and subsequent rapid accumulation of new words probably result from the child's increasing efficiency at acquiring words through the same procedures as before the vocabulary spurt.

The data from the children with WBS did support the universality of a specific link between the onsets of spontaneous exhaustive sorting and the ability to fast map. Eight children demonstrated the onset of both abilities in the same session. The two remaining children demonstrated fast mapping at the session before the one at which they evidenced spontaneous exhaustive sorting.

Semantics

Recent studies of the semantic abilities of individuals with Williams-Beuren syndrome have focused on either very young children or on older children and adolescents. Studies of early lexical development were reviewed above. Here I focus on two other aspects of semantic development that have been addressed in recent studies: spatial language and semantic fluency.

Spatial Language

The area of greatest weakness for most individuals with WBS is visuospatial construction. It often has been argued that people's spatial language offers clues to their nonlinguistic spatial representation (e.g., Bowerman 1996). Landau and Zukowski (2003) stated that, from this perspective, serious difficulties in spatial representation would be expected to result in problems with the use of spatial language. Bellugi and colleagues (2000) have argued that this position is correct. They compared the performance of a group of twenty-eight adolescents and adults with WBS on two spatial language tasks with that of a group of typically developing children (mean CA, eleven years). The first assessment involved a comprehension test for spatial prepositions. The WBS group responded incorrectly to about 11% of the items. In contrast, the TD group performed at ceiling. The second task required the participant to describe the spatial position of a colored object relative to a noncolored object (e.g., *the [colored] tree is beside the [noncolored] house*). The WBS group again performed significantly worse than the TD group, making errors on 30% of the items. These findings suggest that many adolescents and adults with WBS have difficulty with spatial prepositions. However, because the mental age of the control group was well above that of the WBS group, interpretation of the findings is difficult.

Our group compared the performance of forty five- to seven-year-olds with WBS with that of forty-three TD four- to seven-year-olds matched for receptive concrete vocabulary size (PPVT-III raw score) on the TRC (Mervis et al. 2003). Despite very similar receptive vocabulary sizes, the WBS group knew significantly fewer relational concepts than did the TD group. It was possible to closely match a subgroup of thirty-seven participants with WBS to a subgroup of twenty-six TD children for relational vocabulary size (TRC raw score). The two subgroups did not differ significantly in the number of spatial concepts known. However, because Bellugi et al. (2000) have argued that individuals with WBS have specific difficulty with spatial concepts, we decided to compare the WBS group with the TD group for each of the spatial concepts included in the TRC. The WBS group performed at the same level as the TD group on fourteen of the seventeen spatial concepts. On the remaining three (front/back, above/below, middle), the WBS group had significantly more difficulty than the TD group. These results suggest that, although individuals with WBS may have more difficulty than expected with a few spatial concepts, their primary lexical difficulty is with abstract/relational concepts in general, rather than with spatial concepts per se.

Landau and Zukowski (2003) also addressed the question of the possible effect of difficulties with spatial representation on spatial language. In their study, the performance of a group of twelve children with WBS, ages 7 to 14 years (median CA, 9.61 years) was compared with that of a MA-matched TD group (median CA, 5.0 years) and a group of college students. Participants watched a series of eighty video clips depicting events containing spatial relations and described what happened. Descriptions were divided into figure (main character, typically subject of the sentence), ground (typically, object of the preposition), motion and manner of motion (typically, verb), and path (typically, prepositional phrase). Three path types were considered: bounded-to (paths toward a specified object), bounded-from (paths away from a specified object), and via (paths for which the ground object is at neither the beginning nor the end). The children with WBS reliably encoded the figure and ground correctly. Of the 480 descriptions of figure-ground events produced by the WBS group, only 3 involved reversals of the figure and ground (a type of error that Bellugi et al. [2000] had identified). All three groups used the same set of verbs to describe the motions. In describing figure-only events, the college student group usually included a path term. In contrast, both groups of children tended to omit the path term. The most common path descriptions for figure and ground events were the same for the three groups. However, the TD group was significantly more likely than the WBS group to include a path term. The WBS group performed significantly better on the bounded-to events than on the other types. The preposition *over* was used by the WBS group as the default spatial term. Although most of the uses were correct (or ambiguous), some were anomalous. The TD group also used *over* in an anomalous fashion, but much less frequently. Landau and Zukowski concluded that children with WBS show good control over much of the language needed to describe spatial events, including the semantic-syntactic mapping between spatial representation of the event and linguistic structure. Description of the path was the most difficult component for both groups of children. The authors suggested that, for individuals with WBS, this difficulty is due to the interaction of the linguistic system with an impaired nonlinguistic spatial system, the impact of which is most apparent when spatial memory is required. Bounded-from and via paths require memory for two spatial locations; bounded-to paths, which were easier for the WBS group, require memory for only one spatial location. Results of a recent study of the use of spatial language by Hungarian-speaking children with WBS (Lukács et al. 2004) provide further evidence that spatial memory problems contribute to the particular difficulty children with WBS have with bounded-from and via paths. The question remains of whether the pattern found for children with WBS is restricted to this syndrome (or other syndromes characterized by particular difficulty with visuospatial construction) or is characteristic of mental retardation more generally.

Racsmány et al. (2001) used a series of suffix elicitation tasks to study the spatial language abilities of Hungarian individuals with WBS between the ages of six and twenty years. Unlike English, Hungarian is a morphologically rich language. Many spatial concepts are marked as suffixes rather than as separate words. Racsmány and colleagues compared the percentage of correct uses of simple agreement-related (nonspatial) grammatical morphemes, such as the plural or accusative, with that of spatial morphemes marked by suffixes and spatial morphemes marked as postpositions (separate words that follow the verb). Participants correctly marked significantly more of the nonspatial morphemes (87%) than either the spatial suffixes (46%) or the spatial postpositions (49%). Because no contrast group data or data on the normal sequence of morphologic development in Hungarian were provided, it is difficult to interpret these findings. In most languages, basic-agreement morphemes are mastered before spatial morphemes not only by children with WBS but also by TD children. Results of a regression analysis of the WBS data indicated that 93% of the variance in performance on the spatial morphemes elicitation task was explained by a combination of verbal memory capacity and spatial memory capacity. The authors argued that this result indicates that, when learning spatial language, children need to keep in mind both phonological information and spatial information simultaneously. Thus, both verbal and spatial working-memory capacity constrain the acquisition of spatial language.

Semantic Organization

The semantic organization of a category refers to how an individual cognitively relates the members of the category. Typically, this type of organization is measured by word fluency tests, in which a person is asked to name all the items that he or she can think of that are members of the category named by the researcher. The first study of the semantic organization of individuals with WBS was conducted by Bellugi et al. (1992, 1994), who asked six adolescents with WBS, six CA- and IQ-matched adolescents with Down syndrome, and a group of typically developing second-graders to name all the animals that they could in one minute. Based on the findings from this study, Bellugi and colleagues argued that the semantic organization of adolescents with WBS was deviant. In particular, the participants with WBS were more likely to list unusual (defined as low word frequency) animals. This finding was consistent with the researchers' statement that individuals with WBS use unusual words in their spontaneous speech.

More recently, we compared the semantic organization of the *animal* category for a group of twelve nine- and ten-year-olds with WBS relative to that of three contrast groups: CA- and MA-matched children with Down syndrome, MA-matched TD children, and CA-matched TD children (Mervis et al. 1999). Several measures were considered. Fluency was measured by the number of animal names produced. The representativeness of the items produced as members of the *animal* category was determined based on goodness-of-example (GOE) ratings obtained in a procedure similar to that used by Rosch (1973, 1975). College students were asked to use a seven-point scale to rate the animal names generated by the child participants for how well each fit the student's idea or image of *animal*. Three measures of GOE were used: mean rating for all the animal names a child produced; rating for the most representative (typical) animal name the child produced; and rating for the least representative (most atypical) animal name the child produced. Word frequency was measured in two different ways: mean frequency of the animal names in children's texts (standard frequency index [SFI]; Carroll et al. 1971) and proportion of items listed that had an SFI of less than 50 (Bellugi et al.'s criterion for classification as low frequency). Two measures of category composition were used: percentage of animal names produced at the basic level (e.g., dog) and percentage of animal names produced at the subordinate level (e.g., beagle).

On seven of the eight measures, the performance of the three groups matched for mental age (WBS, DS, TD, MA-matched) was similar. For the remaining measure, the GOE rating of the least typical exemplar produced, the WBS and DS groups performed at the same level as the TD CA-matched group. The least typical exemplar produced by these groups was significantly less representative of the *animal* category than the least typical exemplar named by the MA-matched group. The performance of the WBS group also was similar to the CA-matched group for mean SFI value and proportion of basic-level animal names. However, the CA-matched group named, on average, more than twice as many animals as did the WBS group and included a significantly higher proportion of subordinate-level exemplars. In addition, mean GOE rating was significantly higher for the CA-matched group, indicating that, on average, the exemplars listed by the WBS group were more representative of the *animal* category than were the exemplars listed by the CA-matched group.

This pattern of findings indicates that, in many ways, the semantic organization of the *animal* category is similar for the four groups of children. The proportion of animal names listed at the basic level, the mean SFI rating, and the proportion of items for which SFI was less than 50 were equivalent for all four groups. The latter finding contrasts with that of Bellugi et al. (1992, 1994). Our finding (Mervis et al. 1999) that the least representative exemplar produced was reliably less representative for the three older groups than for the MA-matched group, however, fits with Bellugi et al.'s finding that the WBS group produced more unusual animal names than did the TD second-graders. This component of semantic organization seems to be more dependent on amount of experience with animals (as measured by CA) than on cognitive level (as measured by MA). On all the other measures of semantic organization, however, the WBS group performed similarly to the two groups matched for mental age.

Volterra and colleagues (1996) found that the performance of Italian children with WBS on a semantic fluency task was highly similar to that of MA-matched TD controls. The two groups listed equivalent numbers of animals, and most of the animal names were of high word frequency. Temple et al. (2002) reported semantic fluency data for four adolescents with WBS. The number of animals listed fell in the range found for MA-matched TD controls. One person with WBS produced significantly more low-frequency animal names than expected based on MA-matched TD controls; this participant's proportion was in the expected range for TD children of a younger mental age, however. Overall, the performance of individuals with WBS on semantic fluency tasks is appropriate for MA, suggesting that the development of semantic organization in WBS is delayed rather than deviant.

The most recent study of semantic fluency of individuals with WBS was conducted by Levy and Bechar (2003). The performance of seven Israeli children and adolescents with WBS (mean CA, 11.75 years) was compared with that of seven children with mental retardation of unknown etiology, individually matched to the participants with WBS for both CA and IQ, and a group of TD children whose mean CA (7.25 years) corresponded to the mean MA for the WBS and mental retardation groups. Mean number of animal names produced was 13.14 for the WBS group, 15.14 for the mental retardation group, and 16.30 for the TD group. Once again, there was no significant difference between groups in the number of animal names produced, providing further support for the position that semantic organization in WBS is delayed rather than deviant.

Morphology

A major controversy regarding the language abilities of individuals with Williams-Beuren syndrome is centered on morphology, particularly on past-tense morphology in English. There is relatively good agreement about the basic findings on past-tense forms produced by individuals with WBS: at least by late childhood, most individuals with WBS reliably mark the past tense correctly on regular verbs. In contrast, they are likely to overregularize the past tense for irregular verbs—for example, by saying *gived* rather than *gave* or *eated* rather than *ate*. When they are given a nonsense word used as a verb and asked to provide its past tense, the forms provided are almost always regular, even when the nonsense word rhymes with a known irregular verb.

There is considerable disagreement about the interpretation of these findings, however. According to one account (Clahsen and Almazan 1998; Clahsen and Temple 2003; Pinker 1999), data from WBS provide excellent support for the dual-mechanism model of language. In this model, language is composed of a computational (or rule-based) system (module) and a lexicon consisting of stored entries. Regular past-tense forms are derived from the rule-based system; irregular past-tense forms are stored in the lexical entry for the verb stem. Clahsen and his colleagues and Pinker argue that language in WBS is best characterized as composed of a spared computational system accompanied by impairment in lexical representation and/or access. According to a second account (Thomas et al. 2001), data from WBS provide support for a single-route developmental model in which the past tense is learned by building up associations between phonological forms of verb stems and the corresponding past-tense forms. In this model, the phonological representations of individuals with WBS differ from those of typically developing individuals in that individual phonemes (sounds) are more discriminable. Here I review the available data on acquisition of past-tense morphology and other types of morphology by individuals with WBS. Resolution of the dual- versus single-mechanism controversy most likely will require longitudinal studies of both individuals with WBS and TD children.

English Morphology

Past Tense: Regular and Irregular Verbs. The first published study of past-tense morphology production by individuals with WBS was conducted by Clahsen and Almazan (1998). The participants were four adolescents, eleven to fifteen years of age. Based on the Wechsler Intelligence Scale for Children–III (WISC-III), two participants had a mental age of five years (MA-5) and two of seven years (MA-7). Two control groups of TD children were included, one with a CA of five years (CA-5) and the other of seven years (CA-7). Participants were given pairs of sentences and asked to fill in the verb form in the second sentence (e.g., *"Every day I play baseball. Just like every day, yesterday I ____."*) All participants performed very well on the regular verb forms; the participants with WBS formed the correct past tense about 90% of the time. In contrast, the participants with WBS had considerably more difficulty with the irregular verbs; the MA-5 pair produced the correct form 14% of the time, the MA-7 pair 50% of the time. Overregularizations were produced 43% of the time by the MA-5 pair and 29% of the time by the MA-7 pair. The remaining responses consisted of bare verb stems. In contrast, the CA-5 control group produced correct irregulars 79% of the time and over-regularized forms only 8% of the time. All groups performed well on the "regular" nonsense verbs (nonsense words that did not rhyme with any ir-regular English verb); the MA-5 pair produced the correct regular past-tense form 83% of the time and the MA-7 pair 100% of the time. However, the participants with WBS had great difficulty with the "irregular" nonsense verbs (nonsense words that rhymed with irregular English verbs), producing irregular forms only 4% (MA-5) or 7% (MA-7) of the time and overregu-larized forms 57% (MA-5) and 64% (MA-7) of the time. The CA-5 control group produced correct irregular forms 68% of the time. Based on this pat-tern of findings, Clahsen and Almazan argued that the WBS data provide strong support for an intact computational module accompanied by an im-paired lexical module.

Thomas and colleagues (2001) replicated this study with a considerably larger sample, including eighteen individuals with WBS ranging in age from ten to fifty-three years and four TD control groups: CA of six years, eight years, and ten years, and adults. The performance of the WBS group was sim-ilar to that of the CA-6 group. Furthermore, the WBS group's performance was broadly similar to that of the WBS participants in Clahsen and Almazan's study (1998). The primary difference between the findings from the two studies was that, in Thomas et al.'s study, very few irregular past-tense forms were produced for "irregular" nonsense verbs, even by the oldest control groups. This finding replicated that of van der Lely and Ullman (2001) for TD children, suggesting that Clahsen and Almazan's TD sample may have been unusual. Regression analyses indicated that, whereas the WBS group was more delayed than expected based on verbal mental age, the delay was no greater for irregular verb forms than for regular forms, supporting a single-mechanism model of past-tense acquisition.

In a second study, Thomas et al. (2001) used a larger set of verbs varying in word frequency and imageability. The results indicated an effect of word frequency for the WBS group for regular verbs but not irregular verbs and an effect of imageability for irregular verbs but not regular verbs, findings also inconsistent with Clahsen and Almazan's proposed model. Thomas and colleagues also used data from small subsets of their participants to demon-strate that, depending on who was included, results for WBS could vary from those found by Clahsen and Almazan (1998, four participants), to the sug-gestion that individuals with WBS were extremely poor at both regular and irregular past-tense formation, to the suggestion that individuals with WBS were extremely good at both regular and irregular past-tense formation.

In response to Thomas et al. (2001), Clahsen and colleagues (2003) added five adolescents with WBS and a mental age of five or seven years to their original sample, for a total sample size of nine. The resulting group continued to perform at ceiling on the regular past tense and on "regular" nonsense verbs; performance on irregular verbs and "irregular" nonsense verbs improved considerably, especially for the MA-7 group. Clahsen et al. argued that, because the WBS sample performed at the same level as the controls on regular forms but significantly worse (but only by a one-tailed test) than the CA-7 controls on irregular forms, the dual-process model is upheld. This conclusion requires acceptance of the premise that groups of different chronological age that are matched for mental age should perform at the same level on any measure on which they are tested. This premise is problematic, however; when MA-matched groups differ in CA, one would predict significant differences between groups on other measures, particularly those involving verbal memory, with the older group expected to perform significantly worse (Mervis and Robinson 1999, 2003, 2005). If so, one would expect to find significant differences in performance on irregular verbs in the dual-process model, given that these verbs need to be retrieved from the lexical store. This pattern, then, would not support Clahsen et al.'s argument that WBS represents a case of an intact computational module accompanied by an impaired lexical module.

Other Grammatical Morphemes. Researchers have also looked at the use of a few other grammatical morphemes by individuals with WBS whose native language is English. Here I briefly consider data on two such morphemes: past-tense formation for denominal verbs and the comparative form of adjectives. A third morpheme that is common in many other languages, grammatical gender, is not considered here (representative studies include, for French, Karmiloff-Smith et al. 1997 and Monnery et al. 2002 and, for Hebrew, Levy and Hermon 2003).

In English, denominal verbs (verbs formed from nouns) take the regular past tense, regardless of the phonological properties of their stems. As a result, denominal verb stems that are homonyms of irregular verb stems nonetheless take the regular past tense (e.g., *She rang the bell* vs. *The army ringed the city*). Clahsen and colleagues (2003) tested the same nine participants with WBS as noted above, this time on past-tense formation of denominal verbs and their irregular verb homonyms. Both the MA-5 and MA-7 groups performed as well as the control groups on the denominal verbs (means of 84%–95% correct). Interestingly, the MA-7 group performed as well as the CA-7 group on the irregular verb past-tense forms (74% correct for MA-7 and 73% correct for CA-7); in this study, the higher-MA WBS group did not evidence any deficit at all on irregular past-tense formation.

Comparative adjectives are formed in one of three ways: by the addition of -*er* to the adjective stem, by the addition of *more* before the adjective stem, or by suppletive (irregular) forms. Clahsen et al. (2003) tested, again, the same nine adolescents with WBS, along with different control samples of TD children ages five or seven years. Almost all the children performed perfectly on the stems whose comparatives are formed by adding -*er*. However, all but one of the participants with WBS also formed comparatives in this manner when the correct version was *more* plus the stem. Although the TD children were more accurate than the participants with WBS, performance was still poor; 70% or more of the comparatives were formed by using -*er* rather than *more* (the correct form). When tested with nonsense adjectives, the WBS group always formed comparatives by using -*er*. Although most TD participants always used -*er* to form comparatives for nonsense adjectives, a few occasionally used *more*. Performance on suppletive forms was poor for all groups, with the seven-years-olds with WBS performing slightly better than the others. The data presented suggest that, although a few of the TD children performed better than the WBS group, the modal performance of the TD children was the same as for the WBS group.

Hungarian Morphology

Hungarian is a Uralic language, very different from Germanic languages (e.g., English, German) or Romance languages (e.g., French, Spanish). Uralic languages are agglutinative, meaning that they connect long series of morphemes together to combine into a single word information that would require several words and/or other syntactic devices (e.g., word order) in other types of language. Thus, morphology in Hungarian is both extensive and complex. Lukács et al. (2001, 2004) considered the morphological abilities of fifteen Hungarian children and adolescents with WBS (mean CA, 13.2 years; range, 5.9–19.6 years). Two noun morphemes were studied: the plural and the accusative. Consistent with findings for English morphology, Hungarian children with WBS were significantly more likely to produce correct regular plural or accusative nouns than correct irregular plural or accusative nouns. (This same finding holds for two groups of younger TD children acquiring Hungarian as their native language: children matched to the WBS group for vocabulary age based on the Hungarian version of the PPVT and still younger children similar in mental age to the WBS group.) One class of regular accusative morpheme was also overregularized (to a different regular class). Overregularizations were more common among children younger than ten years of age. Lukács and colleagues (2001) also considered the relation between verbal memory (digit span) and morphologic ability. Results based on a median split of digit span indicated that the longer-span group performed significantly better than the shorter-span group on both the regular forms (97% vs. 77%) and irregular forms (90% vs. 61%). The authors noted that the memory-span effect remains even after controlling for chronological age.

Hebrew Morphology

Unlike almost any other language family, roots in Semitic languages such as Hebrew are formed of consonants, with morphology indicated by prefixes, suffixes, and infixes that compose primarily vocalic patterns. Levy and Hermon (2003) compared the morphological abilities of ten Israeli adolescents with WBS, aged twelve to seventeen years, with those of two groups of TD Israeli children with chronological ages similar to the endpoints of the mental age range for the WBS group (five years and eleven years). All three groups performed well on the root-extraction task. This finding was expected because very young TD Hebrew speakers can extract roots (Levy 1988). On the remaining aspects of Hebrew morphology studied, the WBS group performed substantially and significantly worse than the CA-11 group. The WBS group performed at about the same level as the CA-5 group on verb derivation; performance on noun derivation was weaker than that of the CA-5 group, although the difference was only marginally significant (two-tailed $P < 0.07$). These measures tapped regular morphology; irregular forms are rare in Hebrew and were not addressed in this study. Profile analysis was conducted by partial order scalogram analysis (Shye 1985). The resulting plot clearly separated the WBS group from the CA-11 group, with the WBS group interleaved with the CA-5 group. Morphology is clearly not a strength for Israeli children with WBS; overall, morphological ability is about at the level expected for TD children whose chronological age matches the bottom of the mental age range of the WBS group. This result is not restricted to WBS; Levy et al. (2000) have identified the same pattern for children with other neurologic syndromes that result in similar levels of mental retardation.

Syntax

Grammatical ability often has been considered a particular strength of individuals with Williams-Beuren syndrome. In fact, the ability of individuals with WBS to comprehend and produce complex syntax was the primary basis for Bellugi et al.'s claim (e.g., 1988, 1994, 2000) that WBS provides a compelling case for the independence of language from cognition. Examples of complex syntactic constructions comprehended and produced by individuals with WBS include passives, tag questions, conditionals, and relative clauses. These constructions were much less likely to be comprehended or produced by CA- and IQ-matched individuals with Down syndrome, a difference taken as further evidence that the language abilities of individuals with WBS far outstripped their cognitive abilities. More recently, however, it has become clear that individuals with DS have inordinate difficulty with language relative to their overall level of cognitive ability (Mervis et al. 2003; Volterra et al. 2004). Furthermore, most aspects of complex syntax, including those tested by Bellugi et al., are used by TD children by age six years (Guasti 2002). Thus, it is not surprising that adolescents with WBS can comprehend and produce these constructions.

To determine whether the syntactic abilities of individuals with WBS are unusually good for their overall level of cognitive ability, both comparisons with CA- and IQ-matched individuals with other forms of mental retardation and comparisons with TD children of similar mental age are needed. Initial studies using such control groups have considered children acquiring English (Klein 1995; Mervis et al. 2003; Udwin and Yule 1990), German (Gosch et al. 1994), and Italian (Volterra et al. 1996, 2004). The results of these studies, which have focused on children between the ages of four and ten years, have been consistent: children with WBS do not differ significantly from matched children with other forms of mental retardation or from typically developing children matched for MA or for the mean-length-of-utterance measure.

More recent studies have focused on older children and adolescents with WBS and on more complex aspects of syntax, particularly relative and embedded clauses. The potential role of verbal memory in syntactic acquisition by individuals with WBS also has been considered.

Relative Clauses

In their study of the performance of twenty individuals with WBS (mean CA, 18.58 years) on the Test for Reception of Grammar, Karmiloff-Smith et al. (1997) found that 68% of the responses to the final block were incorrect. Every participant failed this block (Grant et al. 2002), which measures center-embedded object-gap relative clauses (e.g., *The boy the dog chases is big*). Comprehension of other types of relative clauses also was relatively weak. This weakness also has been noted by Mervis et al. (1999) for English and by Volterra et al. (1996) for Italian. To determine whether individuals with WBS have difficulty with relative clauses because their grammars do not generate these clauses, Zukowski (2001, 2004) conducted an elicited production study of relative clauses. In this study, the ten participants with WBS (mean CA, 12.42 years; range, 10.0–16.25 years) were individually matched to ten younger TD children (mean CA, 6.0 years; range, 4.5–7.5 years) based on raw scores on the Vocabulary and Matrices subtests of the K-BIT. Zukowski first administered the TROG. As expected based on previous studies, the WBS group had significant difficulty on the blocks measuring relative clauses, with error rates ranging from 40% for the simplest relative clauses (right-branching embedded subject gap; e.g., *The cow chasing the dog is brown*) to 75% for the most complicated (center-embedded object gap). The elicited production task was then administered. In this computer-presented task, the child was shown two identical characters who could be differentiated by their actions (e.g., a girl pointing at her foot vs. an otherwise identical girl pointing at her hand). Each of the characters was then changed (e.g., the first girl turned pink and the second girl turned green). The child was then asked a "double" question (e.g., who turned pink and who turned green?). To answer the questions correctly, the child had to produce embedded clauses. The scenarios were set up to elicit six types of relative clauses (for examples, see Zukowski 2004).

Results of the Zukowski study (2001, 2004) indicated that all the children in both the WBS and TD groups produced at least one subject-gap relative clause, nine of the ten children in each group produced at least one object-gap relative clause, and nine of the ten children with WBS and all the children in the TD group produced at least one right-branching embedded and one center-embedded relative clause. Furthermore, across nine of the ten children with WBS, 94% of the relative clauses produced were grammatically correct. (The remaining child produced a large number of errors.) Thus, the grammars of all the children with WBS were able to produce relative clauses.

However, a more fine-grained analysis indicated that the various types of relative clauses differed greatly in ease of production. The WBS group produced far more subject-gap forms (mean, 22.6 of 48 opportunities) than object-gap forms (mean, 5.1 of 48 opportunities), when these forms were appropriate. In contrast, the MA-matched TD group produced the two types of relative clauses equally often (means, 22.1 and 24.5, respectively). Thus, production of object-gap relative clauses was significantly more difficult for the WBS group than for the MA-matched TD group. Only three of the ten participants in the WBS group produced any center-embedded object-gap relative clauses. Furthermore, 38% of the responses of the WBS group to the scenarios designed to elicit object-gap relatives were composed of semantically anomalous subject-gap constructions, in which the object on which the subject acted was treated as the subject in the child's utterance. This error rate is significantly higher than the 13.5% rate for the TD group. In summary, the findings from Zukowski's research indicate that individuals with WBS can produce relative clauses of all types. However, their performance on the more difficult object-gap constructions is significantly weaker than the performance of the MA-matched TD control group.

Zukowski (2001, 2004) also used the elicited production technique to study the ability to produce another complex syntactic structure, negative questions (e.g., *What drink don't you like? Where don't you want to play?*). The WBS group (45%) and the TD groups (47%) were equally likely to produce grammatically correct negative questions. The remaining responses of the WBS group were somewhat more likely to be ungrammatical (43%) than those of the TD group (29%). The WBS group (31%) was significantly less likely to raise the auxiliary (e.g., producing *Why you didn't eat your cookie?* rather than *Why didn't you eat your cookie?*) than the TD group (9%). Zukowski (2001) noted that the questions produced by the WBS group resembled the responses of the three- and four-year-old TD children studied by Guasti et al. (1995). Thus, the results of Zukowski's research provide no support for prior claims that, for individuals with WBS, syntactic ability is better than expected for level of cognitive ability.

Grant and colleagues (2002) used a different methodology to study the ability of individuals with WBS to produce relative clauses: elicited imitation. In this technique, the participant is asked to repeat exactly the utterance produced by the researcher. The elicited imitation technique considerably reduces the demands of either picture-sentence matching (as in the TROG) or elicited production (as used by Zukowski). The performance of fourteen individuals with WBS (mean CA, 17.92 years) was compared with that of three groups of TD children (mean CA, 5, 6, and 7 years). Mean British Picture Vocabulary Scale (BPVS; the British version of the PPVT-R [PPVT second edition]) raw score was higher for the WBS group than for the oldest TD group, indicating that any problems with sentence imitation were unlikely to be due to vocabulary limitations. Four types of relative clauses were included, designated SS (subject of the relative clause is co-referential with the subject of the main clause; e.g., *The girl chasing the sheep is big*), SO (direct object or prepositional object of the relative clause is co-referential with the subject of the main clause; e.g., *The dog the horse chases is brown*), OS (subject of the relative clause is co-referential with the object of the main clause; e.g., *The dog chases the horse that is brown*), and OO (object of the relative clause is co-referential with the object of the main clause; e.g., *The dog chases the cow that the girl is looking at*). Responses were considered correct if the repetition was verbatim or if it left the meaning and essential structure of the sentence unchanged. (Changes such as inserting or deleting a relative pronoun or changing number or determiner were acceptable.)

Although few of the results reached conventional levels of statistical significance, a consistent and reliable pattern emerged: the WBS group had more difficulty than any of the other groups. The mean number of sentences imitated correctly was lower for the WBS group than for any other group for sentence types OS, SO, and OO and was lower than all the groups except the five-year-olds for sentence type OS. The pattern of difficulty was similar for the four groups (in descending order of difficulty): SO > OS > OO > SS. Note that the difficulty order is not the same as the length order; with the exception of type SS (both shortest and easiest), the longer the sentence, the lower the difficulty. Because initial results indicated that SO sentences were particularly difficult to imitate, a fifth category was added: SO-that (e.g., *The dog that the horse chases is brown*). Addition of *that* increased the rate of correct imitation for the WBS group, even though it made the sentence longer. This probably occurs because the presence of an overt marker makes the relation between the main clause and the embedded clause syntactically clearer, thus making it easier to process a complex sentence when the participant is experiencing conceptual or processing strain (Grant et al. 2002). The WBS group also was more likely than the other groups to insert relative pronouns when repeating sentences that originally did not include a relative pronoun. Overall, their performance was most similar to the TD five-year-old group, once again indicating that syntactic ability is not "intact" for people with WBS.

Relations between Verbal Memory Ability and Grammatical Ability

In typically developing populations, verbal working memory is associated with the acquisition of both vocabulary (Gathercole and Baddeley 1989, 1993) and syntax (Kemper et al. 1989; Norman et al. 1992). Similarly, the nonword repetition task has been proposed as a phenotypic marker for specific language impairment (SLI) (Bishop et al. 1996). These and other studies suggest that verbal working memory plays an active role in the acquisition of words and grammatical structures by diverse populations.

Our research group (Robinson et al. 2003) hypothesized that, given the WBS cognitive profile, verbal working memory may play a *more important* role in the language acquisition of individuals with WBS than in language acquisition by TD children. To address this possibility, we compared the relations between verbal short-term memory (forward digit span), verbal working memory (backward digit span), phonological short-term memory (Montgomery's nonword repetition task [1996]), and receptive grammatical abilities (TROG raw score) for a WBS group (n = 39; mean CA, 10.24 years; range, 4.5–16.7 years) with those of a younger TD group (n = 32; mean CA, 6.01 years; range, 4.08–10.26 years) closely matched for TROG raw score.

As expected, the correlations between the memory measures and TROG raw score were significant for the WBS group. Forward digit span, nonword repetition, and backward digit span shared partial correlations (controlling for CA) of 0.33, 0.48, and 0.52 with TROG, respectively. Taken together, the memory variables accounted for 26% of the variance in TROG raw scores in the WBS group, above and beyond CA. However, regression analysis indicated that forward digit span alone did not uniquely contribute to variance in the scores once CA, nonword repetition, and backward digit span were taken into account. Nonword repetition, by contrast, did account for additional unique variance, even after CA and the other memory measures were controlled for. Thus, phonological memory may account, in part, for the grammatical skills of individuals with WBS. This finding fits with that of Grant et al. (1997), who reported that nonword repetition scores were significantly related to receptive vocabulary. One would therefore expect that the ability to encode and store small speech units, such as bound morphemes and function words, would similarly be related to grammatical ability. The measure of verbal *working* memory accounted for the largest proportion of variance in TROG scores for the WBS group. Even after controlling for CA, forward digit span, and nonword repetition, backward digit span accounted for an additional 10% of variance. Thus, the ability to manipulate verbal items, not just store them, seems to be important to grammatical ability.

After controlling for CA, there were no significant differences between the WBS group and the TD group in the strength of relation between either forward digit span or nonword repetition and TROG raw scores. The WBS group, however, showed a significantly stronger relation between the working-memory measure and receptive grammar than did the TD group. Therefore, it is possible that individuals with WBS may have to rely more heavily than TD children on verbal working-memory abilities in order to puzzle out complex grammatical structures. Comprehending phrases and, presumably, learning grammatical constructions require more than the storage of linguistic items in short-term memory. A child must extract the meaning of a phrase from the context of the utterance and then associate it with the linguistic item that is stored in short-term memory. The interpretation of nonlinguistic cues to meaning involves perceptual, social, and cognitive analysis. For a TD child, much of the process of extracting meaning from context is effortless and not limited by working-memory capacity. For a child with deficits in one or more of the domains necessary to the processing and integration of the nonlinguistic cues, however, more effort and time is required for meaning extraction and therefore working-memory capacity might be more important for language acquisition.

Further evidence that verbal memory ability plays an important role in grammatical ability for children with WBS is provided by a study comparing the performance of a group of thirteen nine- and ten-year-olds with WBS on the subtests of the McCarthy Scales of Children's Abilities (McCarthy 1972) with the performance of a group of thirteen children with Down syndrome closely matched for both CA and MA (as measured by total raw score on the McCarthy Scales) (Klein and Mervis 1999). As expected, the DS group performed significantly better than the WBS group on subtests measuring visuospatial construction. Interestingly, the WBS and DS groups performed virtually identically on subtests measuring verbal ability but not memory ability. However, there were significant and large differences in favor of the WBS group on the subtests that measured verbal memory ability. Consistent with these differences in verbal memory ability, there were large differences in the proportion of children who typically spoke in complete, grammatical sentences: nine of thirteen children with WBS versus four of thirteen children with DS. Thus, despite being closely matched for level of overall cognitive ability and showing virtually identical verbal conceptual ability as measured by the verbal nonmemory subtests of the McCarthy Scales, the WBS and DS groups clearly differed on productive grammatical ability. Comparisons of the original samples of children from which the matched pairs had been selected revealed an even larger difference: nineteen of the twenty-three children with WBS but only four of the twenty-five children with DS typically spoke in complete grammatical sentences.

Developmental Trajectories

In the literature on the language abilities of individuals who have Williams-Beuren syndrome, two types of issues on developmental trajectories have been considered. The first involves comparisons between individuals with WBS and individuals with Down syndrome at an early point in language acquisition and then at a later point. This type of research is concerned with the question of whether the group that initially shows an advantage continues to show an advantage or whether, instead, the relation changes over time. The second type of developmental trajectory research is concerned with the question of whether the pattern of intellectual strengths and weaknesses shown by individuals with WBS is magnified as individuals get older. Research addressing developmental trajectories has often suffered from serious methodological flaws. These are addressed briefly here (for further discussion see Mervis and Robinson 1999, 2003; Mervis 2004).

Between-Group Comparisons: Williams-Beuren Syndrome and Down Syndrome

Singer Harris and colleagues (1997) were the first to claim that there were clear changes in developmental trajectories for vocabulary acquisition by children with WBS and children with Down syndrome. In particular, these authors argued that, before acquisition of a fifty-word expressive vocabulary, children with DS have an advantage over children with WBS. That is, a comparison of the expressive vocabulary sizes of children who produced fewer than fifty words indicated that the children with DS produced significantly more words than the children with WBS. Once the children began to combine words, however, the advantage shifted to the children with WBS. Earlier in the chapter I pointed out the methodological problems with the initial comparison of the two groups of children: expressive vocabulary size was used as both the independent variable and the dependent variable, producing a clear confound. Later studies that matched for either chronological age only or for chronological and mental age showed that, as a group, children with DS never had larger expressive vocabularies than children with WBS.

More recently, Paterson and her colleagues also have argued for a divergence in vocabulary ability between individuals with WBS and individuals with DS (Paterson 2001; Paterson et al. 1999). Their study involved two comparisons: one of very young children and one of young adults. In the child study, the DS and WBS groups were CA and MA matched. Each child was shown pairs of pictures of objects at the same time that she or he heard the name of one of the objects, and the proportion of time spent looking at the correct object was measured. Trials were included only if the parent reported that the child understood the names of both objects in a pair. Results indicated no differences between groups in proportion of time spent looking at the correct picture. On this basis, Paterson an colleagues argued that, during early childhood, vocabulary ability was similar for children with WBS and children with DS. Note that amount of time spent looking at an object whose name the child knows in response to hearing its name is an unusual measure of vocabulary ability. In particular, it does not measure vocabulary size.

For the young adult groups, MA was derived from performance on the British Ability Scales (BAS; the British version of the DAS). Paterson et al. argued that the WBS and DS groups were matched for MA based on the results of a t test indicating $P > 0.05$ (actual $P = 0.07$). Mean CA was six months older for the DS group than the WBS group. The groups were compared on the difference between their CA and the vocabulary age corresponding to their raw score on the BPVS. A significant difference emerged, favoring the WBS group. Accordingly, Paterson et al. argued that, by young adulthood, the trajectories of vocabulary ability have diverged, with the WBS group evidencing a significantly more rapid trajectory than the DS group. There are several serious methodological issues that call this finding into question, however. First, lack of a significant difference between the two adult groups for the MA t test does not guarantee that the two groups are matched. Frick (1995) has argued that groups are definitely *not* matched if $P < 0.20$. Second, given that the individuals in the DS group were, on average, six months older than the individuals in the WBS group, it would not be surprising to find a significant difference in Paterson et al.'s dependent variable, even if the two groups did not differ in vocabulary ability as measured by BPVS raw score. Third, the measures of vocabulary ability at the two ages are not comparable.

Thus, neither the Singer Harris et al. (1997) nor the Paterson et al. (Paterson 2001; Paterson et al. 1999) study has provided evidence of a divergence in vocabulary acquisition trajectories between individuals with WBS and those with DS. The question of whether such a divergence exists remains open.

Within-Group Comparisons: Williams-Beuren Syndrome

As discussed early in this chapter, individuals with WBS typically have a relative strength in language and extreme weakness in visuospatial construction. This pattern could be the result of either consistent or divergent trajectories. Jarrold and his colleagues, based on both cross-sectional (Jarrold et al. 1998) and longitudinal (Jarrold et al. 2001) studies, have argued that the trajectories are divergent. In the cross-sectional study, the performances of sixteen individuals (CA, 6.92–28.00 years) on the BPVS and the BAS Pattern Construction subtest were compared, using age equivalents (MAs) derived from raw scores. Although the difference between the two age equivalents indicated a significant advantage for the vocabulary measure, even for younger children, the difference was considerably larger for older individuals. In the longitudinal study, Jarrold et al. (2001) retested fifteen of the sixteen participants forty months later and compared the difference in age equivalents on the BPVS and the BAS Pattern Construction subtest at both times. The difference was significantly larger at the second time point, a finding that was interpreted as evidence for divergent trajectories for verbal and nonverbal (specifically, visuospatial construction) abilities. However, as noted in the manuals for most standardized assessments, age equivalents are nonlinear, with larger differences required to show an equivalent amount of MA progress at younger ages than older ages (Sattler 2001; other problems with MA are discussed in Mervis and Robinson 1999, 2003).

A more accurate way to address the question of diverging trajectories is to compare standard scores at different ages. Significant changes in standard scores on a particular assessment over time indicate that a participant's developmental trajectory is either increasing or decreasing relative to the rate expected for same-CA peers. Comparisons also could be made between standard scores on two different assessments over time for the same participant or group of participants, provided the assessments were normed on the same sample or on equivalent samples. Longitudinal data comparing standard scores for individuals with WBS have not been published. Cross-sectional comparisons over a wide age range, however, indicate that, on all of the measures considered, the correlation between standard score and CA is not significant, suggesting that, for individuals with WBS as a group, standard scores for language or visuospatial construction measures do not either systematically increase or systematically decrease as a function of CA (Mervis et al. 1999). Furthermore, as noted earlier, large differences in standard scores on verbal and visuospatial construction assessments (e.g., Mullen Scales of Early Learning) are present even for toddlers. In combination, these findings suggest that verbal and visuospatial-construction standard scores do not diverge over time and therefore that, in WBS, verbal and visuospatial construction developmental trajectories are not changing over time. However, given that standard scores are higher for verbal abilities than for visuospatial abilities from a very young age and the difference in standard scores is consistent over time, one would expect that, as Jarrold et al. (1998, 2001) found, rate of progress would be more rapid for language than for visuospatial construction.

Summary and Practical Implications

In 1990, the prevailing view among language researchers was that Williams-Beuren syndrome provided a paradigmatic example of the independence of language from cognition. In particular, WBS was argued to provide strong evidence that excellent language abilities could exist side-by-side with severe mental retardation (Bellugi et al. 1998, 1990, 1992). Jackendoff (1994) stated that, despite significant mental retardation, the language of individuals with WBS "is if anything more fluent and advanced than that of their age-mates" (117). The research reported in this chapter suggests a more nuanced picture. The language abilities of individuals with WBS are indeed a relative strength. Both vocabulary and grammar are considerably more advanced than would be expected for the level of nonverbal cognition as measured by tests of visuospatial construction. Furthermore, both receptive vocabulary and finite verb morphology are more advanced than for children with specific language impairment matched for MLU (Mervis and Klein-Tasman 2000; Rice 1999), and both MLU and grammatical ability are more advanced than for children with Down syndrome who are matched for chronological and mental ages. These findings are consistent with the position of Bellugi et al. (1988, 1990, 1992, 1994).

However, individuals with WBS who have language abilities at the level expected for their CA are rare. Mean levels of performance by individuals with WBS on a variety of standardized assessments of language are consistently in the borderline to mild deficit range. Grammatical ability as measured by spontaneous language is below that of CA-matched typically developing peers. Instead, for individuals with WBS who acquire English as a native language, grammatical ability is at the same level as that of younger TD children matched for general level of cognitive ability. For individuals with WBS acquiring native languages with more complex morphology, some aspects of morphologic ability are typically below the level expected for general level of cognitive ability (e.g., for French, Karmiloff-Smith et al. 1997; for Hebrew, Levy and Hermon 2003). Language abilities are only slightly more advanced than nonverbal reasoning abilities. Nonconcrete language ability is considerably weaker than concrete language ability. For example, abstract relational vocabulary ability is considerably below the level expected for concrete vocabulary ability. Comprehension of figurative language is considerably below the level expected for both concrete vocabulary ability and receptive grammatical ability (Mervis et al. 2003). Finally, not only are language abilities less impressive than previously claimed, but IQ is considerably higher than expected based on initial reports. Mean IQ for individuals with WBS is in the range of mild mental retardation, not the severe to profound mental retardation range reported in Bates's presentation (1990) of Bellugi's research. Therefore, the language abilities of individuals with WBS are much more in line with what would be expected, given their IQ.

In many important ways, acquisition of language by individuals with WBS is best characterized as normal but delayed. For example, although both the onset of vocabulary acquisition and the onset of grammatical acquisition are delayed, the relation between expressive vocabulary size and grammatical complexity is the same as for the general population. Grammatical ability is at the level expected for overall level of cognitive ability. Many of the specific links between particular linguistic abilities and theoretically linked cognitive abilities that hold for TD children and children with DS also are shown by children with WBS. For example, canonical babble, a critical step in the beginning of language acquisition, begins at the same time as rhythmic hand banging. The early object labels of children with WBS name the same child-basic-level categories as for TD children and children with DS. Basic-level categories and category names are acquired before subordinate- or superordinate-level categories and category names. Furthermore, the onsets of spontaneous exhaustive sorting and the ability to fast map new words whose referents were not explicitly identified by the speaker occur at about the same time.

However, several putative links between specific aspects of language development and particular aspects of cognitive development that are evidenced by both TD children and children with DS do not hold for children with WBS. In particular, children with WBS do not comprehend and produce referential pointing gestures before beginning to produce referential language. The onset of referential language typically precedes the onset of comprehension and production of pointing gestures by six months or more. Despite the delay in pointing, parents of children with WBS successfully establish joint attention by other communicative methods, such as labeling the object that is already the focus of the child's attention or tapping the object on which the speaker wishes the child to focus. Such interactions allow children with WBS to begin to acquire language without the ability to comprehend or produce referential pointing gestures.

The finding that the onset of referential language usually precedes the onset of comprehension and production of pointing gestures has important implications for language intervention. The onset of referential communicative gestures often is used as an indicator that children are ready to acquire language; at this point, speech therapy and/or developmental therapy is likely to begin to focus on vocabulary acquisition. Similarly, if children do not come to the attention of intervention agencies until after acquisition of a basic vocabulary, it is assumed that these children have already mastered the referential gesture system. Both of these assumptions are incorrect for children with WBS. Children with WBS are ready for language intervention focused on vocabulary acquisition long before they begin to produce referential communicative gestures. And many young children with WBS who have two hundred or more words in their productive vocabularies still have difficulty both comprehending and producing referential communicative gestures and would benefit from therapy directed at improving their nonverbal communicative abilities.

Another set of specific links that holds for TD children and children with DS, but not for children with WBS, involves the onset of the vocabulary spurt. For children with WBS, the onset of the vocabulary spurt precedes the onsets of both spontaneous exhaustive sorting and fast mapping, typically by six months or more. These three abilities, which have previously been claimed to be linked to the related conceptual realizations that all objects belong to a category and that all objects have basic-level names, are evidenced at about the same time for both TD children and children with DS. I have argued that the onset of the vocabulary spurt may well not indicate the realization that all objects have names. Instead, the vocabulary spurt may simply reflect increasing efficiency in applying vocabulary acquisition strategies that the child already has. Given that individuals with WBS show a relative strength in verbal short-term memory and that four-year-olds with WBS who show logistic vocabulary growth have considerably stronger verbal short-term memory abilities than those with slow linear vocabulary growth, it is possible that increases in verbal memory ability facilitate the vocabulary spurt for children with WBS. Grant et al. (1997) and Lukács et al. (2001) have shown that verbal or phonological memory is strongly related to vocabulary size for older children with WBS.

Strong verbal memory abilities, while effective at enhancing concrete vocabulary acquisition, are not nearly as helpful for facilitating acquisition of more abstract vocabulary. Thus, despite the strong correlation between concrete vocabulary size and abstract vocabulary size, the abstract relational vocabularies of children with WBS are considerably smaller than expected given their concrete vocabulary size. Similarly, adolescents' and adults' understanding of figurative language, although highly correlated with their understanding of concrete language with the same grammatical constructions (Mervis et al. 2003), is much more limited. The end result is that the acquisition of abstract language ability is substantially more delayed than the acquisition of concrete language ability, with large discrepancies remaining even in adulthood. Most children and adolescents with WBS, even if their receptive concrete vocabulary is at their CA level, would benefit from speech or cognitive therapy focused on relational language and, at older ages, on figurative language. In both cases, it is important that the therapy be designed to ensure that the individual is able to generalize the language that has been taught to novel settings outside the therapeutic context. Anecdotal reports suggest that music therapy is helpful for acquisition of relational language, especially if the therapy is structured to facilitate generalization from the original context to a wide variety of additional contexts.

Verbal short-term memory ability also is important to grammatical ability for individuals with WBS. At age four years, the ability to produce multi-word utterances is strongly related to verbal short-term memory ability. For older children and adolescents, verbal short-term memory, phonological memory, and verbal working memory are all related to grammatical ability. This pattern of relations between memory abilities and grammatical ability also is shown by typically developing children. However, the strength of the relation between verbal working memory and grammatical ability is significantly greater for children with WBS than for TD children matched for receptive grammatical level. This finding suggests that individuals with WBS may need to depend more than TD individuals on verbal working memory to figure out complex grammatical structures. In particular, TD children may rely on more advanced conceptual abilities to learn grammar that place fewer demands on working memory, whereas children with WBS, who cannot apply some of these strategies or who take longer to apply them, place a higher demand on verbal working memory to acquire the same grammatical constructions.

Future Directions

Research on the language abilities of individuals with WBS began less than twenty years ago. A great deal has been learned in that time, culminating in the research reported in this chapter. Much of this research has been cross-sectional, often including a wide chronological age range in a single group. Cross-sectional studies will most likely continue to dominate language research on WBS, as they dominate language research on individuals with other developmental disabilities and on typically developing children. Nevertheless, longitudinal studies will become increasingly important as researchers seek to resolve theoretical controversies that are best addressed by data from the same children over time, rather than from different children at different ages. For example, the question of whether the morphological patterns shown by individuals with WBS are best characterized by a dual-mechanism or a single-route model will be best resolved by tracking the course of morphological development (e.g., development of the past-tense morpheme) over many years. Similarly, the question of whether people with WBS acquire their relatively good language abilities through mechanisms that are the same as or different from those used by children with other developmental disabilities or TD children is best addressed by tracking language development in the same set of children over a long period. As a third example, theoretical questions concerning links between lexical and grammatical abilities or between specific language abilities and theoretically related cognitive abilities will be most adequately answered through longitudinal designs.

There have been several magnetic resonance imaging studies of the brains of adults with WBS (see chapter 4), but only a few functional neuroimaging studies involving language tasks have been conducted. As yet, the results are available only as brief summaries in chapters (e.g., Bellugi et al. 1999) or as conference presentations (e.g., Bonner-Jackson et al. 2003; Fonaryova Key et al. 2003). Event-related potential and positron emission tomography methods have been used to study older children and/or adults engaged in tasks involving morphology or semantics. The results indicate differences between the WBS and TD participants in brainwave forms in response to open-class versus closed-class words or to semantically appropriate versus semantically anomalous sentence endings, and differences in the brain regions recruited for semantic fluency tasks. Bonner-Jackson and colleagues noted that these findings could reflect differences in the cognitive strategies used to solve the research tasks, differences in the language production system, and/or altered neural circuitry. They suggested that newer neuroimaging techniques such as diffusion tensor imaging may be helpful in addressing these issues. In contrast to these findings, results of an event-related potential study of the speech perception (a much lower-level component of language) of four-year-olds with WBS suggested that many children with WBS have brainwave forms similar to those of TD children. Furthermore, several measures of the extent of differentiation of a child's brainwaves in response to different consonant sounds were highly correlated with behavioral measures both of language ability and nonverbal ability (Fonaryova Key et al. 2003). These studies are just the start of what is likely to be a large number of neuroimaging studies. Research that combines multiple neuroimaging techniques and/or relates neuroimaging findings to potential behavioral correlates will be especially helpful in addressing questions of the neural substrate of language in WBS, its relation to behavior, processing strategies used by people with WBS, and ways in which the neural substrate is similar to or different from that of people with other developmental disabilities or TD individuals. Developmental studies, preferably beginning in infancy, are crucial for addressing the question of whether the starting state of the neural substrate for language in WBS is the same as for TD individuals.

In this chapter, I have considered lexical, semantic, morphologic, and syntactic aspects of language acquisition and use by individuals with WBS. These areas are likely to continue to be the most heavily researched, and much remains to be learned about them. Language includes two other important areas in which there has been virtually no research on individuals with WBS (and that are therefore not discussed in this chapter). The first is phonology, including speech perception and production. In addition to the Fonaryova Key et al. (2003) study of speech perception discussed earlier in the chapter, one other study of the phonological development of children with WBS has been reported. Velleman et al. (2005) conducted a longitudinal study of early phonological development, focusing on consonant production, mean babble level, and the onset of referential words. Onset and rate of phonological development ranged from severely delayed to normal, paralleling the toddlers' performance on the Mullen Scales of Early Learning (Mullen 1995).

The second area is pragmatics, the everyday use of language. Pragmatics is critical for everyday communication—for example, in following conversational conventions, successful referential communication, and appropriate word choice. The only studies of pragmatics in WBS (Laws and Bishop 2004; Peregrine et al. 2005) have used the Children's Communication Checklist (CCC [Bishop 1998] or CCC-2 [Bishop 2003]), a parent-report measure of child language ability that includes scales measuring pragmatics. The studies found significant pragmatic impairment, including difficulties with nonverbal communication, overreliance on context, overuse of stereotyped language or topics of conversation, and inappropriate initiation of conversation. Problems with social relationships also were identified.

To fully understand language abilities in WBS, studies of both phonology and pragmatics are needed. Research on pragmatics is also needed from an applied perspective; both casual observation of individuals with WBS and parental responses to interviews focusing on adaptive behavior suggest that, although older children and adults with WBS usually speak fluently, difficulties with conversational conventions such as staying on topic are very common.

In conclusion, language ability is a relative strength for individuals with WBS. In many important ways, the acquisition of language proceeds in the same manner as for individuals in the general population. There is increasing evidence, however, that verbal memory—often the strongest ability of individuals with WBS—is more important in the acquisition of language for these individuals than for their TD peers. The importance of verbal short-term memory to the acquisition of vocabulary by children with WBS and the importance of verbal working memory to their grammatical development highlight basic differences between how children with WBS and TD children acquire language. It is an open question as to whether these differences are a matter of extremes on a single continuum or whether children with WBS acquire language through significantly different mechanisms from TD children. Future studies using longitudinal designs and/or neuroimaging techniques in conjunction with behavioral measures should help provide a solid foundation for addressing this question.

ACKNOWLEDGMENTS

This research was supported by grant HD29957 from the National Institute of Child Health and Human Development and grant NS35102 from the National Institute of Neurological Disorders and Stroke. I thank all the participants and their families. I am grateful to the geneticists, cardiologists, and early-intervention agencies who referred individuals with Williams-Beuren syndrome to my research program, as well as to Terry Monkaba, executive director of the National Williams Syndrome Association, who has encouraged and facilitated the conduct of research at regional and national meetings of the Williams Syndrome Association. Portions of this chapter are based on an earlier publication (Mervis, Robinson, Rowe, Becerra, and Klein-Tasman 2003).

REFERENCES

Adamson, L. B. 1995. *Communication development during infancy.* Madison, WI: Brown and Benchmark.
Bates, E. 1990. Early language development: How things come together and how they come apart. Paper presented at the International Conference on Infant Studies, Montreal, Quebec.
Bates, E., and Carnevale, G. F. 1993. New directions in research on language development. *Developmental Review* 13:446–470.
Bates, E., and Goodman, J. C. 1997. On the inseparability of grammar and the lexicon: Evidence from acquisition, aphasia and real-time processing. *Language and Cognitive Processes* 12:507–586.
Bellugi, U., Marks, S., Bihrle, A., and Sabo, H. 1988. Dissociation between language and cognitive functions in Williams syndrome. In *Language development in exceptional circumstances,* ed. D. Bishop and K. Mogford, 177–189. London: Churchill-Livingstone.
Bellugi, U., Bihrle, A., Jernigan, T., Trauner, D., and Doherty S. 1990. Neuropsychological and neuroanatomical profile of Williams syndrome. *American Journal of Medical Genetics* 6:115–125.
Bellugi, U., Bihrle, A., Neville, H., and Doherty, S. 1992. Language, cognition, and brain organization in a neurodevelopmental disorder. In *Developmental behavioral neuroscience: The Minnesota symposium,* ed. M. Gunnar and C. Nelson, 201–232. Hillsdale, NJ: Erlbaum.
Bellugi, U., Wang, P., and Jernigan, T. L. 1994. Williams syndrome: An unusual neuropsychological profile. In *Atypical cognitive deficits in developmental disorders: Implications for brain function,* ed. S. H. Broman and J. Grafman, 23–56. Hillsdale, NJ: Erlbaum.
Bellugi, U., Mills, D., Jernigan, T., Hickok, G., and Galaburda, A. 1999. Linking cognition, brain structure, and brain function in Williams syndrome. In *Neurodevelopmental disorders,* ed. H. Tager-Flusberg, 111–136. Cambridge: MIT Press.

Bellugi, U., Lichtenberger, L., Jones, W., Lai, Z., and St. George, M. 2000. The neurocognitive profile of Williams syndrome: A complex pattern of strengths and weaknesses. *Journal of Cognitive Neuroscience* 12 (suppl. 1): 7–29.

Bishop, D. V. M. 1989. *Test for the Reception of Grammar*, 2nd ed. Manchester, UK: Chapel Press.

———. 1998. Development of the Children's Communication Checklist (CCC): A method for assessing the qualitative aspects of communication impairment in children. *Journal of Child Psychology and Psychiatry* 39:879–891.

———. 2003. *The Children's Communication Checklist*, 2nd ed. London: Psychological Corporation.

Bishop, D. V. M., North, T., and Dolan, C. 1996. Nonword repetition as a behavioural marker for inherited language impairment: Evidence from a twin study. *Journal of Child Psychology and Psychiatry* 37:391–403.

Bonner-Jackson, A., Mervis, C. B., Morris, C. A., Holt, J. L., Meyer-Lindenberg, A., and Berman, K. F. 2003. *The neural substrate of verbal fluency in Williams syndrome*. New York: International Society for Human Brain Mapping.

Bowerman, M. 1996. Learning how to structure space for language: A cross-linguistic perspective. In *Language and space*, ed. P. Bloom, M. A. Peterson, L. Nadel, and M. F. Garrett, 385–436. Cambridge: MIT Press.

Carroll, J. B., Davies, P., and Richman, B. 1971. *Word frequency book*. New York: American Heritage.

Caselli, M., and Casadio, P. 1995. *Il primo vocabolario del bambino*. Milan, Italy: Franco Angeli.

Clahsen, H., and Almazan, M. 1998. Syntax and morphology in children with Williams syndrome. *Cognition* 68:167–198.

Clahsen, H., and Temple, C. 2003. Words and rules in children with Williams syndrome. In *Language competence across populations: Toward a definition of specific language impairment*, ed. Y. Levy and J. Schaeffer, 323–352. Mahwah, NJ: Erlbaum.

Clahsen, H., Ring, M., and Temple, C. 2003. Lexical and morphological skills in English-speaking children with Williams syndrome. *Essex Research Reports in Linguistics* 43:1–27.

Cobo-Lewis, A. B., Oller, D. K., Lynch, M. P., and Levine, S. L. 1995. Relationships among motor and vocal milestones in normally developing infants and infants with Down syndrome. Paper presented at the Gatlinburg Conference on Research and Theory in Mental Retardation and Developmental Disabilities, Gatlinburg, TN.

Dunham, P. J., Dunham, F., and Curwin, A. 1993. Joint-attentional states and lexical acquisition at 18 months. *Developmental Psychology* 29:827–831.

Dunn, L. E., and Dunn, L. E. 1997. *Peabody Picture Vocabulary Test*, 3rd ed. Circle Pines, MN: American Guidance Service.

Edmonston, N. K., and Litchfield Thane, N. 1988. *TRC: Test of Relational Concepts*. Austin, TX: PRO-ED.

Elliott, C. D. 1990. *Differential Ability Scales*. San Antonio, TX: Psychological Corporation.

Fenson, L., Dale, P. S., Reznick, J. S., Thal, D., Bates, E., Hartung, J. P., Pethick, S., and Reilly, J. S. 1993. *MacArthur Communicative Development Inventories: User's guide and technical manual*. San Diego, CA: Singular.

Fenson, L., Dale, P. S., Reznick, J. S., Bates, E., Thal, D., and Pethick, S. 1994. Variability in early communicative development. *Monographs of the Society for Research in Child Development* 59 (5, ser. no. 242): 1–173.

Fonaryova Key, A., Molfese, D. L., Mervis, C. B., and Cunningham, N. 2003. Hemisphere asymmetry for language processing in 4-year-old children with Williams syndrome. Poster presented at the meeting of the International Neuropsychological Society, Honolulu.

Frangiskakis, J. M., Ewart, A. K., Morris, C. A., Mervis, C. B., Bertrand, J., Robinson, B. F., Klein, B. P., Ensing, G. J., Everett, L. A., Green, E. D., Pröschel, C., Gutowski, N., Noble, M., Atkinson, D. L., Odelberg, S. J., and Keating, M. T. 1996. LIM-kinase1 hemizygosity implicated in impaired visuospatial constructive cognition. *Cell* 86:59–69.

Frick, R. W. 1995. Accepting the null hypothesis. *Memory and Cognition* 23:132–138.

Gathercole, S. E., and Baddeley, A. D. 1989. Evaluation of the role of phonological STM in the development of vocabulary in children: A longitudinal study. *Journal of Memory and Language* 28:200–213.

———. 1993. *Working memory and language.* Hillsdale, NJ: Erlbaum.

Gopnik, A., and Meltzoff, A. N. 1987. The development of categorization in the second year and its relation to other cognitive and linguistic developments. *Child Development* 58:1523–1531.

———. 1992. Categorization and naming: Basic level sorting in eighteen-month-olds and its relation to language. *Child Development* 63:1091–1103.

Gosch, A., Städing, G., and Pankau, R. 1994. Linguistic abilities in children with Williams-Beuren syndrome. *American Journal of Medical Genetics* 52:291–296.

Grant, J., Karmiloff-Smith, A., Gathercole, S. A., Paterson, S., Howlin, P., Davies, M., and Udwin, O. 1997. Phonological short-term memory and its relationship to language in Williams syndrome. *Cognitive Neuropsychiatry* 2:81–99.

Grant, J., Valian, V., and Karmiloff-Smith, A. 2002. A study of relative clauses in Williams syndrome. *Journal of Child Language* 29:403–416.

Guasti, M. T. 2002. *Language acquisition: The growth of grammar.* Cambridge: MIT Press.

Guasti, M. T., Thornton, R., and Wexler, K. 1995. Negation in children's questions: The case of English. In *BUCLID 19: Proceedings of the 19th annual Boston University Conference on Language Development,* ed. D. MacLaughlin and S. McEwen, 228–239. Somerville, MA: Cascadilla Press.

Jackendoff, R. 1994. *Patterns in the mind: Language and human nature.* New York: Basic Books.

Jarrold, C., and Baddeley, A. D. 1997. Short-term memory for verbal and visuo-spatial information in Down's syndrome. *Cognitive Neuropsychiatry* 2:101–122.

Jarrold, C., Baddeley, A. D., and Hewes, A. K. 1998. Verbal and nonverbal abilities in the Williams syndrome phenotype: Evidence for diverging developmental trajectories. *Journal of Child Psychology and Psychiatry* 39:511–523.

Jarrold, C., Baddeley, A. D., Hewes, A. K., and Phillips, C. 2001. A longitudinal assessment of diverging verbal and non-verbal abilities in the Williams syndrome phenotype. *Cortex* 37:423–431.

Karmiloff-Smith, A., Grant, J., Berthoud, I., Davies, M., Howlin, P., and Udwin, O. 1997. Language and Williams syndrome: How intact is "intact"? *Child Development* 68:274–290.

Karmiloff-Smith, A., Brown, J. H., Grice, S., and Paterson, S. 2003. Dethroning the myth: Cognitive dissociations and innate modularity in Williams syndrome. *Developmental Neuropsychology* 23:229–244.

Kaufman, A. S., and Kaufman, N. L. 1990. *Kaufman Brief Intelligence Test.* Pines, MN: American Guidance Services.

Kemper, S., Kynette, D., Rash, S., and O'Brien, K. 1989. Life span changes to adults' language: Effects of memory and genre. *Applied Psycholinguistics* 10:49–66.

Klein, B. P. 1995. Grammatical abilities of children with Williams syndrome. Master's thesis, Emory University.

Klein, B. P., and Mervis, C. B. 1999. Cognitive strengths and weaknesses of 9- and 10-year-olds with Williams syndrome or Down syndrome. *Developmental Neuropsychology* 16:177–196.

Laing, E., Butterworth, G., Ansari, D., Gsödl, M., Longhi, E., Panagiotaki, G., Paterson, S., and Karmiloff-Smith, A. 2002. Atypical development of language and social communication in toddlers with Williams syndrome. *Developmental Science* 5:233–246.

Landau, B., and Zukowski, A. 2003. Objects, motions, and paths: Spatial language in children with Williams syndrome. *Developmental Neuropsychology* 23:107–139.

Laws, G., and Bishop, D. V. M. 2004. Pragmatic language impairment and social impairment in Williams syndrome: A comparison with Down's syndrome and specific language impairment. *International Journal of Language and Communication Disorders* 39:45–64.

Levy, Y. 1988. On the early learning of formal grammatical systems: Evidence from studies of the acquisition of gender and countability. *Journal of Child Language* 15:179–187.

Levy, Y., and Bechar, T. 2003. Cognitive, lexical, and morpho-syntactic profiles of Israeli children with Williams syndrome. *Cortex* 39:255–271.

Levy, Y., and Hermon, S. 2003. Morphological abilities of Hebrew-speaking adolescents. *Developmental Neuropsychology* 23:61–85.

Levy, Y., Tennebaum, A., and Ornoy, A. 2000. Spontaneous language of children with specific neurological syndromes. *Journal of Speech Language and Hearing Research* 43:351–365.

Lukács, A., Racsmány, M., and Pléh, C. 2001. Vocabulary and morphological patterns in Hungarian children with Williams syndrome: A preliminary report. *Acta Linguistica Hungarica* 48:243–269.

Lukács, A., Pléh, C., and Racsmány, M. 2004. Language in Hungarian children with Williams syndrome. In *Williams syndrome across languages,* ed. S. Bartke and J. Siegmüller, 187–220. Amsterdam: John Benjamins.

Masataka, N. 2001. Why early linguistic milestones are delayed in children with Williams syndrome: Late onset of hand banging as a possible rate-limiting constraint on the emergence of canonical babbling. *Developmental Science* 4:158–164.

McCarthy, D. 1972. *McCarthy Scales of Children's Abilities.* New York: Psychological Corporation.

Mervis, C. B. 1987. Child-basic object categories and early lexical development. In *Concepts and conceptual development: Ecological and intellectual factors in categorization,* ed. U. Neisser, 201–233. Cambridge: Cambridge University Press.

———. 1999. The Williams syndrome cognitive profile: Strengths, weaknesses, and interrelations among auditory short term memory, language, and visuospatial constructive cognition. In *Ecological approaches to cognition: Essays in honor of Ulric Neisser,* ed. E. Winograd, R. Fivush, and W. Hirst, 193–227. Mahwah, NJ: Erlbaum.

———. 2003. Williams syndrome: 15 years of psychological research. *Developmental Neuropsychology* 23:1–12.

———. 2004. Cross-etiology comparisons of cognitive and language development.

In *Developmental language disorders: From phenotypes to etiologies*, ed. M. L. Rice and S. F. Warren, 153–186. Mahwah, NJ: Erlbaum.

Mervis, C. B., and Bertrand, J. 1993. Acquisition of early object labels: The roles of operating principles and input. In *Enhancing children's communication: Research foundations for intervention*, ed. A. P. Kaiser and D. B. Gray, 281–316. Baltimore: Brookes.

———. 1994. Acquisition of the Novel Name–Nameless Category (N3C) principle. *Child Development* 65:1646–1662.

———. 1997. Developmental relations between cognition and language: Evidence from Williams syndrome. In *Communication and language acquisition: Discoveries from atypical development*, ed. L. B. Adamson and M. A. Romski, 75–106. New York: Brookes.

Mervis, C. B., and Klein-Tasman, B. P. 2000. Williams syndrome: Cognition, personality, and adaptive behavior. *Mental Retardation and Developmental Disabilities Research Reviews* 6:148–158.

Mervis, C. B., and Robinson, B. F. 1999. Methodological issues in cross-syndrome comparisons: Matching procedures, sensitivity (*Se*), and specificity (*Sp*). Commentary on M. Sigman and E. Ruskin, Continuity and change in the social competence of children with autism, Down syndrome, and developmental delays. *Monographs of the Society for Research in Child Development* 64 (ser. no. 256): 115–130.

———. 2000. Expressive vocabulary of toddlers with Williams syndrome or Down syndrome: A comparison. *Developmental Neuropsychology* 17:111–126.

———. 2003. Methodological issues in cross-group comparisons of language and cognitive development. In *Language competence across populations: Toward a definition of specific language impairment*, ed. Y. Levy and J. Schaeffer, 233–258. Mahwah, NJ: Erlbaum.

———. 2005. Designing measures for profiling and genotype/phenotype studies of individuals with genetic syndromes or developmental language disorders. *Applied Psycholinguistics* 26:41–64.

Mervis, C. B., Morris, C. A., Bertrand, J., and Robinson, B. F. 1999. Williams syndrome: Findings from an integrated program of research. In *Neurodevelopmental disorders*, ed. H. Tager-Flusberg, 65–110. Cambridge: MIT Press.

Mervis, C. B., Robinson, B. F., Bertrand, J., Morris, C. A., Klein-Tasman, B. P., and Armstrong, S. C. 2000. The Williams Syndrome Cognitive Profile. *Brain and Cognition* 44:604–628.

Mervis, C. B., Robinson, B. F., Rowe, M. L., Becerra, A. M. and Klein-Tasman, B. P. 2003. Language abilities of individuals who have Williams syndrome. In *International Review of Research in Mental Retardation*, vol. 27, ed. L. Abbeduto, 35–81. Orlando, FL: Academic Press.

Mervis, C. B., Robinson, B. F., Rowe, M. L., Becerra, A. M., and Klein-Tasman, B. P. 2004. Relations between language and cognition in Williams syndrome. In *Williams syndrome across languages*, ed. S. Bartke and J. Siegmüller, 63–92. Amsterdam: John Benjamins.

Monnery, S., Seigneuric, A., Zagar, D., and Robichon, F. 2002. A linguistic dissociation in Williams syndrome: Good at gender agreement but poor at lexical retrieval. *Reading and Writing: An Interdisciplinary Journal* 15:589–612.

Montgomery, J. A. 1996. Examination of phonological working memory in specifically language-impaired children. *Applied Psycholinguistics* 16:355–378.

Mullen, E. M. 1995. *Mullen Scales of Early Learning*. Circle Pines, MN: American Guidance Service.

Mundy, P., and Hogan, A. 1996. *A preliminary manual for the abridged Early Social*

Communication Scales (ESCS). Coral Gables, FL: University of Miami Psychology Department. www.psy.miami.edu/faculty/pmundy/ESCS.pdf

Norman, S., Kemper, S., and Kynette, D. 1992. Adult reading comprehension: Effects of syntactic complexity and working memory. *Journals of Gerontology* 47:258–265.

Paterson, S. 2001. Language and number in Down syndrome: The complex trajectory from infancy to adulthood. *Down Syndrome Research and Practice* 7:79–86.

Paterson, S., Brown, J. H., Gsödl, M. K., Johnson, M. H., and Karmiloff-Smith, A. 1999. Cognitive modularity and genetic disorders. *Science* 286:2355–2358.

Peregrine, E., Rowe, M. L., and Mervis, C. B. 2005. Pragmatic language difficulties in children with Williams syndrome. Poster presented at the biennial meeting of the Society for Research in Child Development, Atlanta.

Pinker, S. 1999. *Words and rules: The ingredients of language*. New York: Basic Books.

Racsmány, M., Lukács, A., Pléh, C., and Király, I. 2001. Some cognitive tools for word learning: The role of working memory and goal preference. *Behavioral and Brain Sciences* 24:1115–1117.

Rice, M. L. 1999. Specific grammatical limitations in children with specific language impairment. In *Neurodevelopmental disorders*, ed. H. Tager-Flusberg, 331–359. Cambridge: MIT Press.

Robinson, B. F., and Mervis, C. B. 1999. Comparing productive vocabulary measures from the CDI and a systematic diary study. *Journal of Child Language* 26:177–185.

Robinson, B. F., Mervis, C. B., and Robinson, B. W. 2003. Roles of verbal short-term memory and working memory in the acquisition of grammar by children with Williams syndrome. *Developmental Neuropsychology* 23:13–31.

Rosch, E. 1973. On the internal structure of perceptual and semantic categories. In *Cognitive development and the acquisition of language*, ed. T. E. Moore, 111–144. New York: Academic Press.

———. 1975. Cognitive representation of semantic categories. *Journal of Experimental Psychology: General* 104:192–233.

Rosch, E., Mervis, C. B., Gray, W. D., Johnson, D. M., and Boyes-Braem, P. 1976. Basic objects in natural categories. *Cognitive Psychology* 8:382–439.

Sattler, J. M. 2001. *Assessment of children*, 4th ed. San Diego: Jerome M. Sattler.

Shye, S. 1985. *Multiple scaling: The theory and application of partial order scalogram analysis*. Amsterdam: North Holland.

Singer Harris, N. G., Bellugi, U., Bates, E., Jones, W., and Rossen, M. 1997. Contrasting profiles of language development in children with Williams and Down syndromes. *Developmental Neuropsychology* 13:345–370.

Temple, C. M., Almazan, M., and Sherwood, S. 2002. Lexical skills in Williams syndrome: A cognitive neuropsychological analysis. *Journal of Neurolinguistics* 15:463–495.

Thomas, M. S. C., Grant, J., Barham, Z., Gsödl, M., Laing, E., Lakusta, L., Tyler, L. K., Grice, S., Paterson, S., and Karmiloff-Smith, A. 2001. Past tense formation in Williams syndrome. *Language and Cognitive Processes* 16:143–176.

Tomasello, M., and Farrar, M. J. 1986. Joint attention and early language. *Child Development* 57:1454–1463.

Udwin, O., and Yule W. 1990. Expressive language of children with Williams syndrome. *American Journal of Medical Genetics Supplement* 6:108–114.

van der Lely, H. K. J., and Ullman, M. 2001. Past tense morphology in specifically language impaired children and normally developing children. *Language and Cognitive Processes* 16:113–136.

Velleman, S. L., Currier, A., Curley, A., and Mervis, C. B. 2005. The early phonology of Williams syndrome. Paper presented at the International Phonology Conference, Denton, TX.

Vicari, S., Caselli, M. C., Gagliardi, C., Tonucci, F., and Volterra, V. 2002. Language acquisition in special populations: A comparison between Down and Williams syndromes. *Neuropsychologia* 40:2461–2470.

Volterra, V., Capirci, O., Pezzini, G., Sabbadini, L., and Vicari, S. 1996. Linguistic abilities in Italian children with Williams syndrome. *Cortex* 32:663–677.

Volterra, V., Capirci, O., and Caselli, M. C. 2001. What atypical populations can reveal about language development: The contrast between deafness and Williams syndrome. *Language and Cognitive Processes* 16:219–239.

Volterra, V., Caselli, M. C., Capirci, O., Tonucci, F., and Vicari, S. 2003. Early linguistic abilities of Italian children with Williams syndrome. *Developmental Neuropsychology* 23:33–59.

Volterra, V., Capirci, O., and Caselli, M. C. 2004. Language in preschool Italian children with Williams and Down syndromes. In *Williams syndrome across languages*, ed. S. Bartke and J. Siegmüller, 163–185. Amsterdam: John Benjamins.

Wang, P. P., and Bellugi, U. 1993. Williams syndrome, Down syndrome, and cognitive neuroscience. *American Journal of Diseases of Children* 147:1246–1251.

Williams, K. T. 1997. *Expressive Vocabulary Test*. Circle Pines, MN: American Guidance Service.

Zukowski, A. 2001. Uncovering grammatical competence in children with Williams syndrome. Ph.D. diss., Boston University.

———. 2004. Investigating knowledge of complex syntax: Insights from experimental studies of Williams syndrome. In *Developmental language disorders: From phenotypes to etiologies*, ed. M. Rice and S. Warren, 99–119. Cambridge: MIT Press.

Specialization, Breakdown, and Sparing in Spatial Cognition

Lessons from Williams-Beuren Syndrome

9

Barbara Landau, Ph.D., James E. Hoffman, Ph.D.,

Jason E. Reiss, M.A., Daniel D. Dilks, M.A., Laura Lakusta, M.A.,

and Gitana Chunyo, B.A.

Just fifteen years have passed since Williams-Beuren syndrome (WBS) first attracted serious attention from cognitive scientists interested in the architecture of the mind. The first reports of this rare syndrome offered it as a possible case of dissociation between the cognitive systems responsible for language and spatial representation—a case that could provide unusual insights into the organization of the mind and brain. If a genetically based syndrome could result in selective, targeted impairment of some cognitive systems while leaving others intact, this would offer a first wedge into the problem of connecting gene and cognition.

The importance of this problem has been met by burgeoning research, which is moving quickly in new directions. As new insights are gained, the grounds for understanding cognition in WBS seem to shift. What began as a relatively simple hypothesis—dissociation of two cognitive systems—has developed into a set of hypotheses that address more closely whether and what kind of deficits exist in each system and even whether the systems as a whole fall apart or do so selectively. What seems clearest is that a complete understanding of the cognitive systems of persons with WBS—like those of individuals undergoing normal development—will require sustained, carefully controlled experimentation and creative theorizing. This understanding should also shed light on the nature of normal development of mind and brain.

In this chapter, we report our recent findings that confirm the initial notion of genetically targeted specialization. Yet these findings are tempered by the fact that the development of cognitive systems, even those that are plausible candidates for specialization, occurs at multiple levels and engages multiple mechanisms. Even one or two small missteps in the delicate sequence of developmental events can lead to cognitive performances that look quite different from the so-called typical profile shown by normally developing children. The critical issue is what these different performances reflect. Do they reflect a qualitatively different architecture that has necessarily evolved from altered genetic potential? Or do they reflect normal structure that evolves from an architecture so highly constrained that it survives despite altered genetic potential? If the latter, then how do we explain obvious differences in performance?

A close inspection of performance reveals a considerable degree of preserved cognitive structure in WBS. Differences in performance—most often reflected in "worse" performance by children with WBS than by mental age–matched (MA-matched) children—appear most strikingly when the task taxes general processes of memory and/or attention. In contrast, similarities in performance reflect intact cognitive architecture; there are often similarities in the qualitative nature of performance and in overall performance, indicating that basic properties of cognitive systems are spared in WBS.

A major key in understanding spatial cognition in Williams-Beuren syndrome—or, for that matter, in normal development—is understanding what natural cognitive architectures are like, what functions they normally serve, and how we might engage them as directly as possible, without adding extra complexity extraneous to the system. When we examine spatial representation in this light, it becomes evident that much of its architecture is spared in WBS. This sparing reflects a normal specialization of spatial cognitive systems that guides development, even under circumstances of genetic deficit.

We present data from our research program on spatial representation and spatial language that supports this notion that much of spatial architecture is spared in WBS, including the cognitive subsystems of object recognition and identification, biological motion perception, and spatial language. At the same time, there are complex, cascading effects of spatial cognition, which can lead from small, well-defined weaknesses to large deficits in performance—deficits due *not* to abnormal architecture but to small misadjustments that culminate in downward-spiraling performance.

The Block Construction Task: Basic Facts about Performance

The spatial deficit associated with Williams-Beuren syndrome is particularly apparent in tasks that require the subject to reproduce a model by drawing it (e.g., the Test of Visual-Motor Integration [VMI; Beery and Buktenica 1967]) or by assembling parts (e.g., the Differential Ability Scales [DAS; Elliott 1990] and the Wechsler Adult Intelligence Scale–Revised [WAIS-R; Wechsler 1981]; see chapter 7). Figure 9.1 shows some typical drawings from our lab by children with WBS and a MA-matched control. The WBS drawings generally preserve the colors and shapes of the component parts of the model but clearly fail to capture their global arrangement. Bellugi et al. (1994) reported similar results for the block construction task: children with WBS tended to choose the correct parts but placed them incorrectly, producing "broken configurations" in which the outline shape of the completed copy did not match the model.

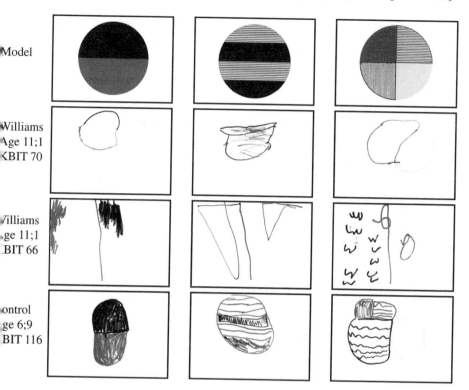

Fig. 9.1. Sample drawings by children with WBS (Williams) and one normally developing child who is matched for mental age. Matching is done with the Kaufman Brief Intelligence Test (KBIT).

One attempt to explain these results proposes that people with WBS are "local processors" who perceive local details but have difficulty perceiving global structure. This is consistent with the broken configurations in block construction tests as well as the tendency to draw the local level of hierarchical figures correctly while failing to represent the global configuration—a pattern described in several reports (Bellugi et al. 1994; Bihrle et al. 1989). It is difficult, however, to attribute errors in these tasks unambiguously to a deficit in perception. Both drawing and block construction tasks require planning and working memory, and these processes could be responsible for a local bias, even if perception of global information were intact. So the key to determining whether there is a deficit in perceptual processing of global spatial relationships or a deficit in further complex operations that are carried out on the products of perception is to devise experiments that can separate the two.

One research group has indeed reported a local bias when subjects with WBS were required to *match* two figures or judge their similarity, tasks that presumably are more diagnostic in terms of a perceptual representation (Deruelle et al. 1999). However, other research has failed to show a general deficit in global perception associated with WBS. For example, Key and colleagues (1998) found that broken configuration errors were relatively rare and occurred at about the same rate for children with WBS and normally developing control children. The most common errors were choosing an incorrect part and placing it in an incorrect location. In addition, Pani et al. (1999) found that, in a visual search task, children with WBS were at least as sensitive as the control children to global configuration effects. We showed that children with WBS were comparable to MA-matched controls in the ability to see biological motion, a task that requires local element motion to be integrated into a global percept. These results suggest that, at minimum, we need further research to disentangle the causes of deficits in representing and/or storing global spatial information.

Aside from these findings, there is evidence that any difference in the representation of global spatial information is probably similar to that seen in younger, normally developing children. For example, our own analyses of copying activities in children with WBS indicate that, while the copies are abnormal for chronological age, they are qualitatively similar to those of normally developing children of roughly three to four years of age (Georgopoulos et al. 2004; Bertrand et al. 1997). The only qualitative difference in copying that we observed was the tendency of children with WBS (who were between seven and fifteen years of age) to create solid-line figures when viewing a figure composed only of individual elements. Thus, for example, when copying a triangle made of small circles, the children tended to draw a solid-line triangle more often than did normally developing MA-matched children. Interestingly, this observation goes against the idea that children with WBS tend to be deficient "global processors"—indeed, their tendency to draw the figure as a solid implies a bias *toward* global reconstruction.

These conflicting findings need to be resolved, but at the very least they suggest that we should dissect tasks into component processes to attribute errors to particular processing stages. We address this later in the chapter, when we return to the question of why block construction is so difficult. First, however, we take a closer look at different kinds of spatial representation—each fundamental in its own right.

Specialization and Sparing of Spatial Cognitive Systems

We have examined several different kinds of spatial systems to determine whether the spatial deficit in Williams-Beuren syndrome is global or shows selective breakdown along the lines of normal cognitive architecture. We describe here three components of this research.

Object Representation

One approach to understanding the patterns of preserved and impaired visual abilities in WBS depends on a distinction between the functions of the brain's dorsal and ventral visual pathways. Ungerleider and Mishkin (1982) originally proposed two systems in the mind and brain: the ventral system, thought to be responsible for representing the shape and identity of an object, and the dorsal system, thought to represent location. More recently, Milner and Goodale (1995) have proposed that the dorsal stream is specialized for guiding action in space and the ventral stream for conscious representation of the products of perception, which are often used in object and face perception.

The proposed functions of the dorsal stream are similar to those functions particularly impaired in WBS, which has led some researchers to propose that WBS is a "dorsal stream deficit" (Atkinson et al. 1997; Wang et al. 1995). For example, at least anecdotally, visual-motor tasks such as reaching for and picking up small objects seem to be problematic for individuals with WBS. Additionally, other tasks that may involve the dorsal stream, such as manipulating elements of spatial arrays (e.g., object assembly, block copying, drawing), also show severe impairment (Bellugi et al. 1992; Mervis et al. 1999). Some researchers have also reported deficits in certain kinds of motion perception (as discussed below), which have also been proposed to be dorsal functions. A natural question, then, is whether these apparent deficits reflect targeted damage to the dorsal stream with symmetric sparing of the ventral stream.

If ventral stream functioning were preserved in individuals with WBS, we would expect to find that their ability to recognize objects is normal and, at least anecdotally, that seems to be the case. But this does not necessarily mean they have normal object recognition systems. Until recently, there was only one study that systematically examined object representation independent of other spatial functions (Wang et al. 1995). In this study of the performances of people with WBS and those with Down syndrome, the two groups were comparable in their ability to name objects shown in a canonical view (i.e., a view usually exposing most of an object's critical parts). However, when shown objects from unusual viewpoints, individuals with WBS performed significantly better than those with Down syndrome.

Though intriguing, these findings do little to tell us whether the object recognition system is normal. For one thing, the lack of difference between the two groups in naming objects with a canonical viewpoint could point to impairment (or normalcy) in both groups. Similarly, the difference in naming objects in noncanonical views could mean that people with WBS have spared functions or that people with Down syndrome are particularly impaired. Aside from these issues is the question of whether the object recogni-

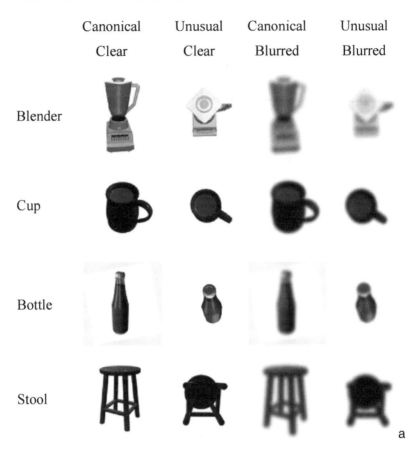

Fig. 9.2. (*a*) Samples of full-color objects used in object-identification studies. Objects are shown in the four experimental conditions: canonical, clear image; unusual, clear image; canonical, blurred image; and unusual, blurred image. Objects are presented on a computer screen for a brief duration (500 msec), and participants are asked to identify them by name. (*b*) Samples of outline drawings of objects used in object-identification studies. Objects are shown in the two experimental conditions: canonical image and unusual image.

tion system in WBS, even if it performs well under some circumstances, might break down more quickly than the normal system when put under pressure.

To investigate this issue, we tested children with WBS, a group of MA-matched controls, and a group of normally developed adults (undergraduate students), who provided a benchmark for optimal performance in this task (B. Landau, J. E. Hoffman, and N. Kurz 2005). All subjects were shown a set of eighty common objects presented in one of four different conditions: (1) canonical viewpoint and clear image, (2) unusual viewpoint and clear image, (3) canonical viewpoint and blurred image, and (4) unusual viewpoint and blurred image. We defined canonical viewpoint as that which exposed

Canonical   Unusual

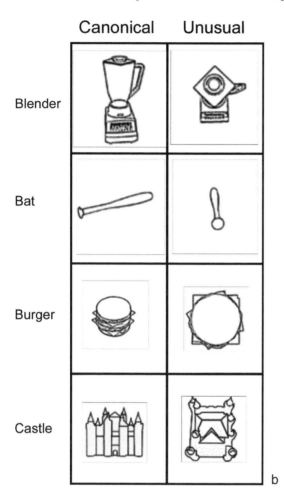

b

most critical parts and was therefore most readily recognized by normally developed adults. Unusual viewpoints were definitely unusual—a stool viewed from the underside, a carrot viewed from the top end, a cheeseburger viewed straight on from the top, and so forth (see fig. 9.2a for examples). The complete set of objects for any subject was drawn from a larger set of 320 images (80 objects × 4 viewing conditions). Images were presented briefly (for 500 msec) on a computer screen, and as each object appeared, participants were asked to name it ("What's that?"). All responses were coded by a rater who did not know whether he was coding a person with WBS or not.

The accuracy of naming responses was generally high, and variation across conditions was quite similar across subject groups. For the objects presented as canonical views and clear images, the adults achieved close to 100% correct, and the children with WBS and the normally developed controls came close, both averaging almost 90% correct. This by itself shows that, even under brief presentation, children with WBS are comparable to normally developed children who are MA-matched, and both groups are performing essentially at ceiling. One critical question is whether in children with WBS, despite their apparently normal performance when viewing canonical, clear images of objects, the object recognition system breaks down more rapidly or more dramatically than for other groups under other presentation conditions. Especially critical are the conditions in which the objects were presented from unusual viewpoints. It has been argued that recognition of objects in noncanonical orientations is more "spatial" and may engage more activity in those areas of the brain normally responsible for spatial processing—that is, the parietal areas (Carpenter et al. 1999; Farah 2000). Thus, individuals with WBS might have special difficulty with recognizing objects viewed from highly unusual perspectives because this might require a mental transformation of the object into a more "normal" perspective before recognition can occur.

However, in our study, an inspection of performance when objects were presented under unusual viewing conditions, whether with clear or with blurred images, indicates that no such breakdown occurred relative to MA matches. WBS children did perform worse than chronologically age-matched children, indicating some compromise in recognition of objects from unusual perspectives. Even in the most difficult conditions, when the objects were presented in unusual perspectives and with blurred images, all groups performed reasonably well, with adults performing at roughly 50% correct and children at roughly 40%.

These results suggest strong sparing of the object recognition system in WBS, at least when the color and texture of objects are visible. It is still possible, however, that children with WBS rely more heavily on surface properties such as color and texture than on more spatial properties such as object shape. To test this, we carried out a second experiment, in which we presented black and white line drawings of common objects for recognition and identification (see fig. 9.2b for examples). The same subject groups were tested using the same procedures. The results were strikingly similar to those of the first experiment. All subject groups performed very well (>80% correct) when identifying objects shown in canonical views, and all subject groups did more poorly for the unusual views. WBS children performed no differently from MA matches but were impaired relative to CA matches. As in the first experiment, the quality of the naming responses was highly similar across subject groups.

Thus, we found no evidence to support the notion of a global breakdown in the object recognition system in children with WBS. Importantly, we documented the capacity of children with WBS to recognize and identify objects from both canonical and unusual perspectives, although unusual perspectives revealed some impairment. If object representation is predominantly a ventral stream function, this evidence would argue in favor of a spared ventral stream. In addition, if recognition under unusual perspectives is carried out by some dorsal stream functions, the findings would argue for some sparing of both ventral but not dorsal stream functions (Dilks et al. 2001).

Biological Motion Perception

If the spatial deficit observed in WBS were due to widespread damage to the dorsal visual system, we would expect to see poor performance in tasks—such as motion perception and visually guided reaching—that are thought to be mediated by this stream. Atkinson and colleagues (1997, 2003) were the first to investigate motion perception in WBS by assessing subjects' ability to detect "motion coherence." Motion coherence tasks require subjects to detect a set of signal dots moving in the same direction, embedded in noise dots moving in random directions. Single cell research in monkeys (Newsome and Paré 1988) and functional imaging work in humans (Braddick et al. 2000) indicate that detection of motion coherence relies at least partly on a dedicated brain area in the dorsal stream (middle temporal visual area in monkeys, area V5 in humans).

Atkinson and colleagues (2003) determined the threshold for detecting motion coherence in people with WBS by varying the number of signal dots relative to the number of noise dots (signal-to-noise ratio, S/N). Performance on this task was compared with that on a companion task that used static line segments to measure "form coherence," which presumably reflects ventral stream processing. These researchers reported that the subjects seemed to fall into one of three distinct subgroups. One group performed poorly on both motion and form coherence tasks, suggesting a possible general deficit in detecting coherence. A second group performed poorly on the motion task but was comparable to controls in perceiving form coherence, a profile found in Atkinson et al.'s earlier work (1997) and also found in younger, normally developing children. The third group achieved normal performance on both tasks. Overall, these results reveal a good deal of variability among WBS subjects in terms of their ability to detect motion coherence, and some children with WBS, who do poorly on this task, seem to be developmentally delayed rather than selectively impaired. In any case, deficits in detecting motion coherence do not seem to be uniformly associated with WBS.

We recently investigated whether children with WBS were impaired on a motion task that involves seeing form-from-motion (FFM)—namely, the perception of so-called biological motion stimuli. These stimuli are produced by filming a person moving in the dark with lights attached to the head and limbs. Viewing these displays leads to a clear perception of a person walking, dancing, and so forth. There are conflicting predictions of how children with WBS should perform on this task. On the one hand, they might find it easy, given their interest in other social stimuli such as faces (Mervis et al. 1999; Tager-Flusberg and Sullivan 2000). On the other hand, this task might be difficult because it requires subjects to integrate the local motion of dots into higher-level units such as arms, legs, and ultimately a person (Johansson 1973). As we noted earlier, some researchers believe that children with WBS have difficulty in integrating local features into global configurations (Bellugi et al. 1994; Bihrle et al. 1989; but see Pani et al. 1999), and therefore we might expect them to have trouble with all FFM tasks, including biological motion.

To test these predictions, we compared children with WBS, MA-matched controls, and normally developed undergraduates on their ability to perceive biological motion (Jordan et al. 2002). In our first experiment, we presented subjects with displays depicting a person engaged in various actions (e.g., slipping on a banana peel, doing jumping jacks; for an example of the stimuli used in this experiment, see http://hoffman.psych.udel.edu/research/emdemo/WilliamsPage.htm). Subjects in all three groups easily identified the activity. Next, we presented subjects with point-light-walker (PLW) displays showing a side view of a person walking (as if on a treadmill; see fig. 9.3, top panel). All three groups were able to discriminate the walker's direction of movement (left or right) at or near perfect levels.

This initial work provided evidence that individuals with WBS can perceive biological motion, but our next study investigated whether this ability was fragile and subject to failure in noisy conditions. To do this, we again showed subjects PLW displays and asked them to indicate the direction the person was headed, but this time the walker was embedded in different types and amounts of noise (see fig. 9.3, middle and bottom panels). The presence of these distractor (or "noise") lights makes the task difficult because the distractors are similar to signal dots in shape, color, and motion and therefore can be mistaken for parts of the "figure" (Cutting et al. 1988).

We examined three types of noise conditions: static noise (static), randomly moving noise (random), and noise having motion paths similar to the signal lights (yoked). The results are shown in figure 9.4. All three groups were at or near ceiling performance in the static condition but made errors in the presence of moving noise (both random and yoked), particularly at high noise levels. In the low noise condition, both the adults and the children with WBS were mildly affected by moving noise whereas the MA-matched controls showed a sharp drop in performance (see fig. 9.4, left panel). In the

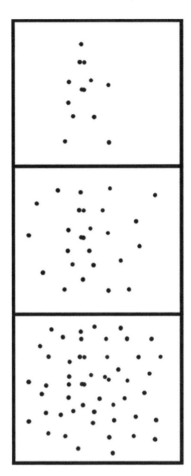

Fig. 9.3. Scale illustrations of the biological motion displays with no noise (top) and in low (middle) and high (bottom) noise conditions. In all cases, the signal and noise lights were white against a black background. People viewed moving displays of these dots and were asked to indicate whether the human figure represented by the dots was moving to the right or left. *Source:* Jordan et al. 2002. Reprinted with permission of Blackwell Publishing.

high noise condition, children with WBS still seemed to perform better than the MA-matched controls, but this difference was not significant. In addition, the adults did only marginally better than the children with WBS (fig. 9.4, right panel). In summary, even with moving noise, children with WBS performed as well as or better than MA-matched controls in their ability to perceive biological motion, and in some cases their performance was comparable to that of normally developed adults, suggesting that biological motion perception is a spared ability in WBS.

Overall, children with WBS do not seem to be generally impaired in perceiving motion, although in some cases they may be developmentally delayed. This finding argues against the hypothesis that WBS is associated with a general deficit in the dorsal stream. Of course, it is still possible that other

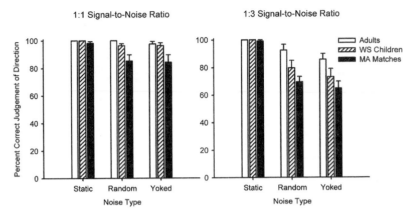

Fig. 9.4. Mean percentage accuracy of reporting the walking direction in biological motion displays for each of three noise conditions (static, random, and yoked) and three subject groups (undergraduates [adults], children with WBS [WS children], and mental age–matched [MA] children). Results are shown separately for low (left) and high (right) noise conditions. Chance performance lies at 50 percent. *Source:* Jordan et al. 2002. Reprinted with permission of Blackwell Publishing.

areas of the dorsal system, such as parietal cortex, are responsible for the spatial deficits observed in WBS. However, our data rule out the strongest form of the hypothesis—that all aspects of motion perception are impaired.

Spatial Language

The severe impairment in some aspects of spatial cognition coupled with the strength in language inevitably leads to the question of how the spatial deficit is reflected in language. The case of spatial language in WBS provides unusual insight into important questions of how space and language interact in normal human architecture. It is usually assumed that, in order to talk about what we see (or hear or feel), we must be able to represent spatial aspects of the world. If these nonlinguistic representations are damaged, one might expect severe impairment in spatial language.

The relationship between spatial language and nonlinguistic representations of space is neither simple nor direct (Landau 2001). Some aspects of spatial representation may be impaired while some spatial language remains intact. First, abundant evidence from brain-damaged adults suggests that individual systems of spatial representation can break down while others are spared (for a review, see Farah 2000). The same could be true for spatial language. We have already argued that the spatial breakdown in WBS is not global; in fact, some aspects of object recognition and some kinds of motion perception seem to be spared. These facts immediately raise the question of whether spatial language might also be a specialized system, which encodes highly selective spatial properties by using formal structures that simply do not exist in nonlinguistic systems (Landau and Jackendoff 1993; Landau 2001, 2002). If it is a specialized and independent system, spatial language might be acquired with impunity even in the face of severe impairments in other aspects of spatial cognition.

We have been testing this hypothesis in a range of studies of spatial language. Before reviewing some of this research, we need to consider the importance of *how* knowledge is measured—that is, the kinds of tasks that are chosen to tap into linguistic knowledge.

Some Observations on Linguistic Competence and Performance. Initial reports on language in people with WBS provided striking evidence for strength in vocabulary comprehension and production and in syntax, as shown by judgments on grammar that tap into subtle grammatical knowledge (Bellugi et al. 1988). More recently, careful studies have confirmed that much of the basic machinery of a mature syntax is present in children with WBS (Zukowski 2001), even though these children show impaired performance on standardized measures of language, such as the Test for Reception of Grammar (TROG; Bishop 1983). We believe that, in large part, such discrepancies are due to the nature of the tasks that are used to measure grammatical competence. We take a slight detour here to illustrate how certain tasks can severely underestimate a child's linguistic knowledge.

Using the TROG, researchers have reported that children with WBS are significantly impaired in processing relative clauses (Volterra et al. 1996; Karmiloff-Smith et al. 1997; Mervis et al. 1999). A sample item from the TROG is shown in figure 9.5. The child is shown four pictures and is asked to point to the picture in which *The circle the star is in is red.* Note that this sentence contains a relative clause not marked by the lexical item *that,* which commonly introduces such clauses.

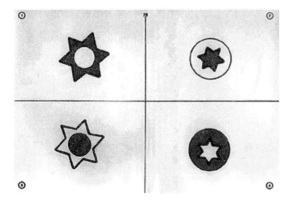

Fig. 9.5. Sample item from the TROG. The child is asked to point to the picture where *the circle the star is in is red. Source:* Bishop 1989.

Clearly, there are many ways in which performance could go awry in this task. Children could be impaired in processing the relative clauses (both subject-relatives and object-relatives), in mapping the syntax to the visual items, in scanning all four items, in making decisions (e.g., they might have looser or more stringent criterion for a *yes*), and so forth. In order to determine whether the impairment reflects a damaged system of grammatical knowledge, one would need a careful test that avoids many of these possibilities, while still tapping into the grammatical structure.

Zukowski (2001) carried out such experiments. She reasoned that accurate production of relative clauses embedded in sentences could be systematically generated only if the appropriate syntactic machinery were intact. She reasoned that the felicitous (i.e., pragmatically appropriate) conditions for eliciting subject- and object-relative clauses were somewhat subtle, and she devised contexts that would likely elicit these clauses from normally developed individuals. She then tested children with WBS who had already been shown to perform very poorly on these items in the TROG. She found that all children who were tested did indeed produce grammatically correct subject- and object-relative clauses, some of which were quite complex. For example, in one case, a subject observed an event depicting one boy sitting on a horse and another, identical boy standing on a horse, followed by each boy turning a different color. When she was asked to describe the event, the subject said, "The boy that's sitting on the horse turned green, and the boy who's standing on a horse turned purple." Zukowski also found some errors of production and some of comprehension, but all of these could be explained by factors related to the mechanisms of production or comprehension per se—not to the presence or absence of the grammatical structures used to generate relative clauses.

Zukowski's work illustrates that, as with all questions of competence and performance, one must be careful to test for the target cognitive function in a way that gives the child his or her "best shot" at being correct. Given the degree of specificity and rich structure required to produce a grammatically correct sentence with a complex relative clause, it would be virtually impossible to generate such a sentence unless the grammatical system were functioning properly. Of course, no cognitive function can ever be completely isolated from the processes that interact with it—we depend on performances to infer competence. This means that, depending on what task we give the child, different competencies might be inferred. Clearly, to discover whether a knowledge system is intact, it is crucial to tap into the system with minimal extraneous demands.

Spatial Language in General. Several reports have hinted that spatial language in people with WBS is impaired. The evidence from these reports is sparse. Using the TROG, Karmiloff-Smith et al. (1997) examined the items that tap comprehension of spatial and other relational terms: longer/bigger/taller, in/on, and above/below. Error for these items was 27.0% for longer/bigger/taller, 14.5% for in/on, and 27.9% for above/below. It is unclear how to interpret these results. Compared with the extremely poor performance on "complex grammatical" items such as embedded clauses (e.g., *The book the pencil is on is red;* 67.9% errors), the spatial items look like strengths. But compared with performance on "simple" grammatical items, such as two-element combinations (e.g., *The dog is sitting;* 1.3% errors), the spatial items look like weaknesses. Aside from this problem, the spatial test items in the TROG cannot be regarded as a serious estimate of spatial language in WBS, because they test comprehension of single terms in single, often ambiguous contexts rather than systematically examining the spatial distribution of the use of a given term (e.g., Landau and Hoffman 2005).

Bellugi and colleagues (2000) reported that children with WBS were more likely than normally developed children to switch figure and ground objects in their sentences—for example, saying *The bowl is in the apple* rather than *The apple is in the bowl.* Unfortunately, interpretations of such performance are open to the same difficulties we observed for relative clauses. Errors on figure/ground assignment could reflect misassignment of semantic roles to their syntactic positions, or they could reflect misalignment of the elements of the sentence during the process of production (Bock and Levelt 1994). The former would reflect a damaged part of the linguistic system, whereas the latter would reflect missteps in the coordination of separate processes involved in production. Without systematic testing, it is impossible to tell which interpretation is correct.

Our strategy in examining spatial language has been to look both broad and deep. We have been examining spatial language broadly by looking at the language that expresses the locations of objects (*above, below, near, far,* etc.) (Zukowski et al. 1999; Landau and Hoffman 2005), the language that expresses the locations of object parts within objects (*top, bottom, side,* etc.) (B. Landau and N. Kurz, unpublished results), and the language that expresses motion events, in which objects move through space over paths (Landau and Zukowski 2003; Lakusta and Landau 2005). Here we focus on motion events, but the findings are similar to those in our other studies of spatial language. They suggest that much (if not all) of the structure of spatial language is spared in WBS and that unusual patterns of performance reflect the operation of nonlinguistic systems as they interact with language.

The Language of Motion Events. English, like other languages, expresses motion events through multiple pieces of structure that combine to express the entire event. According to widely cited linguistic theories, English expresses the motion event by encoding (1) the *figure,* or object that moves, by a noun phrase; (2) the *motion* itself, usually by a verb; (3) the *path* over which the object moves, usually by a preposition; and (4) the *ground,* or *reference* object, for the moving object, another noun phrase (Talmy 1983). For example, in *The dog jumped off the fence,* the *dog* is figure, the *fence* is reference object, *jump* expresses the motion, and *off* expresses the path—one in which the dog moves away from the reference object.

The acquisition of each type of component is complex. For example, expression of each component requires that the child perceive the component (object, motion, path) accurately and then encode it correctly in language. This parsing of the event into motion/manner and path complex differs across languages, so part of the child's task is to determine just how to parse the event for his or her native language. In addition, there are spatial constraints on the expression of path. Linguistically, paths can be divided into three types: *to, from,* and *via* paths (Jackendoff 1983), and different prepositions are appropriate to each path type. Finally, in each path type, the preposition selects for the type of reference object. Some prepositions choose for "container-like" objects (e.g., *in, into*), whereas others choose "surface-like" reference objects (e.g., *on, off*) These constraints function to narrow down which preposition is the correct one for expressing any particular path. In sum, linguistically expressing a motion event requires accurate perception of the event, accurate parsing into the correct elements, and accurate choice of path terms on the basis of spatial and linguistic constraints.

We investigated how much of this structure is available to children and adults with WBS by showing people a set of eighty motion events, in which figures underwent a variety of motions over a variety of paths, and asking, "What happened?" (Landau and Zukowski 2003; Lakusta and Landau 2005). We found that the children with WBS named both figure and reference ob-

Table 9.1.
Twelve Most Frequent Specific Verbs of Motion Used by Children with Williams-Beuren Syndrome and by Control Subjects (percentage use) (after Landau and Zukowski 2003)

Normal Adults		Control Children		Children with WBS	
Verb	%	Verb	%	Verb	%
fall	26.6	fall	31.0	fall	28.1
jump	14.7	jump	17.2	jump	12.7
fly	9.1	fly	11.3	fly	11.5
hop	7.1	hop	7.5	hop	5.6
walk	5.6	walk	4.5	walk	7.3
roll	4.4	roll	5.5	roll	4.2
drive	4.2	drive	1.5	drive	1.9
slide	3.8	slide	1.9	flip	4.4
make a turn	2.6	run	1.4	turn	3.8
spin	1.5	go in "L"	1.5	zigzag	3.5
back up	2.3	ride	1.4	run	2.9
bounce	1.8	bump	1.4	bounce	1.9
Totals	83.7		86.1		87.9

jects with the same nouns used by both other groups. We also found that children with WBS used almost exactly the same manner-of-motion verbs as the normal controls. Table 9.1 shows the top twelve verbs used by each group and their proportions of use. The children accurately perceived the objects and motions and correctly encoded them in language. Given the variety of motion types, we find it especially impressive that children with WBS were able to select the correct verbs.

Overall, expression of the path was also done accurately—the appropriate path term was chosen in most cases, and an impressive variety of path terms was produced (Landau and Zukowski 2003). The selection of path term types—*to, from,* and *via*—by children with WBS matched that of the normally developed controls and adults, indicating that the children correctly determined whether the path itself was most felicitously expressed in terms of its goal, source, or the intermediate (for *via* paths). The only place where we found a difference between children with WBS and the controls was in *whether* the path complex was expressed: *to* paths were almost always expressed by all groups, but both *via* and *from* path types and their reference objects were frequently omitted by children with WBS. For example, if the motion event showed a girl moving past a block, the child with WBS was more likely than the controls to indicate the girl and her movement but not the block (e.g., *The girl was walking*). Or, if the event showed a block falling off a swing, the child was more likely to indicate the block and its motion but no reference object (e.g., *The block fell* or *The block fell off,* but rarely *The block fell off the swing*). Thus, the difference amounted to simply omitting the path complex and/or the reference object alone in events that displayed *via* or *from* path types.

How can we explain this difference? First, note that, although the effect was quite specific, it was reliable. Second, the effect did *not* result in ungrammatical sentences, given that specifying the path complex for such events is linguistically an option. Third, all the pertinent grammatical and semantic structure in the sentences was preserved, showing that children with WBS had control over the linguistic expression of motion events. Hence, the problem in production of *from* paths does not lie with knowledge of language.

Rather, we suggest that the selective omission of path complex in *via* and *from* path types may reflect a fragility in retaining information about the event that is less salient or important to the observer. Specifically, when observers view the motion events, the most salient aspect of the event is the figure object's motion. In cases of *to* paths, the figure moves to end up at the reference object, and in these cases the children with WBS preserved the entire path complex, producing both path and reference object. But in *via* and *from* path types, the figure moves away from or past the reference object and is not spatially coincident with the reference object at the end of the event, when the observer must describe it. In these cases, it seems natural that the observer would either focus only on the moving figure object or might even forget what the reference object was and what path was traversed. People with WBS are known to have fragile visuospatial memories (Jarrold et al. 1999; Wang and Bellugi 1994; Vicari et al. 1996). Therefore, it seems possible that they might have greater difficulty holding in mind these aspects of the event over time. Because the focus of the vulnerability seems to be "sources" (the reference objects located at the beginning of *from* path events), we call it "source vulnerability."

If our hypothesis is correct, the tendency to drop the path complex should be correlated with weaker visuospatial memory. Moreover, this interpretation implies that the weakness is not linguistic per se—there is nothing abnormal about the nature of the linguistic system but only as it interacts with visuospatial memory. Thus, we should be able to create circumstances where *from* path types are produced more easily and regularly. Finally, our interpretation places the vulnerability in the nonlinguistic system that is responsible for representing and storing events. If we are right, we should see the reflex of a "source vulnerability" in nonlinguistic representations of events. Such vulnerability should definitely show up in people with WBS, but it may also be a characteristic of normal event representation and, if so, should appear in the performance of normally developing children and adults. Recent data show this to be the case (Lakusta and Landau 2005).

Summary: Specialization and Sparing

Our research suggests strong sparing and preservation of structure in WBS in three domains: object representation, biological motion perception, and spatial language. In each case, we have taken pains to test people's capacity under stringent conditions that allow us to determine whether the structures underlying normal representations are spared. The findings show that structural properties of these spatial representations are indeed intact. Given these strengths, we can now ask why people with WBS show such severe spatial breakdown in the block construction task.

Revisiting the Block Construction Task: Why the Deficit?

Subjects can show poor performance in the block task for a variety of reasons. Earlier, we speculated that errors in construction tasks could be attributed broadly to two different sources: (1) executive processes that are required for planning and maintaining information in working memory and (2) spatial-perceptual processes that construct and manipulate representations of objects and their spatial relationships. Impairment in the first kind of process is a plausible source of errors in people with WBS, who may have impaired frontal lobe functions (Atkinson et al. 2003) and are moderately mentally retarded. Impairment in the second would be expected on the assumption that WBS selectively impairs spatial capacities. The problem with the block task is that, if we examine only the final outcome of the task, these two factors are inextricably woven together. A deeper understanding of the locus of any deficits can come only through a careful analysis of the task's requirements and decomposition of these into underlying mental processes (see Hoffman et al. 2003 for a full report of this analysis).

A Model for Thinking about Construction Tasks

We assume that insight can be gained into the locus of deficits by examining people's puzzle solutions on a micro-time line—looking at when and how people move individual blocks and where they look during this process. To understand the kinds of insight such an analysis can provide, we turn to the work of Ballard et al. (1997), who studied eye movements of normally developed adults while they solved block construction puzzles such as those shown in figure 9.6. In this task, people have to duplicate a *model* by moving

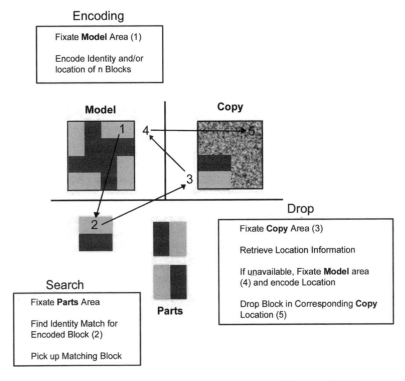

Fig. 9.6. Example of a block construction puzzle, including the model (upper left), the parts bin (lower panel), and the copy area (upper right). *Source:* Hoffman et al. 2003. "Spatial breakdown in . . . ," *Cognitive Psychology* 46(3): 260–301. Reprinted with permission from Elsevier.

blocks from a *parts* area to a *copy* area—much as subjects with WBS must do when confronted with the hallmark block assembly task in the DAS. Intuition suggests that normal, healthy adults might solve such a puzzle by first glancing at the model, then memorizing the identities and locations of several blocks, and then rapidly moving the corresponding parts into place. After this has been done perhaps one or two times, the copy would be complete. Assuming that people can accurately represent the identity of each block and its location, the copy would also be correct.

Surprisingly, Ballard et al. found that observers did not solve the puzzle in this way. Rather, people tended to look at the model *each time* they moved a single block. In fact, subjects often looked at the model *twice* before placing each block—the first time, apparently, to get the *identity* of the block (then picking it up from the parts area) and the second time to determine its *location* (then moving it into its position in the copy area). As Ballard and colleagues point out, subjects who use this two-prong strategy seem to be minimizing the amount of information they must hold in working memory, using the model as a kind of external source that they can continually revisit and eliminating the need to store in working memory multiple block identities and multiple locations of blocks in the puzzle.

By examining the relationship between where people looked and the actions they took (e.g., picking up a block in the parts area, placing it in the copy, removing a piece from the copy), Ballard and colleagues made otherwise covert executive processes amenable to study. We believe their analysis also suggests that failure at copying, such as occurs in people with WBS, could arise at any of several points during the process of constructing a copy. For example, if individuals with WBS have faulty *executive mechanisms* (the mechanisms that might help in planning while solving these puzzles), many of the processes uncovered by Ballard et al. should show impairment. It is executive mechanisms that guide people's sequence of fixations on the different regions of the problem space (the model area, the parts area, the copy area) as they encode the identity and location of model parts, search the parts area, and place blocks in the copy area. Executive processes also determine when a person should check for errors (reflected in back-and-forth fixations between copy and model) and attempt needed repairs. These executive processes can be examined by analyzing the person's sequence of eye fixations across different regions of the problem space, both while placing blocks and while attempting to initiate any repairs.

In addition, if WBS specifically targets *spatial representations,* people with WBS might fail because they cannot create and maintain a representation of the identity and location of the pieces. This problem may be particularly acute for the kind of puzzle shown in figure 9.6, in which the pieces consist of parts in various spatial arrangements. For example, the block in the upper left of the model needs to be represented as something like "a vertical orientation with the dark part on the right." The location of the block in the complete puzzle needs to be represented as "upper left section of the puzzle." If subjects with WBS have trouble representing these kinds of *spatial* relationships, they will often choose incorrect parts and/or place them in incorrect locations in the copy (Key et al. 1998). In separating these two kinds of processes, we can determine whether the deficit is due to executive mechanisms, spatial representations, or some interaction of the two.

Experimental Findings

We examined the eye fixations of children with WBS, MA-matched controls, and normally developed adults while they solved puzzles such as those shown in figure 9.6. Subjects used the computer mouse to select and move parts into a copy area to duplicate a model that was continuously visible on the screen. The copy area contained placeholders for the blocks, which "snapped into place" if they were dropped close to the correct position. Thus global shape errors or "broken configurations" were eliminated as a source of errors.

Normally developing MA-matched controls correctly solved more puzzles than children with WBS, and the difference increased as the puzzles became larger and more complex. For example, children with WBS correctly solved only 15% of the most complex puzzles, compared with 50% for controls. In addition, we found that the controls were more accurate on their *individual block drops* during the complex construction task. This already suggests that errors are made during the construction process, block by block.

The low accuracy of children with WBS, however, was not attributable to faulty executive processes. For smaller puzzles (two and three pieces), all three groups fixated the model equally often, showing that the children with WBS looked back and forth between model and copy normally when the puzzle was relatively simple. For the larger puzzles, both the adults and the control children increased their fixations on the model relative to the simple puzzles, whereas the children with WBS showed a precipitous drop, being much less likely to consult the model—which could easily lead to poor performance. We believe, however, that this reduction in model fixation was a *result* rather than a cause of poor accuracy on these problems. First, drop accuracy was not directly related to degree of model fixation: it was approximately the same whether the individual drops were or were not preceded by fixations on the model. For example, children with WBS fixated the model approximately 95% of the time before their first drop in the nine-piece puzzles and their drop accuracy was 47% (chance was approximately 32%). On the remaining drops, their fixation rate dropped to 48% and their accuracy fell to 41%—only a 6% difference. In other words, their accuracy was low on these puzzles regardless of the degree to which they fixated the model, so the decrease in fixation did not cause poorer performance per se. Rather, for the larger puzzles, the children with WBS seemed to adopt a strategy of moving pieces randomly into the copy area in the hope of creating a correct copy by chance—resulting in poor performance.

We examined other executive processes by looking at the children's error-detection and repair procedures. Again, the children with WBS and both control groups were quite similar, checking their *final* solutions at the same rate. So, when the children with WBS completed a puzzle, they knew they should check their copy against the model for accuracy. Children in the control group also frequently checked their *partial* solutions as they moved through the construction process, which is a reasonable strategy, given the high probability of an error on each drop. Children with WBS, however, checked their partial solutions less often, consistent with our suggestion that they were more likely to attempt a random generation of the puzzle solutions, followed by checking. Finally, both groups of children were unlikely to attempt repairs on correct puzzles, showing that they knew which of their solutions were correct and which were not. For subjects with WBS, 96% of their repair attempts were directed at *incorrect* puzzles. The corresponding figure for controls was 92%. Thus, both groups seemed to recognize when their copies corresponded to the model.

These findings indicate that poor overall performance by children with WBS is not due to impaired executive processes that guide the pickup of information from the model. First, the children accurately solved smaller puzzles by using eye fixations similar to those used by the control children. Second, they checked complete copies and could determine when their copy was wrong, accurately initiating repair procedures. The only ways in which they differed from control children were the degree to which they fixated the model for the most complex puzzles and the degree to which they fixated the model as they moved through the construction process—that is, after partial solutions. Both of these differences may result from their being aware of their own deficit—most strikingly present for the most complex and largest puzzles—and, under these circumstances, they simply adopt a new strategy in which they attempt to solve the puzzle by placing pieces randomly, hoping for some accuracy.

What about deficits in spatial representations? We carried out two experiments to evaluate these. In the *matching* task, the four- and nine-piece puzzles from the first experiment were presented along with a cue (i.e., a disk in the center of a randomly chosen block in the model). Subjects were to choose the block in the parts area that matched the single cued block. Overall, subjects with WBS were correct only 46% of the time, compared with 81% for MA-matched controls. Thus, the subjects with WBS are severely impaired in a task that reduces much of the strategic complexity of the block construction task and depends primarily on representing and matching block identity.

Similarly, the *location* task was designed to evaluate the ability of children to represent the location of blocks in the model without the complexity of the full puzzle. Models were presented with a cue on just one of the blocks, subjects were given a single block, and they had to place this into the copy location corresponding to the cued location in the model. Overall, subjects with WBS were correct on 80% of the trials, compared with 97% for controls. This result suggests that the subjects with WBS are also impaired in representing the location of the block in the model.

As these two experiments indicate, children with WBS are impaired in representing spatial relationships that are important for *identifying* the blocks in the model and coding their *locations*. These impairments seem to be sufficient to account for much of the observed deficit in block construction, because people seem to solve these puzzles "one block at a time" by coding the identity and location of individual blocks. The finding that children with WBS seemed to be good at recognizing whether their copies were correct suggests that, contrary to some reports, their perception of global shape may be intact.

In summary, the results of our microanalysis of the block construction task show, first, that the executive processes used to search for information, check copies against the model, and initiate repairs are all intact in children with WBS. Where they differ dramatically from normally developing MA-matched children is in the quality of their representations of the blocks themselves and of the spatial relationships among them in the model. Their inability to choose the correct matching block and their difficulties in placing even a single block in the copy space reveal a real fragility in the spatial representations that must be engaged during this highly complex task.

This fragility needs to be more precisely characterized, a task in which we are now engaged. One question that arises is why the children perform so poorly in the simple block matching task when they do so well on demanding object recognition and identification tasks (as discussed earlier in the chapter). One possibility is that the complexity of familiar everyday objects is different from the complexity of the blocks used in the construction task. In particular, the key property of the blocks and their distractors is asymmetry. The *target* blocks in the standard construction task are vertically, horizontally, or diagonally asymmetric by color (e.g., split right/left, top/bottom, or top-left/right-bottom, by color). The *distractor* blocks in the full construction task and in the matching task are also vertically, horizontally, or diagonally asymmetric by color. Thus, accuracy on the matching task requires that the subject note the color relationships of the target (i.e., how the block is split, and which side has which color) and match it to another, disregarding blocks that are split differently and those that are split the same but with colors in a mirror-image relationship to the target.

Inspection of all children's errors in the matching task shows that their errors are overwhelmingly choices of the mirror-image mates to the target. For example, given a black/white block split horizontally (black on top, white on bottom), all children may erroneously choose the black/white horizontal split with reversed colors—but rarely the vertically or diagonally split blocks. However, children with WBS make more such errors than MA-matched controls. In addition, the errors are predominantly made on diagonally split blocks, followed by horizontals and verticals in equal proportion. Again, children with WBS make more such errors, but the error types are the same as in normally developing MA-matched children.

Possibly, one locus of deficit in WBS lies in a highly specific characteristic of object recognition that engages the capacity to differentiate mirror-image reversals. Add to this the fact that even our simple matching task requires some degree of visuospatial memory (as one moves from the model to the block choices), and we suggest that the deficit in WBS taps into fragile mirror-image relationships that are further weakened over time.

The fragility in placing single blocks into the copy raises yet other questions. Why should this task be a problem, given the strength seen in recruitment of spatial relationships in other circumstances, such as the description of spatial motion events? We do not yet have an answer, but ongoing experiments in our lab are designed to provide greater detail on how spatial relationships are represented by people with WBS. Some evidence suggests that, as in the case of objects and blocks, specific kinds of relationships may be particularly hard to represent and may undergo rapid decay whenever the task requires any retention in memory.

In sum, we have placed the burden of the deficit in the block construction task on spatial representations and not on the executive processes that control the viewer's selection and use of information. We should also point out that the two aspects of cognition interact in a clear but complex way. As noted above, the executive processes seem remarkably intact for simple puzzles in children with WBS, but with larger (more complex) puzzles, the children seem to adopt a different kind of strategy. Specifically, they no longer consult the model as frequently as with simple puzzles and seem to merely place blocks in the puzzle with no rhyme or reason, hoping for a solution to appear. This strategy is also used by normally developing children when working with more complex puzzles, but the difference is that, for these children, (1) the overall accuracy for individual blocks is much higher and (2) the children check partial solutions more frequently than do children with WBS. The upshot is that normally developing children can correct more frequently along the way and, when they do, they are more often accurate in their corrections, leading to an overall performance that greatly outstrips that of the children with WBS. Thus, although the executive processes of the children with WBS are normal, they are derailed when the puzzles become too difficult. In this way, the complexity of the full block construction puzzle and the striking performance deficits seen in WBS reveal a complex sequence in which a persistent deficit in representing spatial relationships can derail other mechanisms, leading to downward-spiraling performance.

Clinical Implications

Although our work is not applied research, our findings may well have important implications for the treatment and education of people with Williams-Beuren syndrome. One clear implication of our results is that WBS is not characterized by monolithic spatial impairment. We have found remarkable sparing of spatial representational capacities in three separate domains: object representation, biological motion, and spatial language. To the extent that clinicians can build on spared aspects of spatial cognition, they may find ways to help people with WBS compensate for their impairments. The result would be more effective treatment and education.

Our findings may also help in understanding the exact nature of the WBS impairment, further elucidating treatment and education possibilities. Like other researchers, we have found striking shortcomings among children with WBS in the hallmark task of block construction. However, we have also been able to distinguish between the executive (i.e., planning) processes that are used in the task and the spatial representations used to identify blocks and place them in locations. We suggest that only the latter are severely impaired in WBS but that this impairment interacts with executive processes as the puzzles become more complex. Children are aware of their difficulties and so shift executive strategies to essentially abandon what they recognize to be futile strategies of information search. Furthermore, the block task taps many spatial functions, including visual memory for objects and locations, planning ability, and motor control. It also requires maintenance of an overall "plan" that allows periodic checking between a partially constructed model and the final production. As we have pointed out, things can go wrong for the individual with WBS at any point along the route to final solution of the puzzle, and failure does not necessarily indicate failure at all levels. This puts the failure in a new perspective and suggests that the focus for researchers should be to discover more precisely what characterizes the deficit in representing certain kinds of spatial relationships.

Understanding the nature of spatial strengths and deficits in WBS should have implications for treatment and intervention. For example, perhaps we can take advantage of the plasticity of brain connections to provide targeted training that would gradually produce improvement in those brain circuits that are deficient in WBS. Tallal et al. (1996) produced rapid improvement in language-learning impaired children by requiring them to discriminate temporal information in synthetic speech. This training was given in the context of a computer game in which the temporal information was easy to discriminate but became progressively more difficult over time. Presumably, perceptual learning produced changes in neural networks responsible for processing the rapid changes that occur in human speech, and these changes were manifest as improvements in comprehending speech. Subsequent applications of this approach to dyslexia (Temple et al. 2003) resulted in improved reading performance, and the authors observed training-induced changes in language-related brain areas on functional magnetic resonance imaging.

This approach depends on having a good understanding of the underlying causes of any given deficit, which would allow a targeted training regimen to be designed. Therefore, an important goal in research on people with WBS is to achieve a detailed understanding of the nature of their spatial deficits and strengths.

Future Directions

The next ten years of research should emphasize three themes. One is the study of highly specialized spatial and cognitive systems to gain a greater understanding of what is spared. We would especially like to see a serious study of domains that, like the spatial domain, are likely to reflect inherent characteristics of the human brain and mind. Such domains include knowledge of objects, causality, number, and music. If basic structural aspects of the architecture of these knowledge domains are shown to be spared in WBS, we will have ample evidence for the idea that this syndrome does not compromise the qualitative nature of knowledge. Additionally, the survival of some aspects of spatial cognition in people with WBS is a testament to its robust nature and to the likelihood that these aspects of cognition emerge naturally in development, despite genetic deficit. To the extent that other, nonspatial domains follow this pattern, we will have stronger evidence that genetic syndromes need not impinge on basic cognitive architecture. These findings would be important for studies of WBS and, equally, for our scientific theories of human cognition.

The second theme is the need to determine just what goes wrong in WBS cognition. This may be a very difficult task, especially given the inherent complexity of any cognitive task in any domain. However, by investigating fundamental representations and mechanisms—such as visuospatial memory and attention—we might be able to develop a model that speaks to both the strengths and the weaknesses of the WBS cognitive profile. To use spatial cognition as an example, we have shown that the cognitive processes that are specific to functions such as object recognition and biological motion perception (for example) are preserved. Yet, it is possible that the WBS cognitive system might break down quite rapidly as pressure from memory and/or attentional requirements increases. Such breakdown would reflect greater fragility under stress but not a different cognitive architecture.

The final theme is the importance of studying learning itself in people with WBS. Until now, researchers' major task has been to document the pattern of strengths and weaknesses in an attempt to firmly establish the nature of the cognitive profile. Crucial questions about this profile may be answered by studying how people with WBS learn. Because learning has both theoretical and applied ramifications, this theme may be the most important of all.

ACKNOWLEDGMENTS

The research reported here was supported in part by grants 12-FY970670, FY980194, FY0187, and FY0446 from the March of Dimes Foundation and BCS 9808585 and BCS 0117744 from the National Science Foundation. We thank the children and families who have participated in our research and, especially, the Williams Syndrome Association, which has provided unflagging support for our research endeavor.

REFERENCES

Atkinson, J., King, J., Braddick, O., Nokes, L., Anker, S., and Braddick, F. 1997. A specific deficit of dorsal stream function in Williams' syndrome. *NeuroReport* 8:1919–1922.
Atkinson, J., Braddick, O., Anker, S., Curran, W., Andrew, R., Braddick, F., and Wattam-Bell, J. 2003. Neurobiological models of visuo-spatial cognition in children with Williams syndrome: Measures of dorsal-stream and frontal function. *Developmental Neuropsychology* 23:139–172.
Ballard, D. H., Hayhoe, M. M., Pook, P. K., and Rao, R. P. N. 1997. Deictic codes for the embodiment of cognition. *Behavioral and Brain Sciences* 20:723–767.
Beery, K. E., and Buktenica, N. A. 1967. *Developmental Test of Visual-Motor Integration.* Cleveland: Modern Curriculum Press.
Bellugi, U., Marks, S., Bihrle, A., and Sabo, H. 1988. Dissociation between language and cognitive functions in Williams syndrome. In *Language development in exceptional circumstances,* ed. D. Bishop and K. Mogford, 177–189. Hillsdale, NJ: Erlbaum.
Bellugi, U., Bihrle, A., Neville, H., Doherty, S., and Jernigan, T. L. 1992. Language, cognition, and brain organization in a neurodevelopmental disorder. In *Developmental behavioral neuroscience: The Minnesota Symposia on Child Psychology,* ed. M. Gunnar and C. Nelson, 201–232. Hillsdale, NJ: Erlbaum.
Bellugi, U., Wang, P. P., and Jernigan, T. L. 1994. Williams syndrome: An unusual neuropsychological profile. In *Atypical cognitive deficits in development disorders: Implications for brain function,* ed. S. H. Broman and J. Grafman, 23–56. Hillsdale, NJ: Erlbaum.
Bellugi, U., Lichtenberger, L., Jones, W., Lai, Z., and St. George, M. 2000. The neurocognitive profile of Williams syndrome: A complex pattern of strengths and weaknesses. *Journal of Cognitive Neuroscience* 12 (suppl.): 7–29.

Bertrand, J., Mervis, C., and Eisenberg, J. 1997. Drawing by children with Williams syndrome: A developmental perspective. *Developmental Neuropsychology* 13:41–67.

Bihrle, A. M., Bellugi, U., Delis, D., and Marks, S. 1989. Seeing either the forest or the trees: Dissociation in visuospatial processing. *Brain and Cognition* 11:37–49.

Bishop, D. 1983. *Test for Reception of Grammar*. London: Medical Research Council.

———. 1989. *The Test for Reception of Grammar*. Published by the author.

———. 2003. *The Test for Reception of Grammar, version 2 (TROG-2)*. London: Psychological Corporation.

Bock, K., and Levelt, W. 1994. Language production: Grammatical encoding. In *Handbook of psycholinguistics*, ed. M. Gernsbacher, 945–984. San Diego: Academic Press.

Braddick, O. J., O'Brien, J. M. D., Wattam-Bell, J., Atkinson, J., and Turner, R. 2000. Form and motion coherence activate independent, but not dorsal/ventral segregated, networks in the human brain. *Current Biology* 10:731–734.

Carpenter, P. A., Just, M. A., Keller, T. A., Eddy, W. K., and Thulborn, K. 1999. Graded functional activation in the visuo-spatial system with the amount of task demand. *Journal of Cognitive Neuroscience* 11:9–24.

Cutting, J. E., Moore, C., and Morrison, R. 1988. Masking the motions of human gait. *Perception and Psychophysics* 44:339–347.

Deruelle, J., Mancini, M. O., Livel, M., Casse-Perot, C., and de Schoon, S. 1999. Configural and local processing of faces in children with Williams syndrome. *Brain and Cognition* 41:276–298.

Dilks, D., Landau, B., Hoffman, J. E., and Siegfried, J. 2001. Selective impairment of dorsal stream functions in Williams syndrome? Poster session presented at the annual meeting of the Cognitive Neuroscience Society, New York.

Elliot, C. D. 1990. *Differential Ability Scales*. San Diego: Harcourt, Brace, Jovanovich.

Farah, M. J. 2000. *The cognitive neuroscience of vision*. Malden, MA: Blackwell.

Georgopoulos, M. A., Georgopoulos, A. P., Kurz, N., and Landau, B. 2004. Figure copying in Williams syndrome and normal subjects. *Experimental Brain Research* 157:137–146.

Hoffman, J. E., Landau, B., and Pagani, B. 2003. Spatial breakdown in spatial construction: Evidence from eye fixations in children with Williams syndrome. *Cognitive Psychology* 46:260–301.

Jackendoff, R. 1983. *Semantics and cognition*. Cambridge: MIT Press.

Jarrold, C., Baddeley, A., and Hewes, A. 1999. Genetically dissociated components of working memory: Evidence from Down's and Williams syndrome. *Neuropsychologia* 37:637–651.

Johansson, G. 1973. Visual perception of biological motion and a model for its analysis. *Perception and Psychophysics* 14:201–211.

Jordan, H., Reiss, J. E., Hoffman, J. E., and Landau, B. 2002. Intact perception of biological motion in the face of profound spatial deficits: Williams syndrome. *Psychological Science* 13:162–167.

Karmiloff-Smith, A., Grant, J., Berthoud, I., Davies, M., Howlin, P., and Udwin, O. 1997. Language and Williams syndrome: How intact is "intact"? *Child Development* 68:246–262.

Key, A. F., Pani, J. R., and Mervis, C. B. 1998. Visuospatial constructive ability of people with Williams syndrome. Paper presented at the Sixth Annual Workshop on Object Perception and Memory, Dallas, TX.

Kramer, J. J., Bulusewicz, M. J., Kaplan, E., and Preston, K. A. 1991. Visual hierarchical analysis of block design configural errors. *Journal of Clinical and Experimental Neuropsychology* 13:455–465.

Lakusta, L., and Landau, B. 2005. Starting at the end: The importance of goals in spatial language. *Cognition* 96:1–33.

Lakusta, L., Licona, R., and Landau, B. 2002. Interaction between spatial representation and spatial language: The language of events. Paper presented at the Boston University Conference on Language Development, Boston.

Landau, B. 2001. Perceptual units and their mapping with language. In *From fragments to objects: Segmentation and grouping in vision,* ed. T. F. Shipley and P. J. Kellman, 71–118. New York: Elsevier.

———. 2002. Spatial cognition. In *Encyclopedia of the human brain,* ed. V. Ramachandran, 395–418. San Diego: Academic Press.

Landau, B., and Hoffman, J. E. 2005. Parallels between spatial cognition and spatial language: Evidence from Williams syndrome. *Journal of Memory and Language* 53(2):163–185.

Landau, B., Hoffman, J. E., and Kurz, N. 2005. Object recognition with severe spatial deficits in Williams syndrome: Sparing and breakdown. *Cognition,* in press.

Landau, B., and Jackendoff, R. 1993. "What" and "where" in spatial language and spatial cognition. *Behavioral and Brain Sciences* 16:217–265.

Landau, B., and Zukowski, A. 2003. Objects, motions, and paths: Spatial language in children with Williams syndrome. *Developmental Neuropsychology* 23:105–138.

Mervis, C. B., Morris, C. A., Bertrand, J., and Robinson, B. F. 1999. Williams syndrome: Findings from an integrated program of research. In *Neurodevelopmental disorders: Developmental cognitive neuroscience,* ed. H. Tager-Flusberg, 65–110. Cambridge: MIT Press.

Milner, A. D., and Goodale, M. A. 1995. *The visual brain in action.* New York: Oxford University Press.

Mottron, L., Belleville, S., and Menard, E. 1999. Local bias in autistic subjects as evidenced by graphic tasks: Perceptual hierarchization or working memory deficit? *Journal of Child Psychology and Psychiatry and Allied Disciplines* 40:743–755.

Newsome, W. T., and Paré, E. B. 1988. A selective impairment of motion perception following lesions of the middle temporal visual area (MT). *Journal of Neuroscience* 8:2201–2211.

Pani, J. R., Mervis, C. B., and Robinson, B. F. 1999. Global spatial organization by individuals with Williams syndrome. *Psychological Science* 10:453–458.

Tager-Flusberg, H., and Sullivan, K. 2000. A componential view of theory of mind: Evidence from Williams syndrome. *Cognition* 76:59–89.

Tallal, P., Miller, S. L., Bedi, G., Byma, G., Wang, X., Nagarajan, S., Schreiner, C., Jenkins, W. M. and Merzenich, M. M. 1996. Language comprehension in language-learning impaired children improved with acoustically modified speech. *Science* 271:81–84.

Talmy, L. 1983. How language structures space. In *Spatial orientation: Theory, research, and application,* ed. H. Pick and L. Acredolo, 225–282. New York: Plenum.

Temple, E., Deutsch, G. K., Poldrack, R. A., Miller, S. L., Tallal, P., and Merzenich, M. M. 2003. Neural deficits in children with dyslexia ameliorated by behavioral remediation: Evidence from functional MRI. *Proceedings of the National Academy of Sciences USA* 100:2860–2865.

Ungerleider, L. G., and Mishkin, M. 1982. Two cortical visual systems. In *Analysis of visual behavior,* ed. D. Ingle, M. Goodale, and R. Mansfield, 549–586. Cambridge: MIT Press.

Vicari, S., Brizzolara, D., Carlesimo, G. A., Pezzini, G., and Volterra, V. 1996. Memory abilities in children with Williams syndrome. *Cortex* 32:503–514.

Volterra, V., Capirci, O., Pezzini, G., Sabbadini, L., and Vicari, S. 1996. Linguistic abilities in Italian children with Williams syndrome. *Cortex* 32:663–677.

Wang, P. P., and Bellugi, U. 1994. Evidence from two genetic syndromes for a dissociation between verbal and visual-spatial short-term memory. *Journal of Clinical and Experimental Neuropsychology* 16:317–322.

Wang, P., Doherty, S., Rourke, S. B., and Bellugi, U. 1995. Unique profile of visuoperceptual skills in a genetic syndrome. *Brain and Cognition* 29:54–65.

Wechsler, D. 1981. *Wechsler Adult Intelligence Scale–Revised.* New York: Psychological Corporation.

Zukowski, A. 2001. Uncovering grammatical competence in children with Williams syndrome. Ph.D. diss., Boston University.

Zukowski, A., Schwartz, D., and Landau, B. 1999. Spatial language and spatial cognition: Evidence from Williams syndrome. Paper presented at the Boston University Conference on Language Development, Boston.

Social Cognition in Williams-Beuren Syndrome   10

Daniela Plesa-Skwerer, Ph.D.,

and Helen Tager-Flusberg, Ph.D.

One of the most striking and endearing aspects of children and adults with Williams-Beuren syndrome (WBS) is their distinct personality profile. People with WBS have a keen interest in people and empathic concern, and they are extremely sociable, as documented in parental anecdotes, clinical reports, and recent systematic investigations (Jones et al. 2000; Mervis and Klein-Tasman 2000). Given these characteristics, in conjunction with relatively spared language abilities, high expressiveness in verbal communication (Reilly et al. 1990), and an outgoing, affectionate, and friendly personality (Gosch and Pankau 1994), it would seem that people with WBS should be at ease navigating the social world. By adulthood, however, most individuals with WBS have experienced a history of difficulties in social interactions and in establishing and maintaining successful relationships, and many have developed high levels of anxiety and social isolation (Davies et al. 1998; Dykens and Rosner 1999; Udwin and Yule 1991).

For individuals with WBS, difficulties in making friends and in sustaining positive peer relations become apparent by middle childhood, despite an unrelenting strong interest in and affection for people manifested in their social behavior from an early age. As Dykens and Rosner (1999) have pointed out, WBS entails phenotypic complexities that "feature contradictory descriptions of social interaction" (159), such as social withdrawal, anxiety, and peer difficulties, associated with a friendly, pleasant, empathic demeanor.

Thus, recent research on the behavioral and personality profile of people with WBS has produced a complex picture, suggesting a paradoxical combination of high sociability and empathy but poor social relationships and difficulties in social functioning. To explain why such a high propensity toward social interaction results in poor social outcomes, we have been exploring various aspects of social cognition in people with WBS. In this chapter, we present findings from our ongoing research program, which involves a systematic investigation of theory of mind, or "mentalizing," abilities in children, adolescents, and adults with WBS.

Social Cognition and the Importance of "Theory of Mind" in Social Functioning

Definition and Background

Successful social interactions depend on the ability to understand other people's behavior in terms of their mental states, such as beliefs, desires, knowledge, and intentions. Social situations cannot be interpreted appropriately on the basis of overt behavior alone, without representing the mental premises underlying people's actions. Understanding people as intentional, mental beings is at the core of social cognition. The ability to interpret people's behavior within such a mentalistic explanatory framework, using a coherent, causally related set of mental constructs, is referred to in the cognitive science and developmental literature as "theory of mind" or "folk psychology" (Astington et al. 1988; Carruthers and Smith 1996; Perner 1991; Wellman 1990; Whiten 1991). At the heart of this rapidly growing area of investigation on theory of mind have been the questions of *when* and *how* children develop an understanding of people as mental beings whose actions are intentional, caused by mental states (e.g., desires, knowledge, beliefs, goals), and how children reason about the relationships among mental states, reality, and behavior.

Development of Theory of Mind

The earliest signs of social understanding appear in infancy, including preferential gaze toward people rather than objects, imitation, the ability to detect intentional behavior and biological motion, and joint attention (Baldwin and Moses 1994; Meltzoff 1995; Meltzoff and Gopnik 1993; Repacholi 1998). By the time children reach the preschool years, a *representational* understanding of mind emerges in typical development. Holding a representational theory of mind involves the ability to explain and predict human actions by inferring the contents of people's mental states and understanding that mental states can be different from reality and are private and subjective. The understanding that a person's behavior can be predicted or explained on the basis of the person's belief about a situation, which may differ from reality (i.e., a false belief), has been considered a hallmark of a representational theory of mind.

Other types of evidence for a mentalistic construal of persons that emerges in the preschool years consist of children's capacity to use mental states to explain human action (Bartsch and Wellman 1989), ability to use information about a person's perceptual access or knowledge to judge whether an action was intended or accidental (Schult and Wellman 1997; Pillow 1988), and preference for psychological explanations over behavioral descriptions of action scenarios (Lillard and Flavell 1990). These abilities are the main ingredients of a basic theory of mind and have been shown to develop over several years in typically developing children, usually between two and five years of age.

More advanced theory of mind abilities continue to develop through middle childhood and adolescence. By the age of six years, children can begin to reason about one person's thoughts about another person's thoughts or beliefs, which constitutes second-order reasoning (Perner 1988; Perner and Wimmer 1985; Sullivan et al. 1994). Further developments in theory of mind, which take place during middle childhood and early adolescence, include the capacity to use information about personality traits to predict how a person might behave in a new situation or to judge the morality of people's actions based on the intentionality of their behavior (Mant and Perner 1988; Pillow 1991; Yuill and Pearson 1998). Other social cognitive skills related to more advanced theory of mind developments are reflected in the ability to interpret the meaning of utterances in communication by taking into account the speaker's and listener's mental states. This includes being able to distinguish between surface form and intended meaning in communication by appropriately interpreting nonliteral, figurative language; distinguishing between mistakes and lies, or lies and jokes; and understanding irony and sarcasm (Happé 1993; Leekam 1990; Sullivan et al. 1995). Thus, reasoning about social situations while using increasingly advanced social concepts is the result of a complex process that develops over an extended period and builds on the achievements of the first few years, when a basic understanding of the connections between behavior and simple mental states such as desires and beliefs emerges. Given the complexity and temporal course of developing theory of mind abilities, it is also essential to take a developmental approach to the study of social cognition in atypical populations.

Current Perspectives

In current research, there is a consensus that theory of mind encompasses more than just a representational concept of mind. This broader conceptualization has led to new models, which propose that theory of mind is composed of several interacting components, each associated with distinct underlying mechanisms for processing different aspects of social information. One important distinction in theory of mind is between basic *social perceptual* and *social cognitive* components (Tager-Flusberg 2001; Tager-Flusberg and Sullivan 2000). The perceptual component refers to the direct, immediate judgment of a person's mental state, based on information available in faces, voices, and body postures and movements. The cognitive component refers to our capacity to make more complex cognitive inferences about the content of mental states that require integrating information across time and events. Support for this model may be taken from a variety of sources, including developmental and neurobiological research.

The social perceptual component of theory of mind builds on the innate preferences of infants to attend to human social stimuli, especially faces and voices and body gestures. The perceptual component of theory of mind emerges first in development and is available to infants for making a range of mental-state judgments about other people. These immediate perceptual capacities, however, continue to develop as children become more adept at using facial and prosodic information as cues to mental state, culminating, for example, in adults' ability to make very sophisticated judgments from just the eye region of the face (Baron-Cohen et al. 1997). The development of the social cognitive component of theory of mind builds on the earlier-emerging perceptual component. The social cognitive component is involved in making mental-state inferences that depend on integrating information not only from perceptual cues but also from sequences of events over time. The social cognitive component of theory of mind is more closely linked to other cognitive or information-processing systems, such as working memory (needed for integrating information) and language, especially the ability to talk about what other people think or say. The development of the cognitive component of theory of mind begins during the early preschool years when children begin to talk and reason about epistemic states (Bartsch and Wellman 1995). It is firmly in place by four years of age, when young children are able to pass false-belief and other related tasks. More advanced social cognitive knowledge continues to develop in middle childhood and early adolescence, as described earlier. These later developments involve the integration of constructs such as belief and intention and entail more complex social reasoning and inferencing skills.

Thus, in this model, there are two components to a theory of mind, each with its own developmental time course, each dependent on different underlying mechanisms. In everyday life, the social perceptual and social cognitive capacities described here function in a complex interconnected way such that our mental-state judgments, inferences, and reasoning entail both components. At the same time, traditional theory of mind tasks tap into the social cognitive component more exclusively, by eliminating direct social cues to mental state. Our research on theory of mind in WBS has taken this dual-component model as its guide. Specifically, we have explored both the social perceptual and social cognitive components of theory of mind in WBS in an effort to understand what underlies the complex picture of social functioning in both children and adults.

Social Cognition and Theory of Mind in Williams-Beuren Syndrome

Although some researchers have been intrigued by the apparent paradox of hypersociability, empathic manner, and high emotional sensitivity coupled with difficulties in peer relations and social interactions that characterizes the WBS phenotype, few studies have examined systematically how individuals with Williams-Beuren syndrome make sense of the social world and what they understand about the mental states of other people. One early study by Karmiloff-Smith and colleagues (1995) examined theory of mind abilities in people with WBS. The majority of their participants succeeded at most of the tasks, suggesting that theory of mind may be an "islet of relatively preserved ability" (202); however, their study suffered from methodologic limitations that call into question the interpretation of these results (Tager-Flusberg and Sullivan 2000).

Our own studies designed to address the question of sparing in the domain of social cognition in WBS were guided by the following. First, we considered it important to take a developmental approach, choosing tasks appropriate for the participants' developmental level by considering both chronological and mental age. Second, we included appropriate comparison groups matched for age, language, and cognitive level that would enable a reliable assessment of different aspects of theory of mind in WBS. Third, we examined the hypothesis that social cognitive capacities may place a constraint or upper limit on the abilities of individuals with WBS to engage in peer relationships and appropriately interpret social situations. We also hypothesized that a distinction between perceptual and cognitive components of social knowledge or social intelligence may be reflected in the following profile of social information processing in WBS: a relative sparing of abilities based on direct perception of social information coupled with difficulties in the capacity to make more complex cognitive inferences about the content of people's mental states—that is, impairment in social cognitive components of theory of mind.

Basic Theory of Mind Skills in Williams-Beuren Syndrome

The first set of experiments in our research program was designed to explore perceptual and cognitive aspects of theory of mind in children with WBS. The children were generally matched to two comparison groups on age (four to ten years), IQ, and standardized language measures. The comparison groups included children with Prader-Willi syndrome (PWS), another genetically based neurodevelopmental disorder, and children with nonspecific mental retardation (MRU). Each experiment included between fifteen and twenty-five children in each group.

How well do children with WBS understand facial expressions of emotion? In one experiment, we tested their ability to discriminate and match facial expressions of basic emotions in comparison with the performance of children with PWS and MRU (Tager-Flusberg and Sullivan 2000). In a task adapted from Hobson et al. (1988), the stimuli consisted of sixteen photographs in which two men and two women portrayed the emotions *happy, sad, angry,* and *scared* in facial expressions. Children were shown four photographs of a target person displaying the four basic emotional expressions, which were first labeled by the experimenter. Then the child was given the set of photographs of the test people and asked to sort and match their facial expressions with the ones displayed by the target person.

The children with WBS performed the same as the controls in discriminating and matching facial expressions of emotion. Similar patterns of performance were found across different emotion types for all groups: children correctly matched more of the scared items than the other facial expressions and more of the happy than the angry or sad items. *Scared* and *happy* were easier to discriminate and match in all groups, which is consistent with findings from research on normally developing children (Gross and Baliff 1992). These results did not confirm our expectation of superior performance by the children with WBS. However, research on emotion matching has suggested that performance on these kinds of tasks may be mediated by language rather than nonlinguistic or social perceptual abilities. Therefore, tasks with a limited involvement of linguistic mediation might be needed as more sensitive measures of possible sparing in social perceptual capacities in people with WBS.

Another approach to assessing social affective capacities is represented by the ability to empathize with other people's emotions. Empathy is a complex process defined by sharing of the perceived emotion of another (Eisenberg 1986). Although cognitive components are involved in the capacity to understand and represent another person's emotional state, the sensitivity and inclination to respond affectively to another's emotion may depend largely on intuitive social perceptual skills and personality characteristics. Anecdotal reports and clinical behavioral descriptions of individuals with WBS had often noted their empathic concern for other people's emotional states. However, there had been no systematic investigations of empathy in people with WBS.

We compared empathy in young children with WBS and a matched group of children with PWS. We used a simulated distress procedure adapted from Sigman et al. (1992), which they used for their studies of children with autism and other developmental disorders, in which a familiar experimenter feigned hurting herself and displayed appropriate facial and vocal expressions of distress for about half a minute. Children's behavior in response to this episode was videotaped and analyzed for degree of attention (e.g., looking at or away from the experimenter), nonverbal behavior (e.g., withdrawal, comforting, helping), verbal behavior (e.g., affective comments: *You must be upset;* validating statements: *I know it hurts;* or solicitation of help: *Somebody call 911*), facial expressions of affect, and overall degree of concern.

Both the WBS and the PWS group spent about three-quarters of the time recorded looking at the experimenter, clearly observing her distress. However, the children with WBS showed significantly greater empathy as evidenced by their comforting behavior, expressions of sympathy and help, and their overall concern. A more recent study by M. L. Thomas and colleagues (unpublished observations) used the same procedure with four-year-olds and included comparison groups of normally developing children and children with other developmental delays. The children with WBS showed higher levels of empathic behavior relative to both comparison groups. The question of whether the intense empathic response of children with WBS to the distress of another person reflects a spared ability to recognize a broader range of emotional states in other people and respond to them appropriately requires further research involving other types of social situations, more comparable to the complex interactions that characterize everyday life.

A representational theory of mind involves the capacity to draw inferences that link behavior, reality, and mental states and is at the heart of social cognitive achievements in young children. As noted earlier, several different tasks have been developed to test basic theory of mind in children. Our investigations included two standard false-belief tasks (unexpected change of location and unexpected contents), an explanation-of-action task, and a task involving the attribution of intentionality.

To probe the understanding of false belief, children with WBS, PWS, and MRU were given two trials of a standard location-change task enacted with dolls and, if they did not pass both of these trials, two trials of a simpler task (Tager-Flusberg and Sullivan 2000). In one of the stories used for the standard tasks, two characters, a boy, Daniel, and his mother, put the boy's cup in the dishwasher, then the boy goes out to play. While Daniel is outside, his mother moves the cup from the dishwasher to the cupboard. To assess the children's ability to follow the stories, they were first asked memory and reality check questions to ensure recall of the main story events. The critical test questions followed, probing the child's ability to attribute knowledge to the story character (*Does Daniel know where the cup is?*) and to predict the character's behavior on the basis of false belief (*Where will Daniel look first for the cup?*). Results showed that young children with WBS were no better than the two comparison groups in their ability to attribute knowledge and to predict behavior based on false belief. On the knowledge question, significantly more of the children in the MRU group gave correct answers than the children with WBS and, on the false-belief question, significantly more of the children in both control groups than the WBS participants, indicating that children with WBS are not spared on a basic measure of theory of mind relative to other groups of children with mental retardation.

The same groups of children were given a task that required explaining a person's action by appeal to mental states, using a task developed by Tager-Flusberg and Sullivan (1994). The task consists of nine stories designed to elicit children's explanations of a person's action by appeal to desire, emotion, and cognition terms and a control set of three stories that require nonpsychological causal explanations. For instance, in one story, Sally is shown walking through the park, where she sees a dog that starts to bark. Sally then runs away. Children were asked, *Why does Sally run?* The correct response required reference to Sally's mental state, such as fear. Children's justifications of the story character's action were coded as appropriate (i.e., responses including a relevant mental-state term for the target stories and a logical causal explanation for the control stories) and inappropriate (i.e., responses that included nonpsychological explanations for the mental-state stories). Analyses showed similarities among the three groups of participants in the overall number of appropriate mental-state explanations provided for the target stories. In all groups, children provided significantly more appropriate responses for the desire and the emotion stories than for the cognition stories and, overall, provided more desire and emotion terms than cognition terms in their explanations of behavior. No significant group differences were found on any of the measures.

These findings revealed that children with WBS performed at the same level as but no better than matched comparison groups when asked to provide mental explanations for a person's action. The level of performance for all three groups was equivalent to that of typically developing preschoolers, indicating that the participants in this study performed at a level close to their mental or linguistic age rather than chronological age.

Another important ingredient of a basic theory of mind is the ability to distinguish between accidental and purposeful outcomes of actions, based on information about an agent's mental states. We used a task devised by Joseph and Tager-Flusberg (1999) to probe children's understanding of intended action as it relates to the actor's belief or knowledge state, which uses simple narratives. Children were presented with two brief stories acted out with dolls and props, in which the same outcome was the result of one intended and one accidental action. Thus, although the protagonist's action was identical in each of the stories, in one the action was intended but in the other it was the result of the protagonist's lack of perceptual access to a relevant aspect of the situation. For instance, in one story, a boy sees a puddle on the path in front of him, and in the parallel story, a girl's direction of gaze is lateral, so she cannot see the puddle straight ahead. The key difference between the stories is that the boy knows about the puddle, but the girl does not. Both stories end with the protagonist stepping in the puddle. Children were asked a knowledge question (*Who did not know that the puddle was there?*), an intention question (*Which one was trying to step in the puddle?*), a justification question (*How can you tell that the boy/girl was trying to . . . ?*), and, at the end, a perception question (*Who could see the puddle?*). Answers to the perception, knowledge, and intention questions were coded as correct or incorrect, and justification responses to the intention questions were coded into mutually exclusive categories based on whether or not they involved mental-state references in justifying the action.

On this task, the three groups of participants performed similarly, with the majority of children in all groups (70%–80%) correctly answering the perception and knowledge questions, but fewer children correctly answering the intention question. In all three groups, most children's correct intention responses were justified with non-mental-state responses, suggesting that children had significant difficulties in making judgments about intent on the basis of an agent's knowledge state, even when they showed a rudimentary understanding of goal-oriented action and could match goals to outcomes. The children with WBS were no better than the control groups in understanding the relations among perceptual access, knowledge, and intention. These difficulties in understanding intentionality may have a significantly adverse effect on the acquisition of more complex social concepts, such as learning to judge people's responsibility for their actions, understanding commitment and the moral implications of failing to keep promises, or making inferences about motives for behaviors on the basis of enduring personality traits.

Taken together, the results of these studies on basic theory of mind abilities revealed no evidence of relative sparing in the domain of social cognition for children with WBS compared with matched controls.

Advanced Theory of Mind Skills in Williams-Beuren Syndrome

By adolescence, most individuals with WBS can successfully complete the basic theory of mind tasks described above. However, further social cognitive developments that emerge during middle childhood are crucial for social adaptation, especially in forging peer relationships.

The experiments designed to probe more advanced theory of mind concepts included a second-order reasoning task, a test of the ability to distinguish between lies and jokes, and a task that involved using trait information to attribute intentionality. These tasks all draw on the types of social capacities that lead to a relatively sophisticated interpretation of social interaction. The experiments described here included adolescents with WBS, who were again compared with matched groups of adolescents with PWS and MRU.

To examine second-order reasoning by individuals with WBS and comparison groups of matched controls, we used a task developed by Sullivan and colleagues (1994) (Sullivan and Tager-Flusberg 1999). Children were presented with two stories, each involving a simple deception context in which one character intends to deceive another to conceal a gift. For example, in one story, a father wants to surprise his daughter, Molly, with her much desired birthday gift—a bike. He tells Molly that he got her a video game for her birthday; however, unbeknownst to her father, Molly discovers the bike in the garage. Later in the story, the father talks to the girl's grandmother, who asks him whether Molly knows what she is getting (second-order knowledge) and what she thinks she is getting (second-order belief). A correct response involves attributing to the father a false belief about his daughter's belief about the birthday gift (i.e., understanding that the father thinks that Molly does not know about the bike [second-order knowledge] and thinks that Molly believes she is getting a video game [second-order belief]). To ensure understanding of the story events, the child was presented with several control questions and received corrective feedback before being asked the critical test questions. Children were also asked to justify their responses to the second-order belief question. Justification responses were considered appropriate if they demonstrated an appreciation of the deception involved in the story or contained references to the characters' knowledge states and exposure to relevant information.

There were no significant differences between groups in second-order reasoning skills. For the majority of participants in all groups, the second-order knowledge question was easier than the second-order belief question. The groups also did not differ significantly in the use of different types of justifications for their correct responses on second-order belief, although about a third of the participants in all groups gave inappropriate justifications for their correct belief responses. These results underscore the fragility of second-order reasoning in children and adolescents with developmental disabilities and show that individuals with WBS are not spared in this aspect of social cognitive reasoning.

The ability to understand a speaker's intended meaning is essential for successful social communication. The interpretation of nonliteral language, such as lies and sarcasm, entails understanding the mental states of the speaker and of the listener. By middle childhood, normally developing children are able to distinguish between lies and ironic jokes (Leekam 1990; Winner and Leekam 1991), by considering the intentions and related knowledge states of the speaker. Children and adults with WBS are inclined to use colorful descriptions in their speech, including metaphors and idioms, as well as prosodic features to express the speaker's attitude in social communication. However, little is known about their ability to interpret intended meaning in nonliteral language, when they must take into account the mental states of the speaker and listener.

We investigated the ability of children and adolescents with WBS to distinguish between different forms of falsehood—lies and ironic jokes—using a task developed by Sullivan et al. (1995). Four stories were presented to the participants in two pairs of lie/joke trials (Sullivan et al. 2003). In each story, an adult knows that a child has not completed a required chore, and the child utters a factual falsehood (e.g., *I did a great job cleaning the dishes*). In two of the stories, the child does not know that the adult knows the facts (e.g., has seen the dishes unwashed); thus, the child intends to deceive and utters a *lie*. In the other two stories, the child knows that the adult has seen the facts; thus, the child's utterance is intended to be an *ironic joke*. The critical piece of information needed to interpret correctly the child's utterance as a lie or as a joke is the child-protagonist's second-order belief about the adult's knowledge of the truth.

The majority of our participants were unable to take into account the mental states of the protagonists and correctly interpret the intended meaning of the utterance. Instead, they tended to judge most of the critical utterances as lies, because the protagonist's statement did not match reality. There were no significant differences on the lie/joke task among our participants with WBS, PWS, and MRU, again suggesting that adolescents with WBS show no sparing in the ability to distinguish between different forms of nonliteral utterances and have difficulties taking into account the mental states of speaker and listener when judging intended meaning in communication. Such difficulties have potentially detrimental effects for interpreting the kinds of complex social communicative interactions that mark everyday peer relationships.

Another social cognitive skill essential for appropriately interpreting people's behavior in social situations is the ability to use trait information about a person to attribute intentionality. We devised a task in which trait information is given about a character's social or temperamental personality characteristics (e.g., kind—social/positive; mean—social/negative; cheerful—temperament/positive; shy—temperament/negative). In each of the eight stories, the main character is present when a mishap occurs (e.g., milk is spilled over a sandwich). The participant was asked to judge whether an act resulting in the mishap was intentional or not, based on trait information about the protagonist involved in the specific situation. As with the higher-order theory of mind tasks described above, the participants with WBS were equivalent to controls in using trait information to make intentionality attributions. For all groups, more of the justifications for the social trait stories than the temperament trait stories included trait information, showing that they understood that these kinds of traits are more relevant to making the intentionality attribution. However, the adolescents with WBS showed no special ability in or sensitivity to socially relevant trait information compared with either the PWS or MRU participants.

Overall, most of the participants with WBS had difficulties with higher-order social cognitive tasks. However, these difficulties were similar to those demonstrated by other groups of children with other developmental disorders, suggesting that social cognitive limitations may interfere with the acquisition of more advanced social concepts and may delay the reorganization of individuals' social knowledge after acquiring a basic ability to interpret people's behavior using mental-state information.

Social Perceptual Capacities

Most of the tasks presented above presume the capacity to make inferences about unseen mental states and place relatively high information-processing demands on the participant. If we assume that social intelligence in older individuals also involves more intuitive, social affective components that are not heavily dependent on cognitive or language abilities, it is important to examine how people with WBS perform on tasks that evaluate their social perceptual capacities.

We conducted a study comparing adults with WBS, matched adults with PWS, and age-matched normally developed adults on a task that involved direct perception of mental states expressed in the eye region of the face (Tager-Flusberg et al. 1998). The "eyes task" was developed by Baron-Cohen and colleagues (1997) as a test of social sensitivity in adults. The task consisted of twenty-five photographs of the eye region of the face of men and women, presented one a time, accompanied by two labels. The labels were mental-state terms in pairs of semantic opposites (e.g., concerned-unconcerned, friendly-hostile). The participant was asked to choose which of the two labels best described the mental-state expression in the photograph.

Compared with age-matched adults with PWS, the adults with WBS performed significantly better, and nearly half performed in the same range as normally developed adults. These results suggest sparing of social perceptual capacities in adults with WBS; however, we consider the results somewhat preliminary because of methodologic limitations in the task. Specifically, participants were given only two choices for each photograph, and the choices were usually between terms of opposite valence. Thus, a correct choice could be made just by recognizing the positive/negative valence of the expression displayed, without a real understanding of the content of the mental-state terms involved. A more sensitive test of social perceptual abilities in the format of the "eyes task" would require selecting between mental-state terms of the same valence and having more than two choices for each expression presented (Baron-Cohen et al. 2001). Clearly, more research is needed to explore sensitivity to social cues, such as emotional expressions, in adolescents and adults with WBS.

Conclusions and Clinical Implications

The apparent paradox of hypersociability and emotional sensitivity associated with difficulties in social interactions that marks the Williams-Beuren syndrome phenotype prompted us to develop a research program that focuses on the systematic investigation of the different levels and components of social capacities or theory of mind in people with WBS. Our main findings show that children and adults with WBS may demonstrate an unusual, spared capacity to empathize with others, and perhaps also to read social cues. However, they performed poorly on theory of mind tasks that involve inferring mental states as a basis for people's behavior.

Although we consider the findings from our studies on social perceptual abilities somewhat preliminary, we did find clear evidence for difficulties in social cognitive abilities that involve inferences and in attending to many pieces of information in narratives that entail characters whose mental states are relevant for interpreting knowledge, false belief, intention, or intended meaning in communication. The poor performance of the children and adolescents with WBS on theory of mind tasks might be related to attention problems, well documented in this population, that could have hindered their ability to integrate the task information and formulate an inference about the contents of others' mental states.

These findings have significant implications for considering the social difficulties of children and adults with WBS. Children with WBS often show social disinhibition, distractibility, and overfriendliness with strangers (Gosch and Pankau 1997; Sarimski 1997). They sometimes prefer to interact with adults rather than peers, and they enjoy talking, although they are not always able or inclined to adjust their conversation to the communicative interests or needs of the interlocutor (Pezzini et al. 1999). People with WBS tend to be highly expressive in their speech. Their verbal expressiveness, reflected primarily in the use of social affective and prosodic devices, is another means for engaging others in social interaction (Reilly et al. 1990). As we have noted in this chapter, both anecdotal reports and experimental investigations suggest that children and adolescents with WBS show distinctive emotional sensitivity, especially empathy toward a person in distress. However, their empathic concern and overfriendliness do not preclude difficulties with peer relations and a relatively high rate of emotional and behavioral problems (Dykens and Rosner 1999; Einfeld et al. 1997). Higher levels of anxiety compared with the general population are common in people with WBS, many of whom develop depression as adults. These mood disorders may in part be related to the accumulation of unsuccessful social experiences (Einfeld et al. 1997; Gosch and Pankau 1997; Morris and Mervis 1999).

We suggest that underlying many of these difficulties are delays in social cognitive development beyond what we would expect from the general cognitive and linguistic level of individuals with WBS. Children and adolescents with WBS have social concepts (e.g., understanding of personality traits, friendship, commitment) that are significantly less advanced than those of their normally developing peers, which makes peer relationships difficult for them and leaves them vulnerable to teasing and ridiculing by others.

Future Directions

Over the next several years, studies on social cognition will continue to explore the strengths and limitations of children, adolescents, and adults with WBS. There are still many questions to address in this important area of research:

- What are the specific sources of difficulty underlying poor performance on social cognitive tasks, such as false belief?
- Would people with WBS perform better on social cognitive tasks that involved dynamic stimuli of real people?
- What kinds of social perceptual capacities are relatively or absolutely spared in WBS?
- How well do children and adults with WBS understand emotions in other people?
- Is performance on experimental tasks that tap social cognition directly related to everyday social functioning?
- How do children and adults with WBS understand friendships?
- What are the relationships between emotional arousal, empathy, and personality in WBS, and how are they related to social adaptation?

As research begins to find answers to these and related questions, we will have a clearer understanding about the possible sources of social difficulties related to social cognition in WBS. Ultimately, the goal is to develop new behavioral and educational interventions that will improve social cognitive skills and social adaptation for children and adults with WBS. Through this kind of research, we may be better able to help guide people with WBS toward more productive and fulfilling lives, thus maximizing their adaptation in the community.

ACKNOWLEDGMENTS

The research reported here was supported by grant RO1 HD 33470 from the National Institute of Child Health and Human Development.

REFERENCES

Astington, J. W., Harris, P. L., and Olson, D., eds. 1988. *Developing theories of mind.* Cambridge: Cambridge University Press.
Baldwin, D. A., and Moses, L. J. 1994. Early understanding of referential intent and attentional focus: Evidence from language and emotion. In *Children's early understanding of mind: Origins and development,* ed. C. Lewis and P. Mitchell, 133–156. Hillsdale, NJ: Erlbaum.

Baron-Cohen, S., Jolliffe, T., Mortimore, C., and Robertson, M. 1997. Another advanced test of theory of mind: Evidence from very high-functioning adults with autism or Asperger syndrome. *Journal of Child Psychology and Psychiatry* 38:813–822.

Baron-Cohen, S., Wheelwright, S., Hill, J., Raste, Y., and Plumb, I. 2001. The "Reading the Mind in the Eyes" Test revised version: A study with normal adults, and adults with Asperger syndrome or high-functioning autism. *Journal of Child Psychology and Psychiatry* 42:241–251.

Bartsch, K., and Wellman, H. 1989. Young children's attribution of action to beliefs and desires. *Child Development* 60:946–964.

———. 1995. *Children talk about the mind.* New York: Oxford University Press.

Carruthers, P., and Smith, P. K. 1996. *Theories of theories of mind.* Cambridge: Cambridge University Press.

Davies, M., Udwin, O., and Howlin, P. 1998. Adults with Williams syndrome. *British Journal of Psychiatry* 172:273–274.

Dykens, E. M., and Rosner, B. 1999. Refining behavioral phenotypes: Personality-motivation in Williams and Prader-Willi syndromes. *American Journal on Mental Retardation* 104:158–169.

Einfeld, S., Tonge, B., and Florio, T. 1997. Behavioral and emotional disturbance in individuals with Williams syndrome. *American Journal on Mental Retardation* 102:45–53.

Eisenberg, N. 1986. *Altruistic emotion, cognition and behaviour.* Hillsdale, NJ: Erlbaum.

Gosch, A., and Pankau, R. 1994. Social-emotional and behavioral adjustment in children with Williams-Beuren syndrome. *American Journal of Medical Genetics* 52:291–296.

———. 1997. Personality characteristics and behavior problems in individuals of different ages with Williams syndrome. *Developmental Medicine and Child Neurology* 39:527–533.

Gross, A. L., and Baliff, B. 1992. Children's understanding of emotion from facial expressions and situations: A review. *Developmental Review* 11:368–398.

Happé, F. 1993. Communicative competence and theory of mind in autism: A test of relevance theory. *Cognition* 48:101–119.

Hobson, R. P., Ouston, J., and Lee, A. 1988. What's in a face? The case of autism. *British Journal of Psychiatry* 79:441–453.

Jones, W., Bellugi, U., Lai, Z., Chiles, M., Reilly, J., Lincoln, A., and Adolphs, R. 2000. Hypersociability in Williams syndrome. *Journal of Cognitive Neuroscience* 12 (suppl. 1): 30–46.

Joseph, R., and Tager-Flusberg, H. 1999. Preschool children's understanding of the desire and knowledge constraints on intended action. *British Journal of Developmental Psychology* 17:221–243.

Karmiloff-Smith, A., Klima, E., Bellugi, U., Grant, J., and Baron-Cohen, S. 1995. Is there a social module? Language, face processing and theory of mind in individuals with Williams syndrome. *Journal of Cognitive Neuroscience* 7:196–208.

Leekam, S. 1990. Jokes and lies: Children's understanding of intentional falsehood. In *Natural theories of mind: Evolution, development and simulation of everyday mindreading,* ed. A. Whiten, 159–174. Oxford: Basil Blackwell.

Lillard, A., and Flavell, J. 1990. Young children's preference for mental states versus behavioral descriptions of human action. *Child Development* 61:731–741.

Mant, C. M., and Perner, J. 1988. The child's understanding of commitment. *Developmental Psychology* 24:343–351.

Meltzoff, A. N. 1995. Understanding the intentions of others: Re-enactment of in-
    tended acts by 18-month-old children. *Developmental Psychology* 31:838–
    850.
Meltzoff, A., and Gopnik, A. 1993. The role of imitation in understanding persons
    and developing a theory of mind. In *Understanding other minds: Perspectives
    from autism*, ed. S. Baron-Cohen, H. Tager-Flusberg, and D. J. Cohen, 335–
    366. Oxford: Oxford University Press.
Mervis, C. B., and Klein-Tasman, B. P. 2000. Williams syndrome: Cognition, per-
    sonality, and adaptive behavior. *Mental Retardation and Developmental Dis-
    abilities Research Review* 6:148–158.
Morris, C. A., and Mervis, C. B. 1999. Williams syndrome. In *Handbook of neuro-
    developmental and genetic disorders in children*, ed. S. Goldstein and C. R.
    Reynolds, 555–590. New York: Guilford Press.
Perner, J. 1988. Higher-order beliefs and intentions in children's understanding of
    social interaction. In *Developing theories of mind*, ed. J. W. Astington, P. L.
    Harris, and D. R. Olson, 271–294. Cambridge: Cambridge University Press.
———. 1991. *Understanding the representational mind*. Cambridge: MIT Press.
Perner, J., and Wimmer, H. 1985. "John thinks that Mary thinks that . . .": Attribu-
    tion of second-order beliefs by 5- to 10-year-old children. *Journal of Experi-
    mental Child Psychology* 39:437–471.
Pezzini, G., Vicari, S., Volterra, V., Milani, L., and Ossella, M. T. 1999. Children with
    Williams syndrome: Is there a single neuropsychological profile? *Develop-
    mental Neuropsychology* 15:141–155.
Pillow, B. 1988. The development of children's beliefs about the mental world. *Mer-
    rill-Palmer Quarterly* 34:1–32.
———. 1991. Children's understanding of biased social cognition. *Developmental
    Psychology* 27:539–551.
Reilly, J., Klima, E., and Bellugi, U. 1990. Once more with feeling: Affect and lan-
    guage in atypical populations. *Development and Psychopathology* 2:367–391.
Repacholi, B. M. 1998. Infants' use of attentional cues to identify the referent of an-
    other person's emotional expression. *Developmental Psychology* 34:1017–
    1025.
Sarimski, K. 1997. Behavioral phenotypes and family stress in three mental retarda-
    tion syndromes. *European Child and Adolescent Psychiatry* 63:26–31.
Schult, C. A., and Wellman, H. 1997. Explaining human movements and actions:
    Children's understanding of the limits of psychological explanation. *Cogni-
    tion* 62:291–324.
Sigman, M. D., Kasari, C., Kwon, K., and Yirmiya, N. 1992. Responses to the nega-
    tive emotions of others by autistic, mentally retarded, and normal children.
    Child Development 63:796–807.
Sullivan, K., and Tager-Flusberg, H. 1999. Second-order belief attribution in
    Williams syndrome: Intact or impaired? *American Journal on Mental Retar-
    dation* 104:523–532.
Sullivan, K., Zaitchik, D., and Tager-Flusberg, H. 1994. Preschoolers can attribute
    second-order beliefs. *Developmental Psychology* 30:395–402.
Sullivan, K. Winner, E., and Hopfield, N. 1995. How children tell a joke from a lie:
    The role of second order mental state attributions. *British Journal of Devel-
    opmental Psychology* 13:191–209.
Sullivan, K., Winner, E., and Tager-Flusberg, H. 2003. Can adolescents with
    Williams syndrome tell the difference between lies and jokes? *Developmental
    Neuropsychology* 23:87–105.
Tager-Flusberg, H. 2001. A re-examination of the theory of mind hypothesis of

autism. In *The development of autism: Perspectives from theory and research,* ed. J. Burack, T. Charman, N. Yirmiya, and P. Zelazo, 173–193. Mahwah, NJ: Erlbaum.

Tager-Flusberg, H., and Sullivan, K. 1994. Predicting and explaining behavior: A comparison of autistic, mentally retarded and normal children. *Journal of Child Psychology and Psychiatry* 35:1059–1075.

———. 2000. A componential view of theory of mind: Evidence from Williams syndrome. *Cognition* 76:59–89.

Tager-Flusberg, H., Boshart, J., and Baron-Cohen, S. 1998. Reading the windows to the soul: Evidence of domain-specific sparing in Williams syndrome. *Journal of Cognitive Neuroscience* 10:631–639.

Udwin, O., and Yule, W. 1991. A cognitive and behavioral phenotype in Williams syndrome. *Journal of Clinical and Experimental Neuropsychology* 13:232–244.

Wellman, H. 1990. *The child's theory of mind.* Cambridge: MIT Press.

Whiten, A., ed. 1991. *Natural theories of mind: Evolution, development and simulation of everyday mindreading.* Oxford: Basil Blackwell.

Winner, H., and Leekam, S. 1991. Distinguishing irony from deception: Understanding the speaker's second order intention. *British Journal of Developmental Psychology* 9:257–270.

Yuill, N., and Pearson, A. 1998. The development of bases for trait attribution: Children's understanding of traits as causal mechanisms based on desire. *Developmental Psychology* 34:574–586.

Theoretical Implications of Studying Cognitive Development in Genetic Disorders

The Case of Williams-Beuren Syndrome

Annette Karmiloff-Smith, Ph.D., Daniel Ansari, Ph.D.,

Linda Campbell, B.Sc., Gaia Scerif, Ph.D.,

and Michael Thomas, Ph.D.

Some fifteen years ago, the study of certain genetic disorders seemed to offer the promise of three important theoretical outcomes: (1) the demonstration of dissociations between different cognitive functions, particularly the dissociation of language from cognition; (2) the proof of the existence of innately specified modules in the human mind; and (3) the direct mapping of mutated genes to specific impairments in higher-level cognitive modules. This initial excitement was understandable. For example, although the genes involved in autism, dyslexia, and specific language impairment had yet to be identified, the existence of a genetic component to all of these developmental disorders was well documented by twin studies (Bishop 2001). When cognitive dissociations seemed to obtain for each of these clinical groups, they were used to make sweeping claims about how the genome might prespecify the functional modularity of the human mind: a defective theory of mind module in autism (Leslie 1992; Baron-Cohen 1998), an impaired phonological module in dyslexia (Frith 1995), and a faulty grammatical module in certain forms of specific language impairment (Gopnik 1990).

But it was particularly the neurodevelopmental disorder Williams-Beuren syndrome (WBS) that attracted the attention of linguists, philosophers, psychologists, and neuroscientists and led to strong claims about cognitive dissociations, modularity, and direct genotype/phenotype mappings. Indeed, adults and older children with WBS were found to have impressively proficient language output alongside impaired general cognitive abilities. To certain researchers, this suggested a dissociation between language and general cognition, eloquently illustrated by the following statements:

> Williams syndrome presents a remarkable juxtaposition of impaired and intact mental capacities . . . linguistic functioning is preserved in

Williams syndrome while problem solving ability and visuospatial cognition are impaired (Rossen et al. 1996).

Although IQ is measured at around 50, older children and adolescents with WBS are described as hyperlinguistic with selective sparing of syntax, and grammatical abilities are close to normal in controlled testing. This is one of several kinds of dissociation in which language is preserved despite severe cognitive impairments (Pinker 1991).

And, as more became known about the genetic basis of the syndrome, direct links were heralded between specific genes and the phenotypic outcome (Frangiskakis et al. 1996).

In this chapter we argue that, in their excitement at discovering a syndrome with such an uneven cognitive profile in the phenotypic end state, researchers lost sight of one fundamental explanatory factor in both typical and atypical populations: the actual process of ontogenetic development. This lacuna is, in our view, rather general and holds for much of the work on developmental disorders. Paradoxically, even when researchers study children, they tend to fall back on the *adult* neuropsychological model of the mature brain, failing to take account of how the gradual process of development from infancy onward contributes to the phenotypic outcome (Karmiloff-Smith 1992, 1997, 1998; Thomas and Karmiloff-Smith 2003). Here, we develop this argument with respect to studies of language, social cognition, face processing, spatial cognition, and number in adults and children with WBS. We also challenge attempts at direct genotype/phenotype mappings to higher-level cognitive outcomes. We believe that such mappings will prove to be very indirect, necessitating the identification of low-level impairments in the infant and child phenotype that interact with development over time to differentially affect the adult phenotypic outcome.

The Williams-Beuren Syndrome Phenotype
in Older Children and Adults

The pioneering work of Bellugi and her collaborators first drew attention to the potential theoretical interest of the Williams-Beuren syndrome cognitive phenotype. Studies of four adolescents/young adults with WBS revealed their impressive linguistic prowess, with an ability to produce long and complex monologues sprinkled with erudite-sounding words (Bellugi et al. 1988). This proficiency with language coexisted with serious problems with nonverbal tasks, in particular those calling on spatial processing. People with WBS were shown to perform at floor level, for example, on the Benton Line Orientation Task but to score within the normal range on the Benton Face

Processing Task (Bellugi et al. 1988). This striking contrast between facial and spatial processing led researchers to claim, as they had done for language, that face processing in WBS was "intact," purporting to demonstrate, together with prosopagnosia in adult neuropsychological patients, that face processing was an independently functioning module.

People with WBS were also found to display other signs of an uneven cognitive profile. Their sociability was unusual. Indeed, unlike many individuals with learning difficulties, this was a clinical group who showed extreme friendliness, a lack of shyness, and a proclivity for interaction with others. Williams-Beuren syndrome was soon hailed as the genetic disorder that the nativist school of thought had been waiting for: a seemingly clear-cut dissociation between preserved and impaired cognitive abilities, which could not be explained by the notions of domain-general deficits (e.g., speed of processing) that had hitherto characterized other genetic disorders such as Down syndrome. Such arguments were particularly embraced with respect to the language of people with WBS (Pinker 1991, 1999).

Language in the WBS End State

One of the key interests in WBS lay in the potential of this disorder to establish a developmental independence between language and cognition. It is certainly the case that, compared with language development in other genetic syndromes with equivalent general cognitive abilities, language in WBS seems much more advanced. In an analysis of the expressive language of four children with WBS, Clahsen and Almazan (1998) reported the presence of complex syntactic structures and grammatical morphemes that were almost always used correctly. Several studies have pursued comparisons between language in WBS and in Down syndrome (DS), presumably with the view that DS can serve as a baseline of what one might expect of language development in the presence of mental retardation, against which the achievements of people with WBS may be measured (Bellugi et al. 2000; Jarrold et al. 1999; Mervis and Robinson 2000; Singer Harris et al. 1997). Bellugi and collaborators (2000) go so far as to suggest that WBS and DS "test the outer limits of the dissociations that can occur between language and cognition" (11).

Subsequently, however, detailed investigations demonstrated that language performance is not at normal levels in WBS and at the very least shows a developmental delay in infancy and toddlerhood of some two to three years (Singer Harris et al. 1997; Laing et al. 2002). Most recent studies that compare the performance of individuals with WBS with typically developing children now use a control group matched for *mental age*, to which their performance levels are more closely tied. This implicitly concedes that language development in WBS is not independent of general cognitive ability. Although the language performance of individuals with WBS is relatively impressive (compared with other syndromes with associated low IQs), evidence of atypicalities has accumulated in all areas of language and at all stages of language development, including vocabulary, grammar, pragmatics, and (as we shall see later) the precursors to language development in infants (Thomas and Karmiloff-Smith 2002a).

Despite growing evidence to the contrary, but following the early broad claims of a dissociation between language and cognition in WBS, some researchers then presented a more refined claim, arguing that WBS represents a dissociation *in the language system itself* (Clahsen and Almazan 1998, 2001; Clahsen and Temple 2003; Pinker 1999; Thomas and Karmiloff-Smith 2005). In this account, grammar is now postulated to develop normally while, simultaneously, lexical or word-specific knowledge develops atypically. The purported developmental fractionation between grammar and lexicon in this genetic developmental disorder is viewed as evidence that such a distinction is innately specified (Pinker 1999). However, there are empirical difficulties with the fractionation claim (Thomas and Karmiloff-Smith 2003, 2005). For instance, several studies report that, in children with WBS, grammar development (as assessed by standardized tests of receptive grammar) lags behind vocabulary development (similarly assessed by receptive vocabulary tests) (Clahsen and Almazan 1998; Grant et al. 1997; Karmiloff-Smith et al. 1997; Volterra et al. 1996). And in a study of younger children, the level of productive grammatical complexity turned out to be exactly what one would expect given these children's vocabulary sizes, suggesting no dissociation of grammar and the lexicon in the early phases of language development (Singer Harris et al. 1997).

It is true that children and adults with WBS can show sophisticated use of syntax in line with their overall mental (rather than chronological) age (Clahsen and Almazan 1998; Zukowski 2001). Moreover, this behavior can occur in parallel with anomalies of vocabulary usage. However, the characterization of this pattern as a clean dissociation between grammar and the lexicon is misleading. The anomalies of vocabulary seem to be in part strategic and in part the consequence of a combination of shallow lexical-semantics and relatively stronger phonological processing (Thomas et al. 2001). By contrast, the development of morphology and syntax has been found to demonstrate atypical patterns. Morphologic problems include difficulties in gender assignment reported in several languages (Spanish: Cáceres et al., unpublished results; French: Karmiloff-Smith et al. 1997; Italian: Volterra et al. 1996) and differences in inflectional morphology (Thomas et al. 2001). Some errors in the acquisition of morphology were qualitatively different from those ever encountered in normal development (Capirci et al. 1996). In older children, studies of syntax indicate a greater delay for grammar acquisition than vocabulary acquisition (Grant et al. 2002; Zukowski 2001). (See chapter 8 for a detailed discussion of language abilities in WBS.)

Social Cognition in the WBS End State

The history of studies of social cognition followed a pattern similar to that for language. Anecdotal reports initially indicated that people with Williams-Beuren syndrome were very friendly, capable of empathy with respect to displays of emotions in others, and generally very sociable. Early studies, albeit with small populations and no control group comparisons, seemed to bear this out (Karmiloff-Smith et al. 1995). However, when more substantial empirical work was undertaken (Tager-Flusberg and Sullivan 2000), it rightly challenged the original work in this field. Despite the excellent empirical data provided by Tager-Flusberg and Sullivan's study, however, the theoretical model that they used seemed to follow that of adult neuropsychology, whereby they sought dissociations between components of theory of mind: "The results from this and other studies on WBS support the view that the social-cognitive and social-perceptual component of a theory of mind are dissociable. In WBS only the latter components, which are linked to distinct neurobiological substrates, are spared" (59).

The assumption of a "sparing" or "preservation" of a function, like that of "intactness," implies that part of a system has developed normally and independent of the rest of the (impaired) system. Yet this logic belies what we know about early brain development in both typical and atypical children, and it is becoming increasingly clear that social cognition in WBS does not develop normally (Jones et al. 2000), with early signs of the atypicality from infancy onward (Laing et al. 2002)—as the original work by Tager-Flusberg and Sullivan indirectly intimated. Both social cognition and language development in WBS remain theoretically very interesting, but not from the perspective of clean dissociations across systems or between separate components of a given system identified in the normal adult. We must always keep in mind that WBS is a *developmental* disorder from the very outset.

Face and Visuospatial Processing in the WBS End State

The challenge to the existence of an "intact" social module also characterized subsequent work on face processing. A large number of studies have now established that, although older children and adults with WBS achieve scores in the normal range on some face-processing tasks (Bellugi et al. 1988; Udwin and Yule 1991), their superficial success is not underpinned by the same cognitive processes as those found in normal processing. Usually we tend to process faces configurally; our brains rapidly analyze the spatial *relations* between facial elements. By contrast, people with WBS have been shown either to process faces holistically as a gestalt (Tager-Flusberg et al. 2003) or to analyze faces featurally: they do not focus on the second-order relations between elements of a face (Karmiloff-Smith et al. 2004). Several studies have now pinpointed this difference between normal face processing and that displayed by individuals with WBS, both behaviorally (Rossen et al. 1996; Karmiloff-Smith 1997; Deruelle et al. 1999; Karmiloff-Smith et al. 2004) and electrophysiologically (Mills et al. 2000; Grice et al. 2001). It turns out that this difference holds not only for facial stimuli. Deruelle and her collaborators (1999) showed for non-face displays that people with WBS were also more inclined to use featural than configural processing. In other words, WBS cannot be claimed to involve an "intact" face-processing module and a deficient space-processing module. In fact, *both* facial and spatial processing reveal a similar underlying impairment in configural processing, but the particular characteristics of the problem of recognizing faces allow the WBS system to achieve some degree of behavioral success in this domain by focusing on features. In short, when examined in detail, a superficially proficient face-processing ability proves to be associated with an atypical developmental trajectory (Karmiloff-Smith et al. 2004).

Number Processing in the WBS End State

In the uneven cognitive profile of WBS, the domain of numerical cognition has hitherto been relatively neglected. This is surprising given the high number of anecdotal reports suggesting that individuals with WBS suffer from a marked impairment of number skills (Bellugi et al. 1988; Udwin et al. 1996). Based on studies of neuropsychological patients and on functional neuroimaging of healthy controls, it has been argued that numerical cognition is subserved by two functionally and anatomically dissociated systems of processing, one verbal (symbolic) and the other nonverbal (analog) (Dehaene 1997). The system claimed to be responsible for the analog representation of quantity is thought to be part of the brain system that also underpins spatial cognition. Against the background of the WBS phenotype, with its relative strengths in language and marked impairments in nonverbal, particularly spatial, cognition, it might be tempting to use the adult neuropsychological model of the mature brain to hypothesize that individuals with WBS will show a neat dissociation between a strength in the verbal skills involved in numerical processing and an impairment in the spatial aspects of number. Such a hypothesis is appealing, but it rests on an untenable assumption drawn from adult neuropsychology. By contrast, we have repeatedly argued that dissociations of subsystems in the mature normal brain cannot be used to assume an absence of crucial interactions between the systems during development, before the systems reach their normal end state. For example, during development, the "semantics" of exact language-based numbers may need to be grounded by the analog representation of quantity, before this system can function independently. The point is that, without an account of the *developmental emergence of function*, the precise hypotheses for developmental disorders of cognition remain unclear.

Work is now focusing on the complexities of the atypical developmental trajectory of number development in WBS (Ansari and Karmiloff-Smith 2002; Ansari et al. 2003). Our findings suggest that the final picture of numerical cognition in WBS is highly unlikely to be simply that of one number system developing normally with the other impaired.

In sum, the phenotypic end state in Williams-Beuren syndrome cannot be characterized in terms of independently functioning "intact and impaired modules," as many have claimed. Rather, language, face processing, and social cognition, originally hailed as the three spared domains in WBS, all have subtle as well as more obvious impairments when studied in greater depth. Superficial behavioral proficiency—that is, scoring in the normal range on broad measures—does not necessarily entail cognitive or neural "intactness." The very concept of "intactness" is not only empirically wrong in this case but is theoretically misguided, because it masks the absence of a proper *developmental* account. This holds as much for normal development as for the atypical case (Karmiloff-Smith 1992, 1998). In our view, then, the WBS findings are hardly surprising: a *developmental* disorder is not the same as the case of an adult neuropsychological patient who originally developed normally and then, once the brain was in the mature adult state, suffered injury. In its mature state, the adult brain can be differentially damaged under some circumstances. But this in no way licenses the taking for granted that such specialization and localization of cognitive function is a characteristic of the start state of the infant brain in either normal or atypical development.

The Williams-Beuren Syndrome Phenotype in Early Childhood

The huge amount of research on older children and adults with Williams-Beuren syndrome has not been matched by equivalent work on infants and very young children. This may be because, in the theoretical frameworks mainly used to theorize about WBS, the study of such young individuals was thought to be unnecessary. Indeed, the use of WBS to argue for innate modules simply takes for granted that the uneven pattern of behavioral proficiencies and impairments in adults arises from a similar differential pattern in infancy, followed by independent, linear development in each of the cognitive domains identified in the adult phenotype. This is theoretically untenable and, as work on infants and toddlers with WBS began to appear, it became obvious that the assumption is also empirically flawed.

Language in the WBS Start State

A first set of semi-observational studies examined six toddlers with WBS with respect to several key relationships between the emergence of early language and other cognitive markers in normal development (Mervis and Bertrand 1997). In these studies, referential pointing, a precursor to referential language in typically developing toddlers, appeared *after* the onset of such language in young children with WBS. Given that one of the main routes to acquisition of vocabulary is joint attention to an object being labeled, this implies either an alternative route to vocabulary acquisition or a less referential use of language in WBS (Laing et al. 2002). In typically developing toddlers, vocabulary growth undergoes a sudden rapid expansion that coincides with a new ability to exhaustively sort objects by semantic category—implying that the vocabulary spurt is associated with a change in the understanding of the meanings of words. However, in toddlers with WBS, the vocabulary spurt was found to occur *before* demonstration of spontaneous exhaustive sorting (Mervis and Bertrand 1997). Subsequent experimental studies in our lab with infants and toddlers with WBS showed that they were as delayed as their matched counterparts with DS in vocabulary, despite adults with WBS clearly outstripping adults with DS in the phenotypic outcome (Paterson et al. 1999; see also Nazzi et al. 2003).

Social Cognition in the WBS Start State

Studies of very young children's social communication also reveal atypical start states in WBS (Laing et al. 2002). Typically developing toddlers, matched on mental age to a group of toddlers with WBS, were examined on several tasks involving joint attention and social referencing. The toddlers with WBS were proficient on items measuring dyadic attention (one-on-one interaction) but, compared with the normally developing toddlers, were seriously impaired with respect to triadic attention (the triangle of person-to-person-to-object interaction), failing to understand the referential function of pointing. It is triadic attention that is crucial to early vocabulary development, and the finding suggests that, when it does take off in WBS, vocabulary learning is subsumed by an atypical developmental pathway.

Face and Visuospatial Processing in the WBS Start State

Studies of infants and toddlers with WBS in the domains of face and visuospatial processing are almost nonexistent, although these are beginning to be undertaken. A current study of face processing in infants and toddlers with WBS (K. Humphreys et al., personal communication) suggests that these young children do not show a difference between featural and configural processing such as is evident in the adult phenotypic outcome. Rather, these preliminary data suggest that both featural and configural processing may be atypical in the start state in WBS, and it must be a function of development that this clinical group tends to rely increasingly heavily on the analysis of features.

Number Processing in the WBS Start State

Typically developing preverbal infants can discriminate between numerosities, suggesting that a nonverbal, analog system of number representation is available early in normal development. The development of symbolic, exact number representation such as the understanding of counting principles, however, develops over a protracted period of time (Fuson 1988; Wynn 1992). Current views suggest, however, that both these systems play a role in the development of number abilities (Carey 2001; Ansari and Karmiloff-Smith 2002).

Given the adult numerical phenotype and the weakness of visuospatial processing in WBS, one might expect infants with the syndrome to be particularly impaired in the analog system of numerical representation. Against the background of recent evidence, however, there are reasons to challenge this assumption. Paterson and collaborators (1999) compared the ability of infants with WBS to discriminate between three and two objects with the ability of adults with WBS to judge the relative magnitude of Arabic numerals and dots. Infants with WBS were found to be successful at discriminating between small sets of objects, whereas infants with DS, matched for chronological or mental age, could not. By contrast, adults with WBS were found to be even more impaired than adults with DS in number discrimination tasks (Paterson et al., in press). These findings suggest that the development of numerical cognition in WBS is atypical and does not mirror the trajectory observed in typically developing controls.

In summary, we argue that a more fruitful approach to studying various aspects of cognition in WBS is to chart from the earliest stages in infancy through to adulthood the trajectories of basic, low-level competencies that interact with development and lead over time to proficient or impaired systems of representation. Detecting subtle deviations of these foundational competencies will help identify the developmental precursors and trajectories of impairments in higher-level outcomes of cognition. Asynchronies and atypical relationships between representations in one domain and those in others should reveal how each aspect of cognition interacts with the overall WBS cognitive phenotype.

Why Development Is Crucial in Exploring Genotype/Phenotype Relations

Throughout the chapter we have emphasized the need for studies of the infant origins of subsequent phenotypic outcomes and have shown that one cannot simply assume that the uneven pattern of the adult end state also characterizes the early start state. This is particularly important when exploring relations between genotype and phenotype. One of the exciting aspects of the study of Williams-Beuren syndrome is that both the genotype and the phenotype have been well identified. The genotype is the deletion of some twenty-five genes on one copy of chromosome 7 at q11.23 (Frangiskakis et al. 1996; Donnai and Karmiloff-Smith 2000; Tassabehji et al. 1996). Yet most attempts to relate the expression of particular deleted genes to behavioral outcomes have been based on the adult phenotype. Frangiskakis and collaborators, for example, argued that the deletion of the LIM kinase 1 gene (*LIMK1*), which is expressed in the brain, is a major contributor to the spatial deficits in WBS. Subsequent work on other patients with a *LIMK1* deletion but without either WBS or any spatial impairments challenged this assumption empirically (Tassabehji et al. 1999; Karmiloff-Smith et al. 2003). But the direct mapping is also questionable on theoretical grounds. *LIMK1* is expressed in the brain early in development, so, to understand its implications for the resulting phenotype, researchers need to identify atypical developmental processes during embryogenesis and postnatal brain development, which may prove to be only indirectly related to spatial cognition. Such causal factors could lie in differences in developmental timing, neuronal formation, neuronal density, firing thresholds, biochemical efficiency, transmitter types, dendritic arborization, synaptogenesis, and pruning. Another reason for caution is that the effects of one or several genes on a particular function are unlikely to leave other functions unchanged throughout development, because imbalances in one brain system may drive changes in other systems (Johnson 2001).

Computational Models of the Williams-Beuren Syndrome Phenotype

Although we have stressed the importance of focusing on the *developmental process itself* in our exploration of the causes of developmental deficits, this is of course easier said than done. It is far from clear how exactly to characterize the developmental process. Indeed, one of the weakest areas of developmental psychology is its precise stipulation of mechanisms of change in representational systems that account for the developmental changes in behavior that we witness. This is the case in typical cognitive systems, let alone atypical ones.

The characterization of mechanisms of development is much aided by the use of computational models. The study of simple learning systems, such as connectionist networks, allows for a more precise specification of the learning problem presented by a given cognitive domain, the training environment in which it is presented, and the computational mechanisms available in the cognitive system to acquire the relevant behavior (Thomas and

Karmiloff-Smith 2002b). Connectionist models contain a range of computational constraints that affect the subsequent trajectory of development when the system is exposed to a training environment, as well as its ultimate success in acquiring a target behavior. These computational constraints include the system's architecture, its levels of resources, the input and output representations used to specify the target domain, and the nature of the learning algorithm (Karmiloff-Smith 1992). Initial differences in computational constraints such as these provide candidate lower-level explanations for how a developmentally disordered system may arise (Karmiloff-Smith and Thomas 2002; Thomas and Karmiloff-Smith 2002b).

Two examples of our own work illustrate the potential contribution of computational modeling to the study of developmental disorders. First, one may seek to simulate a precise pattern of empirical data for a given developmental disorder, which we sought to capture for the acquisition of the English-language past tense in WBS (Thomas and Karmiloff-Smith 2002a). Individuals with WBS have been reported as exhibiting difficulties in generalizing inflection patterns from words they know to novel items (Thomas et al. 2001) and, in some studies with smaller subject numbers, selective difficulties with irregular past tenses (Clahsen and Almazan 1998). We took one model of the acquisition of the past tense in normal development and sought to alter the initial constraints in line with empirical data on possible differences in phonological and semantic processing in WBS. The model was able to rule out certain hypotheses while establishing that phonological differences could reduce generalization to novel terms and that semantic differences could produce difficulties in acquiring irregular past-tense forms. In addition, the model demonstrated for the first time precisely how different computational constraints interact in a system during the process of development: the atypical trajectory found in past-tense formation in WBS may arise from the combination of more than one altered constraint in the language system.

Second, one may use computational models to examine more general theoretical issues concerning the effect of developmental processes acting on systems that have initial computational anomalies. In a second model (Thomas and Karmiloff-Smith 2003), we were interested in exploring whether applying disruptions to the *start state* of a learning system tended to produce the same deficits in performance as applying those same disruptions to the *end state* of a normally trained model. The results of the modeling indicated that start-state damage to a system and end-state damage could in some circumstances cause similar impairments, but at other times the patterns were very different. The relationship depended on whether the system could use the developmental process to compensate for damage applied in the start state, by attenuating or even overcoming the effects of early anomalies. But in other cases, early deficits generated greater impairments than damage to the end state, particularly in the case where the early deficits comprised the clarity of the initial representations needed to drive development. By contrast, the end-state system, with its established knowledge, was robust to noisy representations. Importantly, this work convincingly demonstrated that, in developmentally disordered systems, dissociations between impaired behavior and behavior in the normal range cannot be unambiguously interpreted without an understanding of the developmental conditions that pertained in the underlying system.

In short, computational models can help in exploring the contribution of the developmental process to developmental deficits, but they also serve to emphasize the crucial importance of having a precise and truly developmental account of a given cognitive ability before seeking to interpret behavioral deficits in a developmental disorder.

Implications of the Study of Williams-Beuren Syndrome for Future Work on Other Developmental Disorders

In our view, the need to focus on infant precursors and the ways in which low-level deficits interact with development in Williams-Beuren syndrome is an important lesson for other disorders. As an illustration of the clinical implications for future work, we take here the example of two developmental disorders, velocardiofacial syndrome (known also as DiGeorge syndrome or 22q syndrome) and fragile X syndrome. Both of these syndromes have an uneven profile, with language being relatively better than visuospatial processing, as is the case for WBS.

Velocardiofacial Syndrome

More common than WBS, velocardiofacial syndrome (VCFS) is a genetic disorder occurring in approximately 1 in 4,000 live births (Shprintzen et al. 1978). It is a complex disorder characterized by multiple congenital anomalies affecting multiple tissues and organ systems, many of which are embryologically derived from neural crest cells. It is often associated with learning disability and high rates of psychiatric disorder, particularly schizophrenia (Murphy et al. 1999). Not until 1992 were the causative submicroscopic deletions on chromosome 22q11.2 identified (Scambler et al. 1992). At least fifty genes map to the region deleted in VCFS, a considerably larger deletion than in WBS. Several genes have been considered candidates for the cognitive phenotype in VCFS, including the gene coding for catechol-*O*-methyltransferase (Egan et al. 2001; Campbell et al. 2003).

The last decade has witnessed a rise in the number of cognitive approaches to the syndrome (Wang et al. 2000), but not to the extent of the work on WBS. In addition, the conclusions remain limited because of ascertainment biases, small sample sizes, and the lack of adequately matched control groups. Traits that are frequently observed in a majority of individuals and characterize the cognitive phenotype of VCFS include mild to significant delay on major developmental milestones such as speech, language, cognition, and motor skills (Gerdes et al. 1999). It has been reported that individuals with VCFS, like those with WBS, have a significant discrepancy between verbal IQ and performance IQ in favor of the verbal (Swillen et al. 1997). However, one study of older children showed the opposite pattern of impairments, with receptive language clearly more impaired than expressive language (Glaser et al. 2002), indicating that the developmental trajectory in VCFS is likely to be far from straightforward. Like children with WBS, those with VCFS struggle with mathematics. A functional magnetic resonance imaging study confirmed atypical patterns of brain activation in children with VCFS when they were performing a numerical task (Eliez et al. 2001). Interestingly, both VCFS and WBS groups showed higher reading performance than mathematics performance, suggesting that the latter domain is more vulnerable in developmental disorders (Ansari and Karmiloff-Smith 2002).

With increasing knowledge of the structural brain anomalies in VCFS, researchers have focused their studies increasingly on specific brain areas and their functions, drawing inspiration from adult neuropsychological models. However, it is important to keep in mind that the 22q11.2 deletion results in widespread neuroanatomic anomalies, and all our earlier arguments about the crucial role of development in the phenotypic outcome for WBS obviously hold for this syndrome too.

Fragile X Syndrome

One developmental disorder that might offer a more direct window on the mapping between genotype and phenotype is a single-gene disorder, fragile X syndrome (FXS) (de Vries et al. 1997). The vast majority of cases are due to the silencing of the fragile X mental retardation-1 gene (*FMR-1*). The absence of its product, the Fragile X Mental Retardation protein, is the sole direct genetic contribution to the fragile X phenotype (Verkerk et al. 1991). Individuals with the syndrome present with mild to severe mental retardation (Hagerman and Cronister 1996), and the adult phenotype is characterized by an uneven cognitive profile (e.g., relative strengths in language and visual perception accompanied by relative weaknesses in attention and visuospatial cognition) (Cornish et al. 2001). Does this imply that the lack of a single gene product can be directly linked to selective deficits in certain cognitive domains, leaving others to develop normally? We again submit that the very question is flawed because it ignores the developmental nature of FXS by assuming direct links between mutated genes and those higher-level cognitive functions in which behavioral deficits are most evident and by postulating dissociations between spared and impaired domains.

The adult phenotype in FXS is best considered as the end point of cascading effects on the structural and functional constraints on brain development. It is likely that many brain circuits for which *FMR-1*–related neural processes have even distal effects will develop atypically to some extent. However, these particular low-level properties, although not specific to any single cognitive function, may be less relevant to the task demands imposed by some cognitive domains and some processes in each domain, and thus these will develop to display less overt impairment. And in FXS, as in WBS, even domains of relative strength are characterized by subtle differences from typically developing controls, both when one considers discrete life-span time points and when one analyzes performance in terms of developmental trajectories. This is particularly evident for the language of adults with FXS, an area of relative proficiency. For example, although adults' vocabulary knowledge surpasses their abilities in other domains, productive and receptive vocabulary in infancy and early childhood are often delayed (Roberts et al. 2001). In FXS, as in WBS, the focus on relative weaknesses in one domain should not overshadow atypicalities, however subtle, in other domains (Karmiloff-Smith et al. 2002).

These considerations also apply to the processing abilities in which adults with FXS exhibit difficulties, such as selective attention and executive control (Cornish et al. 2001). Inspired by the neurodevelopmental perspective discussed thus far, Scerif and colleagues (2004) asked whether problems with selective attention are already present from toddlerhood and whether they are selectively due to executive difficulties. Our findings indicate that, like older children with the syndrome, toddlers with FXS produce more perseverative behaviors than typically developing toddlers, suggesting that executive attention is already an area of difficulty from toddlerhood onward. The difficulties may become increasingly apparent through development, highlighting yet again the need for a truly developmental approach to the study of this syndrome.

Conclusions and Future Directions

At several points in this chapter, we have emphasized the need to explore developmental disorders across domains in which individuals later display not only impairment but also superficial proficiency. In general, many studies of developmental disorders simply focus on the deficient domains, relying on rather summary, standardized measures of the domains considered to be "normal," "intact," and so forth. But our work has repeatedly shown that, for developmental disorders, it cannot be taken for granted that superficially normal behavioral scores necessarily imply normal cognitive or neural processes. Equal focus should be placed on in-depth studies of domains of seeming proficiency as of those showing clear-cut deficits. We have also repeatedly stressed the importance of a truly developmental approach, in which one attempts to chart the full atypical developmental trajectories of each domain from infancy through to adulthood. This has important implications for both future research and clinical/educational practice. Finally, we have argued that genotype/phenotype relations are best explored at the level of basic processing mechanisms seen in early infancy that subsequently have cascading but differential effects on the developing systems.

When reading the literature on developmental disorders, particularly on Williams-Beuren syndrome, it is crucial to pay attention to the nature of the control groups used. As we have mentioned, the comparison with Down syndrome tends to exaggerate the proficiencies of people with WBS. Another tendency in the literature is worth recalling: that of forgetting, when summarizing results, the basis on which participants were matched. So, although the clinical group has been matched on mental age, researchers tend to claim that for one task the WBS performance reaches the same level as that of the controls and is thus intact and for another task it is lower than controls, and this supports a dissociation between intact and impaired functioning. This of course overlooks the fact that *both* domains are considerably delayed at or below mental age level, not at chronological age level. A more accurate account would be that both domains are very delayed, with one simply less delayed than the other. The temptation to treat relative differences as absolute ones, to ignore real developmental levels, and to use the adult neuropsychological model of intact and impaired modules continues to permeate the study of developmental disorders and, in our view, impedes a deeper understanding of atypical developmental trajectories.

In an earlier publication, Karmiloff-Smith (1998) noted that "brain volume, brain anatomy, brain chemistry, hemispheric asymmetry, and the temporal patterns of brain activity are all atypical in people with Williams syndrome. How could the resulting cognitive system be described in terms of a normal brain with parts intact and parts impaired, as the popular view holds?" (393). This expresses a view that we have been stressing throughout this chapter. Moreover, note that *intact* refers to a *normally developed system* that has "no relevant component removed or destroyed" (Webster's Collegiate Dictionary, 11th ed.). This being so, in the context of developmental disorders, all uses of *is intact* should be replaced either with *has developed normally,* in connection to a cognitive system (if this is indeed what researchers are implying), or with *scores within the normal range,* in connection to a piece of behavior (where researchers are implying no processing account). Use of terms such as *intact, spared,* or *preserved* often obscures the fact that researchers are characterizing deficits in developmental disorders without having any realistic developmental account in mind. We need to remember that adult neuropsychological models can serve as no more than a point of departure in the study of developmental disorders. The journey it-self requires that we constrain our interpretation of atypical trajectories by precise models of mechanisms of change and that we embrace the inherently developmental nature of the genetic disorders that we study.

ACKNOWLEDGMENTS

This chapter was written with the support of grants from the Medical Research Council and PPP Healthcare (U.K.) and Fogarty/National Institutes of Health (U.S.) to Dr. Karmiloff-Smith; a University College London Ph.D. studentship to Dr. Scerif; a Williams Syndrome Foundation Ph.D. studentship to Dr. Karmiloff-Smith for Dr. Ansari; and PPP Foundation grant PAG TX1 ref no. 1206/188 to Drs. Kieran Murphy, Campbell, Karmiloff-Smith, et al.

REFERENCES

Ansari, D., and Karmiloff-Smith, A. 2002. Atypical trajectories of number development: A neuroconstructivist perspective. *Trends in Cognitive Sciences* 6:511–516.

Ansari, D., Donlan, C., Thomas, M., Ewing, S., Peen, T., and Karmiloff-Smith, A. 2003. What makes counting count? Verbal and visuo-spatial contributions to typical and atypical number development. *Journal of Experimental Child Psychology* 85:50–62.

Baron-Cohen, S. 1998. Modularity in developmental cognitive neuropsychology: Evidence from autism and Gilles de la Tourette syndrome. In *Handbook of mental retardation and development,* ed. J. A. Burack, R. M. Hodapp, and E. Zigler, 334–348. Cambridge: Cambridge University Press.

Bellugi, U., Marks, S., Bihrle, A., and Sabo, H. 1988. Dissociations between language and cognitive functions in Williams syndrome. In *Language development in exceptional circumstances,* ed. D. Bishop and K. Mogford, 177–189. London: Churchill-Livingstone.

Bellugi, U., Lichtenberger, L., Jones, W., Lai, Z., and St. George, M. 2000. The neurocognitive profile of Williams syndrome: A complex pattern of strengths and weaknesses. *Journal of Cognitive Neuroscience* 12 (suppl.): 1–29.

Bishop, D. V. 2001. Genetic and environmental risks for specific language impairment in children. *Philosophical Transactions of the Royal Society of London. Series B, Biological Sciences* 1407:369–380.

Campbell, L. E., Stevens, A. F., Azuma, R., Morris, R. G., Karmiloff-Smith, A., Owen, M. J., Murphy, D. G. M., and Murphy, K. C. 2003. A cognitive investigation of children and adolescents with velo-cardio-facial syndrome (VCFS). *Biological Psychiatry* 53 (8, suppl.): 115.

Capirci, O., Sabbadini, L., and Volterra, V. 1996. Language development in Williams syndrome: A case study. *Cognitive Neuropsychology* 13:1017–1039.

Carey, S. 2001. Cognitive foundations of arithmetic: Evolution and ontogenesis. *Mind and Language* 16:37–55.

Clahsen, H., and Almazan, M. 1998. Syntax and morphology in Williams syndrome. *Cognition* 68:167–198.

———. 2001. Compounding and inflection in language impairment: Evidence from Williams syndrome (and SLI). *Lingua* 111:729–757.

Clahsen, H., and Temple, C. 2003. Words and rules in Williams syndrome. In *Towards a definition of specific language impairment in children*, ed. Y. Levy and J. Schaeffer, 323. Mahwah, NJ: Erlbaum.

Cornish, K. M., Munir, F., and Cross, G. 2001. Differential impact of the FMR-1 full mutation on memory and attention functioning: A neuropsychological perspective. *Journal of Cognitive Neuroscience* 13:144–151.

Dehaene, S. 1997. *The number sense*. Oxford: Oxford University Press.

Deruelle, C., Macini, J., Livet, M. O., Casse-Perrot, C., and deSchonen, S. 1999. Configural and local processing of faces in children with Williams syndrome. *Brain and Cognition* 41:276–298.

de Vries, B. B., van den Ouweland, A. M. W., Mohkamsing, S., Duivenvoorden, H. J., Mol, E., Gelsema, K., van Rijn, M., Halley, D. J. J., Sandkuijl, L. A., and Oostra, B. A., Tibben, A., and Niermeijer, M. F., for the Collaborative Fragile X Study Group 1997. Screening and diagnosis for the fragile X syndrome among the mentally retarded: An epidemiological and psychological survey. *American Journal of Human Genetics* 61:660–667.

Donnai, D., and Karmiloff-Smith, A. 2000. Williams syndrome: From genotype through to the cognitive phenotype. *American Journal of Medical Genetics* 97:164–171.

Egan, M. F., Goldberg, T. E., Kolachana, B. S., Callicott, J. H., Mazanti, C. M., Straub, R. E., Goldman, D., and Weinberg, D. R. 2001. Effect of COMT Val108/158 Met genotype on frontal lobe function and risk for schizophrenia. *Proceedings of the National Academy of Sciences U S A* 98:6917–6922.

Eliez, S., Blasey, C. M., Menon, V., White, C. D., Schmitt, J. E., and Reiss, A. L. 2001. Functional brain imaging study of mathematical reasoning abilities in velocardiofacial syndrome (del 22q11.2). *Genetics in Medicine* 3:49–55.

Frangiskakis, J. M., Ewart, A., Morris, C. A., Mervis, C. B., Bertrand, J., Robinson, B. F., Klein, B. P., Ensing, G., Everett, L. A., Green, E. D., Proschel, C., Gutowski, N. J., Noble, M., Atkinson, D. L., Odelberg, S. J., and Keating, M. T. 1996. LIM-kinase1 hemizygosity implicated in impaired visuospatial constructive cognition. *Cell* 86:59–69.

Frith, U. 1995. Dyslexia: Can we have a shared theoretical framework? *Educational and Child Psychology* 12:6–17.

Fuson, K. C. 1988. *Children's counting and concepts of number*. New York: Springer.

Gerdes, M., Solot, C., Wang, P. P., Moss, E., LaRossa, D., Randall, P., Goldmuntz, E., Clark, B., Driscoll, D. A., Jawad, A., Emanuel, B. S., McDonald-McGinn, D. M., Batshaw, M. L., and Zackai, E. 1999. Cognitive and behaviour profile of pre-school children with chromosome 22q11.2 deletion. *American Journal of Medical Genetics* 85:127–133.

Glaser, B., Liron, S., Dahoun, S., Morris, M., Antonarakis, S., Reiss, A., and Eliez, S. 2002. Language abilities and brain function in children with velo-cardiofacial syndrome. Paper presented at the 8th Annual Meeting of the Velo-Cardio-Facial Syndrome Educational Foundation, Inc., Northampton, U.K.

Gopnik, M. 1990. Genetic basis of grammar defect. *Nature* 346:6.

Grant, J., Karmiloff-Smith, A., Gathercole, S. A., Paterson, S., Howlin, P., Davies, M., and Udwin, O. 1997. Phonological short-term memory and its relationship to language in Williams syndrome. *Cognitive Neuropsychiatry* 2:81–99.

Grant, J., Valian, V., and Karmiloff-Smith, A. 2002. A study of relative clauses in Williams syndrome. *Journal of Child Language* 29:403–416.

Grice, S. J., Spratling, M. W., Karmiloff-Smith, A., Halit, H., Csibra, G., de Haan, M., and Johnson, M. H. 2001. Disordered visual processing and oscillatory brain activity in autism and Williams syndrome. *NeuroReport* 12:2697–2700.

Hagerman, R. J., and Cronister, A. 1996. *Fragile X syndrome: Diagnosis, treatment, and research.* Baltimore: Johns Hopkins University Press.

Jarrold, C., Baddeley, A. D., and Hewes, A. K. 1999. Genetically dissociated components of working memory: Evidence from Down's and Williams syndrome. *Neuropsychologia* 37:637–651.

Johnson, M. H. 2001. Functional brain development in humans. *Nature Reviews Neuroscience* 2:475–483.

Jones, W., Bellugi, U., Lai, Z., Chiles, M., Reilly, J., Lincoln, A., and Ralphs, A. 2000. Hypersociability in Williams syndrome. *Journal of Cognitive Neuroscience* 12 (suppl.): 30–46.

Karmiloff-Smith, A. 1992. *Beyond modularity: A developmental perspective on cognitive science.* Cambridge: MIT Press/Bradford Books.

———. 1997. Crucial differences between developmental cognitive neuroscience and adult neuropsychology. *Developmental Neuropsychology* 13:513–524.

———. 1998. Development itself is the key to understanding developmental disorders. *Trends in Cognitive Science* 2:389–398.

Karmiloff-Smith, A., and Thomas, M. S. C. 2002. Developmental disorders. In *The handbook of brain theory and neural networks,* 2nd ed., ed. M. A. Arbib, 292–294. Cambridge: MIT Press.

Karmiloff-Smith, A., Klima, E., Bellugi, U., Grant, J., and Baron-Cohen, S. 1995. Is there a social module? Language, face processing and theory of mind in subjects with Williams syndrome, *Journal of Cognitive Neuroscience* 7:196–208.

Karmiloff-Smith, A., Grant, J., Berthoud, I., Davies, M., Howlin, P., and Udwin, O. 1997. Language and Williams syndrome: How intact is "intact"? *Child Development* 68:246–262.

Karmiloff-Smith, A., Scerif, G., and Thomas, M. 2002. Different approaches to relating genotype to phenotype in developmental disorders. *Developmental Psychobiology* 40:311–322.

Karmiloff-Smith, A., Grant, J., Ewing, S., Carette, M. J., Metcalfe, K., Donnai D., Read A. P., and Tassabehji, M. 2003. Using case study comparisons to explore genotype-phenotype correlations in Williams-Beuren syndrome. *Journal of Medical Genetics* 40:136–140.

Karmiloff-Smith, A., Thomas, M., Annaz, D., Humphreys, K., Ewing, S., Brace, N., van Duuren, M., Pike, M., Grice, S., and Campbell, R. 2004. Exploring the Williams syndrome face processing debate: The importance of building developmental trajectories. *Journal of Child Psychology and Psychiatry* 45:1258–1274.

Laing, E., Butterworth, B., Ansari, D., Gsoedl, M., Longhi, E., Panagiotaki, G., Paterson, S., and Karmiloff-Smith, A. 2002. Atypical development of language and social communication in toddlers with Williams syndrome. *Developmental Science* 5:233–246.

Leslie, A. M. 1992. Pretence, autism and the theory-of-mind module, *Current Directions in Psychological Science* 1:18–21.

Mervis, C. B., and Bertrand, J. 1997. Developmental relations between cognition and language: Evidence from Williams syndrome. In *Research on communication and language disorders: Contributions to theories of language development,* ed. L. B. Adamson and M. A. Romski, 75–106. New York: Brookes.

Mervis, C. B., and Robinson, B. F. 2000. Expressive vocabulary ability of toddlers with Williams syndrome or Down syndrome: A comparison. *Developmental Neuropsychology* 17:111–126.

Mills, D. L., Alvarez, T. D., St. George, M., Appelbaum, L. G., Bellugi, U., and

Neville, H. 2000. Electrophysiological studies of face processing in Williams syndrome. *Journal of Cognitive Neuroscience* 12:47–64.

Murphy, K., Jones, L. A., and Owen, M. J. 1999. High rates of schizophrenia in adults with velo-cardio-facial syndrome. *Archives of General Psychiatry* 56:940–945.

Nazzi, T., Paterson, S., and Karmiloff-Smith, A. 2003. Early word segmentation by infants and toddlers with Williams syndrome. *Infancy* 4:251–271.

Paterson, S., Brown, J. H., Gsödl, M., Johnson, M. H., and Karmiloff-Smith, A. 1999. Cognitive modularity and genetic disorders. *Science* 286:2355–2358.

Paterson, S. J., Girelli, L., Butterworth, B., and Karmiloff-Smith, A. In press. Are numerical impairments syndrome specific? Evidence from Williams syndrome and Down's syndrome. *Journal of Child Psychology and Psychiatry.*

Pinker, S. 1991. Rules of language. *Science* 253:530–535.

———. 1999. *Words and rules.* London: Weidenfeld and Nicolson.

Roberts, J. E., Mirrett, P., and Burchinal, M. 2001. Receptive and expressive communication development of young males with fragile X syndrome. *American Journal of Mental Retardation* 106:216–230.

Rossen, M. L., Klima, E. S., Bellugi, U., Bihrle, A., and Jones, W. 1996. Interaction between language and cognition: Evidence from Williams syndrome. In *Language, learning, and behavioural disorders: Developmental, biological, and clinical perspectives,* ed. J. H. Beitchman, N. Cohen, M. Konstantareas, and R. Tannock, 367–392. New York: Cambridge University Press.

Scambler, P. J., Kelly, D., Lindsay, E., Williamson, R., Goldberg, R., Shprintzen, R., Wilson, D. I., Goodship, J. A., Cross, I. E., and Burn, J. 1992. Velo-cardio-facial syndrome associated with chromosome 22 deletions encompassing the DiGeorge locus. *Lancet* 339:1138–1139.

Scerif, G., Cornish, K., Wilding, J., Driver, J., and Karmiloff-Smith, A. 2004. Visual selective attention in typically developing toddlers and toddlers with fragile X and Williams syndrome. *Developmental Science* 7:116–130.

Shprintzen, R. J., Goldberg, R. B., Lewin, M. L., Sidoti, E. J., Berkman, M. D., Argamaso, R. V., and Young, D. 1978. A new syndrome involving cleft palate, cardiac abnormalities typical facies and learning disabilities: Velo-cardio-facial syndrome. *Cleft Palate* 15:15–62.

Singer Harris, N. G., Bellugi, U., Bates, E., Jones, W., and Rossen, M. 1997. Contrasting profiles of language development in children with Williams and Down syndromes. *Developmental Neuropsychology* 13:345–370.

Swillen, A., Devriendt, K., Legius, E., Eyskens, B., Dumoulin, M., Gewillig, M., and Fryns, J. P. 1997. Intelligence and psychosocial adjustment in velo-cardio-facial syndrome: A study of 37 children and adolescents with VCFS. *Journal of Medical Genetics* 34:453–458.

Tager-Flusberg, H., and Sullivan, K. 2000. A componential view of theory of mind: Evidence from Williams syndrome. *Cognition* 76:59–90.

Tager-Flusberg, H., Pless-Skewer, D., Faja, S., and Joseph, R. M. 2003. People with Williams syndrome process faces holistically. *Cognition* 89:11–24.

Tassabehji, M., Metcalfe, K., Fergusson, W. D., Carette, M. J., Dore, J. K., Donnai, D., Read, A. P., Proschel, C., Gutowski, N. J., Mao, X., and Sheer, D. 1996. LIM-kinase deleted in Williams syndrome. *Nature Genetics* 13:272–273.

Tassabehji, M., Metcalfe, K., Karmiloff-Smith, A., Carette, M. J., Grant, J., Dennis, N., Reardon, W., Splitt, M., Read, A. P., and Donnai, D. 1999. Williams syndrome: Use of chromosomal microdeletions as a tool to dissect cognitive and physical phenotypes. *American Journal of Human Genetics* 63:118–125.

Thomas, M. S. C., and Karmiloff-Smith, A. 2002a. Modelling language acquisition in atypical phenotypes. *Psychological Review* 110:647–682.
———. 2002b. Modelling typical and atypical cognitive development. In *Handbook of childhood development*, ed. U. Goswami, 575–599. Oxford: Blackwell.
———. 2003. Are developmental disorders like cases of adult brain damage? Implications from connectionist modelling. *Behavioral and Brain Sciences* 25:727–788.
———. 2005. Can development disorders reveal the component parts of the human language faculty? *Language Learning and Development* 1:65–92.
Thomas, M. S. C., Grant, J., Gsödl, M., Laing, E., Barham, Z., Lakusta, L., Tyler, L. K., Grice, S., Paterson, S., and Karmiloff-Smith, A. 2001. Past tense formation in Williams syndrome. *Language and Cognitive Processes* 16:143–176.
Udwin, O., and Yule, W. 1991. A cognitive and behavioural phenotype in Williams syndrome. *Journal of Clinical and Experimental Neuropsychology* 13:232–244.
Udwin, O., Davies, M., and Howlin, P. 1996. A longitudinal study of cognitive and education attainment in Williams syndrome. *Developmental Medicine and Child Neurology* 38:1020–1029.
Verkerk, A. J. M. H., Pieretti, M., Sutcliffe, J. S., Fu, Y.-H., Kuhl, D. P. A., Pizzuti, A., Reiner, O., Richards, S., Victoria, M. F., Zhang, F., Eussen, B. E., Van Ommen, G.-J. B., Blonden, L. A. J., Riggins, G. J., Chestain, J. L., Kurst, C. B., Galjaard, H., Caskey, C. T., Nelson, D. L., Oostra, B. A., and Warren, S. T. 1991. Identification of a gene (FMR-1) containing a CGG repeat coincident with a breakpoint cluster region exhibiting length variation in fragile X syndrome. *Cell* 65:905–914.
Volterra, V., Capirci, O., Pezzini, G., Sabbadini, L., and Vicari, S. 1996. Linguistic abilities in Italian children with Williams syndrome. *Cortex* 32:663–677.
Wang, P. P., Woodin, M. F., Kreps-Falk, R., and Moss, E. M. 2000. Research on behavioral phenotypes: Velocardiofacial syndrome (deletion 22q11). *Developmental Medicine and Child Neurology* 42:422–427.
Wynn, K. 1992. Children's acquisition of the number words and the counting system. *Cognitive Psychology* 24:220–251.
Zukowski, A. 2001. Uncovering grammatical competence in children with Williams syndrome. Ph.D. diss., Boston University.

Psychopathology in Persons with Williams-Beuren Syndrome

12

Elisabeth M. Dykens, Ph.D., and Beth A. Rosner, Ph.D.

Persons with mental retardation are at an increased risk for developing psychiatric disorders and behavioral or emotional problems (Gostason 1985; Rutter et al. 1976). Once thought of as having concerns related only to their cognitive deficits, these individuals show the full range of psychiatric problems seen in the general population, from mild adjustment disorders to severe psychosis. In addition, some behaviors seem distinctive to those with mental retardation, such as self-injury and stereotypies.

The past twenty years have seen the growth of the field of "dual diagnosis," or coexistence of mental retardation with a psychiatric disorder or behavioral or emotional dysfunction. Research on psychopathology in persons with Williams-Beuren syndrome (WBS) is an outgrowth of this work. Following an overview of the dual diagnosis field, we review the few existing studies on psychopathology in WBS and describe the methodologic and conceptual challenges in conducting dual diagnosis studies in persons with WBS. We also translate the findings on psychopathology in WBS into specific recommendations for intervention and treatment. Throughout, we emphasize the need to assess the efficacy of these recommendations and to promote successful adaptive outcomes for individuals with WBS and their families.

Dual Diagnosis

Major advances in the dual diagnosis field have occurred in two areas: measuring psychopathology and assessing its prevalence in various populations. Mental health workers now have numerous psychopathology rating scales and screening tools at their fingertips, and many of these tools were developed specifically for persons with mental retardation. The widely used and well-normed screening instruments include the Aberrant Behavior Checklist (Aman and Singh 1994), Reiss Screen (Reiss 1988), and Developmental

Behaviour Checklist (Einfeld and Tonge 1992). Although each measure features slightly different domains or factor structures, these scales are increasingly used in research and to screen clients in service settings (Dykens 2000). With these and other tools in hand, researchers in dual diagnosis have a better sense of the prevalence of psychopathology in persons with mental retardation. Overall rates of behavioral, emotional, or psychiatric problems vary from a low of 10% to 15%, as found in large-scale review studies of state records (Borthwick-Duffy and Eyman 1990; Jacobson 1982), to a high of 87% in clinic-referred samples (Philips and Williams 1975). Recent estimates using robust epidemiologic samples fall between these two extremes and suggest that 30% to 40% of children and adults with mental retardation have significant psychopathology (Einfeld and Tonge 1996; Reiss 1990; Rutter et al. 1976).

Two major aspects of dual diagnosis work, however, have yet to be fully developed. First, the vast majority of studies have examined mixed or heterogeneous groups of persons with mental retardation (Dykens and Hodapp 2001). As a result, we know more about psychopathology in persons with mental retardation in general than in persons with genetic etiologies, including those with WBS. Second, most research on psychopathology in persons with mental retardation is descriptive only and has not taken the next step: to rigorously examine why persons with mental retardation are at increased risk for psychopathology to begin with (Dykens 2000).

Several possible explanations have been discussed over the years, and most fall within the "biopsychosocial" spectrum (Dykens and Hodapp 2001). These include biochemical, neurologic, and genetic abnormalities, sensory impairments, atypical personality-motivational styles, increased risks of experiencing failure, reinforcement of negative behaviors, poor communication and assertiveness skills, compromised social intelligence, social stigma, peer rejection and ostracism, family stress, parental psychopathology, and low levels of family support.

Although this is a solid beginning, researchers have yet to evaluate the causal direction or relative importance of each of these many risk factors for psychopathology. As such, the dual diagnosis field lacks a comprehensive model to explain the higher rates of psychopathology in the population of people with mental retardation. Although one could simply apply models of psychopathology developed for the general population, doing so would obfuscate possible etiologic factors that stem from the experience of having a disability. Further, the population of persons with mental retardation encompasses hundreds of known and unknown etiologies, which complicates any search for a single explanation for high rates of psychopathology in this population.

One way around these complexities is to examine psychopathology in persons with distinctive etiologies, including those with genetic disorders such as WBS. Such etiology-specific studies have important implications, in the short term for treatment and in the long term for making novel connections between genes, brain, and behavior (Dykens 2000; O'Brien and Yule 1995). Links have now been made, for example, between Prader-Willi syndrome and obsessive-compulsive behavior (Dykens et al. 1996), Down syndrome and adult-onset depression and Alzheimer's disease (Lott and Head 2001), and velocardiofacial syndrome and psychosis (Murphy and Owen 2001). Studying psychopathology in these and other syndromes may provide a window into the genetic and environmental contributions to psychiatric disorders in persons with or without developmental delay.

Williams-Beuren syndrome seems to be another disorder that exemplifies the promise of an etiology-specific approach to understanding psychopathology in persons with mental retardation. The data on psychopathology in WBS, although relatively sparse, begin to round out our current understandings of the syndrome's behavioral phenotype and to pave the way for improved interventions and treatment.

Maladaptive Behavior in Williams-Beuren Syndrome

The cognitive-linguistic profile in WBS has been a focus of intense behavioral study (see chapter 7). Other aspects of behavior in WBS, however, remain less well scrutinized, including the types and rates of maladaptive behaviors associated with this disorder. Relatively few studies have examined psychopathology, but the findings are remarkably consistent and point to several sets of general findings.

First, persons with WBS are indeed at risk for clinically significant levels of behavioral or emotional problems. Using the Developmental Behaviour Checklist, Einfeld and colleagues (1997) found that 60% of their sample of sixty-four children and adolescents with WBS exceeded the clinical cutoff criteria for a mental disorder. We found slightly lower rates in a sample of forty-one children and adults tested with the Child Behavior Checklist; 20% had clinically elevated scores, and 20% had scores that were of "borderline" clinical significance (E. M. Dykens and B. A. Rosner, unpublished data). Although variable, these percentages nevertheless demonstrate that at least a sizeable proportion of persons with WBS are at risk for significant maladjustment.

Second, studies have generally identified two patterns of difficulties in WBS: externalizing and internalizing problems. Far fewer studies have examined how these problems relate to specific psychiatric diagnoses in persons with WBS.

Externalizing Behaviors

As depicted in table 12.1, high rates of externalizing symptoms have been reported across studies. These symptoms include inattention, impulsivity, hy-

Table 12.1.
Rates of Maladaptive Behavior across Studies of People with Williams-Beuren Syndrome (percentage)

Externalizing	
Inattention	91–96[a]
Impulsivity	75
Attention seeking	71–73
Prefering adults over peers	68–86[a,b]
Hyperactivity	63–71[a]
Temper tantrums	48–74
Disobedience	32–60
Fights, aggressive behavior	25–47
State/Bodily Regulation	
Eating difficulties	45–70[a,b,c]
Wetting self—day	27–61[b,c]
Sleep difficulties	24–50[b,c]
Internalizing	
Obsessions, preoccupations	70–85[a,b]
Fears	68–73[b]
Lability	64
Irritability	62–68
Worries	50–70[b,c]
Anxiety	45–89[b,c]
Somatic complaints	30–67[b]
Feeling worthless	30
Sadness, depression	10–17

Note: Percentages reported in Davies et al. 1998; Dilts et al. 1990; Dykens and Rosner 1999, Einfeld et al. 1997; Gosch and Pankau 1994, 1997; Udwin 1990; Udwin et al. 1987.
[a]Differs from control in Einfeld et al. 1997.
[b]Differs from controls in Dykens and Rosner 1999.
[c]Differs from controls in Udwin et al. 1987.

peractivity, attention-seeking behavior, tempter tantrums, and disobedience (Davies et al. 1998; Einfeld et al. 1997; Dykens and Rosner, unpublished data; Dilts et al. 1990; Gosch and Pankau 1994; Udwin et al. 1987). Such behaviors are consistent with the "difficult" temperament profile that has been described in children with WBS (Tomc et al. 1990). When compared with typically developing children, children with WBS display greater activity, intensity, and distractibility; more negative mood; and lower persistence, adaptability, and threshold to arousal. As opposed to the usual profile of a "difficult" child, however, children with WBS tend to approach other people instead of withdrawing. Also, severe aggressive behaviors, such as destroying objects and hitting others, are less common in individuals with this disorder than in other types of mental retardation(Gosch and Pankau 1994; Udwin 1990).

Externalizing symptoms such as hyperactivity and aggression may become less frequent or less intense with age. Using a cross-sectional design, Gosch and Pankau (1997) reported that adults with WBS tend to be less restless, quarrelsome, and impertinent than children with WBS. They found, for example, that restlessness and difficulty with sitting still was observed in 64% of forty-eight children younger than ten years of age and in only 19% of twenty-seven adults aged twenty years and older. Aggressive behaviors were also found to decrease with age. On the other hand, 90% of seventy adults showed distractibility (Davies et al. 1998).

These trends are corroborated by Einfeld and colleagues (2001), who conducted the as yet sole longitudinal study of maladaptive behavior in WBS. Observing fifty-three children and adolescents with WBS and controls over a five-year period, they found that, relative to controls, youngsters with WBS no longer had elevated "overactivity" or "tantrums" at the second testing five years later. Both cross-sectional and longitudinal data thus suggest a gradual reduction in externalizing behaviors during the child to adolescent years.

A more unusual externalizing behavior, social disinhibition, has also long been noted in WBS. Beginning with observations from the cardiologists and physicians who first recognized WBS (Williams et al. 1961; Beuren et al. 1962), persons with WBS have been consistently cast as very friendly and engaging with others. More recently, other aspects of sociability in WBS have been examined, including the tendencies toward an empathic, kind-spirited orientation and to accurately read the facial expressions of others (table 12.2; see also chapter 10).

For many people with WBS, these positive social features are also associated with extreme lack of social inhibition. Being too friendly with strangers was noted in 82% of a sample of thirty-six children with WBS (Gosch and Pankau 1997) and in 94% of seventy adults with WBS (Davies et al. 1998).

Table 12.2.
Features of Social Interaction in People with Williams-Beuren Syndrome across Studies (percentage)

Positive Features[a]	
Kind-spirited	100
Caring	94
Seeks company of others	90
Feels terrible when others are in pain	87
Often initiates interactions with others	87
Enjoys social activities	83
Forgiving	83
Unselfish	83
Very happy when others do well	75
Never goes unnoticed in a group	75
Strong desire to help others	66
Negative Features	
Problems with friends[b]	96
Unreserved with strangers[c]	79
Solitary[d,e]	71, 84
Overfriendly with strangers[d]	73
Chatters incessantly[d]	58
Few friends[a]	76
Highly sensitive to rejection[a]	67
Low tolerance for teasing[a]	65
Talks too much[a]	53

[a]Dykens and Rosner 1999, N = 60.
[b]Gosch and Pankau 1994, N = 19.
[c]Davies et al. 1998, N = 70.
[d]Udwin 1990, N = 119.
[e]Udwin et al. 1987, N = 44.

On formal testing as well, persons with WBS have abnormally high tendencies to approach strangers (Bellugi et al. 1999). This behavior can lead to significant problems in their everyday life (see table 12.2), including job loss, difficulty making and sustaining friendships, and increased risks of exploitation and abuse. Although the exact rates of exploitation and abuse are unknown, lack of social inhibition, coupled with a strong desire for friends, renders many individuals with WBS vulnerable to poor social judgment and to being sexually, interpersonally, and financially exploited by others (Dykens and Hodapp 1997).

Internalizing Behaviors

Many people with WBS also struggle with a host of internalizing difficulties. As shown in table 12.1, studies are consistent in pointing to high rates of anxiety, obsessions, worries, fears, and somatic complaints in both children and adults with WBS (Einfeld et al. 1997, 2001; Dykens and Rosner 1999; Udwin 1990; Davies et al. 1998; Udwin et al. 1987). These anxieties and worries often center around future events, imagined or real disasters, and health or somatic concerns. The rates of these types of symptoms in WBS are high even when compared with others with mental retardation (Einfeld et al. 1997; Udwin et al. 1987). Although other internalizing problems such as lability and irritability are also often found, they seem to occur at a rate similar to that in other groups with developmental delay.

Taking a closer look at fears and anxiety in a large group of 120 children and adults with WBS, we found that participants with WBS had significantly more fears than individuals with other types of mental retardation. Relative to the comparison group, increased fears were found in WBS participants in every domain of the Fear Survey Schedule for Children–Revised (FSSC-R; Ollendick et al. 1989). Further, elevated fears were found when using either parents or children/adults with WBS as informants and when persons with WBS were asked about their fears in open-ended questions and in a standardized interview (Dykens 2003).

As many as fifty different fears were reported in 60% to 97% of the WBS sample. As shown in table 12.3, specific fears ranged widely in content, from bee stings and fire to animals and carnival rides. In sharp contrast, only two frequent fears were seen in the comparison group—medical injections and bee stings, in 53% and 55%, respectively. Table 12.3 also highlights the top ten most intense fears named by participants with WBS, with injections leading the list and falling from high places ranked tenth.

Fears in persons with WBS may follow an unusual trajectory with age. In the general population, typically developing children show age-related declines in immediate, tangible fears of injury, small animals, separation, the dark, and "spooky things" (Gullone et al. 1996). With advancing age, how-

Table 12.3.
A Sample of Frequent Fears in Persons with Williams-Beuren Syndrome and Control Subjects

Fear	WBS Group (%)	Control Group (%)	Rank Order of 10 Most Intense Fears for WBS Group
Being teased	92	22	5
Shots, injections	90	53	1
Getting sick	89	11	
Loud sirens, noises	87	30	2
Getting punished, reprimanded	85	25	
Arguments between others	85	32	6
Fire, getting burned	82	32	9
Bee stings	79	55	3
Falling from high places	79	28	10
Being criticized	78	11	
Thunderstorms	78	36	7
Getting lost	76	14	
High places	75	45	
Roller coaster, carnival rides	75	43	4
Earthquakes	74	21	8
Having to go to the hospital	74	46	
Being left behind	73	14	
Parents getting sick	71	77	
Making mistakes	79	10	

ever, children and adolescents experience increases in more abstract, antici-patory fears and in fears involving social and performance issues (Spence and McCathie 1993). In contrast, children with WBS do not seem to show de-clines in tangible or spooky fears (Dykens 2003). Indeed, the mean scores for these types of fears (FSSC-R) were 30.07 in six- to twelve-year-olds, 32.04 in thirteen- to eighteen-year-olds, and 31.66 in eighteen- to forty-eight-year-olds. These same participants also had the expected increases in more ab-stract, anticipatory fears, with scores of 20.74 in children, 23.61 in adoles-cents, and 26.23 in adults. Unlike in the general population, then, fears in persons with WBS in this study were highest among adults.

Although speculative, it may be that some of the salient fears in persons with WBS relate to other aspects of the WBS phenotype (Dykens 2003). For example, fears of falling from high places or of amusement park rides may relate to poor visuospatial functioning, joint contractures, and the problems with balance and gait experienced by many individuals with WBS (Chapman et al. 1996). Fears of loud sounds such as thunder and sirens may directly re-late to the high rate of hyperacusis reported in this disorder (Van Borsel et al. 1997). Medical fears may stem from earlier experiences with cardiac, renal, and other medical complications. Even fears of arguments and of be-ing teased, criticized, punished, or left alone may relate to the heightened so-cial sensitivity and empathic streak found in many individuals with WBS (Dykens and Rosner 1999).

In contrast to high rates of anxiety and fears, other internalizing symp-toms such as sadness and depression are less common in persons with WBS.

Studies suggest that 10% to 17% of individuals with WBS have depressive symptoms, predominantly sadness (Davies et al. 1998; Dykens and Rosner 1999). It is unknown how many of these individuals have full-blown affective illness and how these rates would compare with the 2% to 10% rates of affective disorder among persons with mental retardation in general (Dykens and Hodapp 2001). Unlike externalizing behaviors, as noted above, internal, depressive symptoms seem to increase with age (Gosch and Pankau 1997; Dykens and Rosner 1999; Pober and Dykens 1996). Adolescents and young adults may complain of sadness, feelings of worthlessness, mood swings, and irritability. Moreover, depressive symptoms may be masked by the syndrome's friendly and engaging personality style, and these symptoms should therefore be evaluated and carefully monitored, especially in young adults.

Correlates of Externalizing and Internalizing Problems

Further studies are needed that identify the types and rates of externalizing and internalizing problems in larger samples of children and adults with WBS. These descriptive studies, however, should not be accomplished at the expense of research that examines these problems in more depth. For example, whereas several studies report increased risks of inattention or anxiety, few have examined how these problems relate to features in the persons with WBS themselves, in their environments, and in the complex interactions between the two. What child, family, or environmental variables place persons with WBS at risk for problems, and what variables serve as protective factors?

We propose that researchers should examine correlates of maladaptive behaviors in persons with WBS, including specific child, family, and other factors. It is likely that externalizing and internalizing problems in individuals with WBS are variably related to such child factors as age, gender, past and current health status, sleep problems, and genetic status. For example, perhaps individuals with serious medical problems are more prone to somatic complaints or worries. Further, externalizing difficulties may lessen with age, whereas internalizing problems such as anxiety or fears seem to increase with age. Older females with WBS may be especially vulnerable to heightened anxiety and fears (Dykens 2003), a finding consistent with the twofold higher rate of anxiety disorders among girls and women than among males in the general population (Lewinsohn et al. 1998).

Similarly, sleep disturbance may emerge as an important moderator of daytime behavioral problems in persons with WBS. In particular, as many as 50% of individuals with WBS experience difficulties falling asleep and staying asleep, and these problems may be greater than in other persons with mental retardation (Einfeld et al. 1997; Gosch and Pankau 1994; Udwin et al. 1987; see also chapter 13). Sleep disturbances are associated with elevated tantrums and inattention in persons with mental retardation in general

(Wiggs and Stores 1996) and in those with specific syndromes. In persons with Smith-Magenis syndrome, for example, increased nap length is associated with decreased aggression and attentional problems (Dykens and Smith 1998). Further, treatment of the underlying sleep disorder in Smith-Magenis syndrome has led to improved concentration and reduced behavioral problems in several cases (De Leersynder et al. 2001).

It is not certain how genetic status affects psychopathology in persons with WBS, especially with vulnerabilities to anxiety or fears. Clues may be found in ongoing work that examines how deleted or altered genes are associated with hypersociability and visuospatial deficits in WBS (Korenberg et al. 2001).

In addition to child-related variables, families and schools might also play a role in moderating anxiety and behavioral problems in persons with WBS. For example, how might parents or teachers exacerbate or diminish problematic behavior? Do these interactional styles around problem behaviors associated with WBS differ from parent-child or teacher-student interactions in other types of mental retardation? An additional correlate, necessary for psychiatric diagnoses, is the degree to which problem behaviors are associated with impairment in adaptive functioning. To what extent do inattentiveness and distractibility significantly interfere with day-to-day functioning at home or at school, perhaps leading to a diagnosis of attention deficit hyperactivity disorder (ADHD)? Is the degree of anxiety in WBS sufficient to meet criteria for an anxiety disorder?

Psychiatric Diagnoses

Several researchers have raised concerns about the applicability of traditional psychiatric diagnoses, as found in the *Diagnostic and Statistical Manual* (DSM; American Psychiatric Association) or the International Classification of Diseases (ICD; World Health Organization) systems, for those with mental retardation (Sovner 1986). Some of these concerns relate to the psychiatric interview itself, such as the tendency for persons with mental retardation to show acquiescence and other response biases. Further, many persons with mental retardation are less able to express abstract thoughts and feelings or answer questions about the onset, duration, frequency, and severity of various symptoms (Moss 1999).

Many persons with mental retardation may also manifest symptoms in altered, simplistic, or "masked" ways, including behavioral shifts from baseline states (Reiss 1994). If so, then the "goodness of fit" between psychiatric criteria based on persons in the general population and those with mental retardation may be questionable. Further, traditional diagnostic systems may not reflect the diversity of problems experienced by those with mental retardation. Self-injurious and stereotypical behaviors, for example, seem distinctive to those with mental retardation, and such symptoms are not readily captured by any particular psychiatric diagnosis.

As such, some workers have adapted traditional DSM or ICD criteria for persons with developmental delay, especially for internalizing disorders such as depression (King et al. 1994; Szymanski et al. 1998). Still others have developed interview schedules specifically for persons with mental retardation, such as the Psychiatric Assessment Schedule for Adults with Developmental Disability (PASS-ADD; Moss et al. 1996, 1997).

A common denominator across the DSM, ICD, and PASS-ADD systems is that they assess the extent to which symptoms cause distress or are associated with significant adaptive impairment. Such data add an important dimension to studies on maladaptive behavior and to the behavioral phenotypes of mental retardation syndromes. Few studies, however, have applied these psychiatric nosologies to persons with WBS.

Such inattention to psychiatric diagnoses may reflect "diagnostic overshadowing," or the tendency for some researchers and clinicians to attribute psychiatric symptoms in people with mental retardation to their cognitive delays (Reiss et al. 1982). In addition to the dismissal of psychiatric symptoms as a by-product of a low IQ, we find that certain assumptions about people with genetic syndromes may also contribute to their being underdiagnosed. For example, the impression that most children with Down syndrome are friendly and sociable has been implicated in the underdiagnosis of autism in this population (Dykens and Volkmar 1997). It is unclear whether a similar phenomenon occurs in WBS—in this case, the syndrome's characteristic overly-friendly facade may mask underlying feelings of sadness, anxiety, or other problems.

Regardless of the reason, studies on psychopathology in WBS have yet to adopt use of psychiatric nosology. A handful of researchers, however, have examined two psychiatric diagnoses in more detail: autism and specific anxiety disorders.

Autism

Six cases have been published of individuals with co-morbid WBS and autism (Gillberg and Rasmussen 1994; Reiss et al. 1985). These diagnoses may be attributed to that fact that both disorders involve mental retardation, but WBS and autism have certain features that set them apart from one another. For example, the neocerebellum and limbic systems are relatively spared in WBS and aberrant in autism (Rumsey 1996), and facial and affect recognition are a strength in WBS and a characteristic deficit in autism. Strengths and deficits in face recognition may tap different cortical streams (Elgar and Campbell 2001), and WBS and autism can also be differentiated neurophysiologically, as they show different abnormalities in electroencephalographic oscillatory brain activity (Grice et al. 2001). Given the contrasting symptoms and neurologic patterns, WBS is of keen interest to researchers of autism.

Anxiety Disorders

The types and rates of anxiety disorders were investigated in a cohort of fifty-one persons with WBS, aged five to forty-nine years (Dykens 2003). Diagnoses were based on data derived from the Diagnostic Interview Schedule for Children–Revised (DICA-R; Reich et al. 1991), with corroborating evidence from the Child Behavior Checklist (CBCL). As DICA-R interviews were administered only to parents, the findings were considered to be probable or best estimates of lifetime psychiatric diagnoses (Leckman et al. 1982).

As summarized in table 12.4, several anxiety disorders were not generally seen: separation anxiety disorder, avoidant disorder, and obsessive-compulsive disorder. In contrast, many participants, 57%, were excessively worried about future events, 51% were described as worriers, and 35% were noted to become sick from worry. Eighteen percent experienced symptom-related adaptive impairment, meeting DSM-III-R criteria for an overanxious disorder, as well as fatigue, restlessness, and irritability, thereby meeting DSM-IV criteria for generalized anxiety disorder.

A more striking finding, however, was that the majority of participants manifested symptoms of specific phobia (Dykens 2003). A full 96% showed marked, persistent, anxiety-producing fears for six months or longer, and 84% also avoided their fearful stimuli or endured them with great distress. Thirty-five percent also had symptom-related adaptive impairment and thus met the criteria for a specific phobia. One-half of the eighteen participants who met the full criteria for phobia had more than one phobia subtype. The natural environment subtype was seen in 94% (72% of these had fears of thunderstorms, 55% of high places), 44% had other types (50% were afraid

Table 12.4
Percentage of 51 WBS Participants Showing Best-Estimate Anxiety Disorder Diagnoses and Symptoms

Separation anxiety disorder	4
Obsessive-compulsive disorder	2
Avoidant disorder	0
Overanxious disorder/general anxiety disorder	16–18
Excessively worried about future	57
A "worrier"	51
Becomes sick from worry	35
Shows an inability to relax	25
Sleep problems, fatigue, restlessness, difficulty concentrating, irritability	18
Impaired adaptive functioning	16
Specific phobia	35
Marked, persistent, anxiety-producing fears	96
Avoids fearful stimuli or endures with distress	84
Impaired adaptive functioning	35

of being alone, 35% had miscellaneous fears), and 22% had the animal sub-type. Interestingly, despite their fears in other arenas, no participants met the criteria for social phobia. Consistent with their hypersociability, social fears such as public speaking or meeting someone new for the first time were simply absent from the sample as a whole.

Although 35% of participants with WBS met the full criteria for phobia, the majority of participants, 84%, had what might be considered "subclinical" phobia. These persons met all the criteria for phobia (i.e., marked fears with symptom-related avoidance or distress) except the impaired adaptive behavior component. In contrast, rates of full-blown or subclinical phobia are much lower in samples with mental retardation in general or in typically developing persons. Phobia is seen in 0.6% to 4.3% of persons with mental retardation with mixed causes and in 2.3% to 2.4% of typically developing adolescents (table 12.5). Rates of clinical or subclinical phobia in persons with WBS, then, are much higher than other groups with or without mental retardation.

Why did some participants with WBS not show adaptive impairment related to their fears? Perhaps some are similar to persons with phobias in the general population, who generally adapt well, in part because of infrequent contact with certain fear-inducing stimuli (Craske 1999). Alternatively, parents may underestimate their offspring's fears (Dykens 2003). Thus, while parents had an average score (rating their child) on the fear survey (FSSC-R) of 118.83, their offspring's average score was 161.02. Similarly, parents may also underestimate fear-related distress or impairment, and such ratings may increase when the persons with WBS are interviewed directly.

Lastly, we find that many parents of offspring with WBS or other genetic disorders have the tendency to attribute symptoms in their children solely to the syndrome, thereby avoiding the issue of psychiatric diagnosis. Parents may, for example, assert that worries or fears are "just the syndrome," and,

Table 12.5.
Rates of Phobia Reported in Previously Published Studies

Study	Sample	Criteria	Phobia (%)
Cooper 1997	207 MR adults	ICD-10	4.3
Grizenko et al. 1991	176 MR adolescents-adults	DSM-III-R	0.6
Moss et al. 1996	100 MR adolescents-adults	PASS-ADD	1.0
Anderson et al. 1987	792 TD children	DISC	2.4
Milne et al. 1995	487 TD adolescents	K-SADS	2.3 clinical
			14.5 subclinical
Dykens 2003	51 WBS	DICA-R	35 clinical
			84 subclinical

Abbreviations: MR, mental retardation; TD, typically developing; ICD-10, International Classification of Diseases (10th revision); DSM-III-R, Diagnostic and Statistical Manual (3rd ed., revised); PASS-ADD, Psychiatric Assessment Schedule for Adults with Developmental Disability; DISC, Diagnostic Interview Schedule for Children; K-SADS, Schedule for Affective Disorders and Schizophrenia in School-Age Children; DICA-R, Diagnostic Interview Schedule for Children–Revised.

while this is partly accurate, such symptoms may also be symptomatic of a psychiatric disorder. We refer to this tendency as "syndrome overshadowing" and find that some parents, as well as teachers and clinicians, minimize or even dismiss symptoms by attributing them to the syndrome.

In brief, many persons with WBS seem vulnerable to certain anxiety disorders, notably generalized anxiety disorder and specific phobia. These findings, although preliminary, demonstrate the promise of using psychiatric diagnoses as one way to better characterize behavioral problems commonly seen in this disorder. Similar studies are needed for other classes of diagnoses—including disruptive behavior disorders such as ADHD, affective disorders, and even personality disorders. These data, along with more global descriptors of maladaptive behavior, may serve as guideposts for interventions aimed at improving how persons with WBS learn, live, work, and play.

Intervention Issues

Little research has examined the effectiveness of syndrome-specific treatments in Williams-Beuren syndrome or in other genetic disorders involving mental retardation (Dykens and Hodapp 1997). Several workers recommend interventions for different syndromes based on well-established findings about the behavioral phenotypes of those syndromes (Dykens et al. 2000; Hodapp and Fidler 1999). Yet most of these interventions, though well-grounded in data, have yet to be rigorously assessed. The lack of treatment efficacy studies occurs across the behavioral gamut—from recommended strategies for enhancing reading, language, and social skills to recommendations for psychotropic medications or other therapies that target maladaptive behavior. We review here some intervention strategies that may help to ease or reduce some of the maladaptive and social-emotional challenges faced by people with WBS. Their efficacy, however, needs to be empirically tested.

Externalizing Problems

Typical recommendations for students without mental retardation but with ADHD are often helpful for children with WBS who suffer from inattention and distractibility. Overall, small classroom settings that minimize auditory and visual distractions are beneficial, as are reducing the flow of persons through the class, keeping extraneous material to a minimum, and placing the student's desk in a cubicle or in the front of the classroom. Behavior-modification techniques such as ignoring and redirecting off-task behaviors and rewarding on-task behaviors are also effective. Preliminary open and double-blind pharmacologic studies are encouraging, showing positive responses to methylphenidate for six children with WBS (e.g., decreased impulsivity, irritability, and inattention and activity levels) (Bawden et al. 1997; Power et al. 1997).

Social Issues

In the light of their social problems, many children and adults with WBS benefit from social skills training (Davies et al. 1998; Dykens and Rosner 1999). Although curricula vary, social skills lessons of particular relevance for persons with WBS include how to make and keep friends (e.g., approaching others, taking turns, starting and ending conversations), how to be appropriately wary of strangers, and, for adults, how to deal with romantic attachments. Using a team or "buddy" system to practice social skills may work in school settings, and older adolescents and adults may do well with group therapy aimed at promoting social skills and self-esteem. Although the syndrome's characteristic verbal skills and abilities to recognize others' emotions bode well for group therapies, groups may not be appropriate for persons who are overly anxious or easily distracted. Finally, although socially oriented jobs may be appropriate for some adults with WBS, these individuals will need high levels of sustained support from job coaches to succeed in these settings.

Internalizing Problems

At times, the obsessive thinking, worrying, or fretting about a specific topic or object shown by many persons with WBS can be appropriately tapped to facilitate learning. Examples might include using time with a favored object as a reward for on-task behavior or weaving the topic of interest into lessons to be learned (e.g., reading books about airplanes, using worksheets cut in the shape of an airplane). Yet for many individuals, being fascinated by airplanes, classmates, disasters, or future events gets in the way of learning or of the performance of everyday activities. In these cases, it often helps to set boundaries around the topic or activity and to keep such activities circumscribed to a certain time of day or to a specific place.

Anxieties and fears also respond well to containment tactics. Many children and adults become easily carried away with their fears and seek constant reassurances from parents and teachers. Although reassurances are important, limits are often necessary so that fears and adult attention-seeking are not inadvertently rewarded. After providing a brief period of comfort and reassurance, for example, many teachers and parents find it effective to move on to another topic or activity. If anxieties and fears persist or are associated with considerable distress or adaptive impairment, pharmacotherapy or cognitive-behavioral approaches may be helpful (Dykens 2000).

In the general population, many children and adults with phobic symptoms respond well to cognitive-behavioral techniques such as cognitive restructuring, somatic exercises to reduce physical tension, and systematic exposure (Craske 1999; Ollendick and King 1998). Exposure therapy entails systematic and repeated confrontation with phobic stimuli. A hierarchy of anxiety-provoking situations is usually developed, and exposures progress gradually from the least to most feared task. Exposures may be imagined or shown in a film or through live modeling, with the treatment of choice being live, in vivo exposure. For example, exposures for a child with WBS who has a fear of thunderstorms could begin with the therapist reading a weather report for rain and then progressing to showing the child a videotape of a storm.

Researchers have yet to establish the efficacy of these interventions alone or in combination with pharmacotherapy in treating phobic individuals with mental retardation (King et al. 1990). Nevertheless, the circumscribed goals and relatively short duration of most cognitive-behavioral treatments, combined with the well-developed expressive language and interpersonal strengths of many persons with WBS, bode well for positive therapeutic outcomes.

Although depression does not seem common, persons with WBS should be screened to ensure that the syndrome's charming facade does not mask underlying feelings of sadness or low esteem. Given their investments in people, many children and adults with WBS may be overly sensitive to loss, be it the death of a relative or household pet or letting go of previous relationships with teachers, friends, or therapists. Ruminating about these losses may reemerge in times of stress; if so, reassuring and then redirecting the individual may help him or her to dwell less on past losses.

Finally, in the light of the interests in music shown by some persons with Williams-Beuren syndrome (see chapters 15 and 16), some individuals may respond well to music therapy. Music therapy takes advantage of a variety of musical strategies to promote nonmusical cognitive or emotional goals, such as decreasing anxiety or improving attention, confidence, and self-esteem. The efficacy of music therapy has been shown in studies of anxious persons without mental retardation (Kerr et al. 2001), but its usefulness is less clear for those with mental retardation (Duffy and Fuller 2000). Increased musical activities were associated with less anxiety and fewer fears in two cohorts of persons with WBS (Dykens et al. 2003), suggesting that musical interventions may be efficacious in some cases.

Future Directions

In many ways, research on psychopathology in persons with Williams-Beuren syndrome is at a cross-road much like that in dual diagnosis research as a whole. In both instances, there are several good descriptive studies on maladaptive behavior, using well-established assessment tools. The time is ripe for researchers to shift gears and begin to delve deeper into these problems—including correlates of maladaptive behavior and risk and protective factors that span the "biopsychosocial" spectrum from genetic status to family stress and support. Throughout, a developmental perspective is particularly important, as the trajectories of problems in WBS seem both similar to and discrepant from those in the general population.

Future work could also be enriched by adding psychiatric assessments to data derived from behavioral checklists. This complementary approach would make our understandings of various symptoms more complete and open the door for researchers and clinicians to adapt well-established treatments to the unique qualities of persons with WBS. Finally, studies are sorely needed that test the efficacy of syndrome-based interventions and that optimize the quality of life for persons with WBS and their families.

ACKNOWLEDGMENTS

The authors thank Robert M. Hodapp, Ph.D., for his helpful comments on an earlier draft of this chapter, as well as the many families and persons with Williams-Beuren syndrome who have participated in our research. This work was supported by grant R0135681 from the National Institute of Child Health and Human Development.

REFERENCES

Aman, M. G., and Singh, N. N. 1994. *Aberrant Behavior Checklist—community supplementary manual.* East Aurora, NY: Slosson Educational Publications.

Anderson, J. C., Williams, S., McGee, R., and Silva, P. 1987. DSM-III disorders in preadolescent children. *Archives of General Psychiatry* 44:69–76.

Bawden, H. N., MacDonald, G. W., and Shea, S. 1997. Treatment of children with Williams syndrome with methylphenidate. *Journal of Child Neurology* 12:248–252.

Bellugi, U., Marks, S., Bihrle, A., and Sabo, H. 1988. Disassociation between language and cognitive functions in Williams syndrome. In *Language development in exceptional circumstances,* ed. D. Bishop and K. Mogford, 177–189. Edinburgh: Churchill-Livingstone.

Bellugi, U., Adolphs, R., Cassady, C., and Chiles, M. 1999. Towards the neural basis for hypersociability in a genetic syndrome. *Cognitive Neuroscience* 10:1653–1657.

Beuren, A. J., Apitz, J., and Harmjanz, D. 1962. Supravalvular aortic stenosis in association with mental retardation and a certain facial appearance. *Circulation* 26:1235–1240.

Borthwick-Duffy, S. A., and Eyman, R. K. 1990. Who are the dually diagnosed? *American Journal on Mental Retardation* 94:586–595.

Chapman, C. A., du Plessis, A., and Pober, B. R. 1996. Neurologic findings in children and adults with Williams syndrome. *Journal of Child Neurology* 11:63–65.

Cooper, S. A. 1997. Epidemiology of psychiatric disorders in elderly compared with younger adults with learning disabilities. *British Journal of Psychiatry* 170:375–380.

Craske, M. G. 1999. *Anxiety disorders: Psychological approaches to theory and treatment.* Boulder, CO: Westview Press.

Davies, M., Udwin, O., and Howlin, P. 1998. Adults with Williams syndrome. *British Journal of Psychiatry* 172:273–276.

De Leersynder, H., de Blois, M., Vekemans, M., Sidi, D., Villain, E., Kindermans, C., and Munnich, A. 2001. B_1-adrenergic antagonists improve sleep and behavioural disturbances in a circadian disorder, Smith Magenis syndrome. *Journal of Medical Genetics* 38:586–590.

Dilts, C. V., Morris, C. A., and Leonard, C. O. 1990. Hypothesis for development of a behavioral phenotype in Williams syndrome. *American Journal of Medical Genetics* 6 (suppl. 6): 126–131.

Duffy, B., and Fuller, R. 2000. Role of music therapy in social skills development of children with moderate intellectual disability. *Journal of Applied Research in Intellectual Disabilities* 13:77–89.

Dykens, E. M. 2000. Annotation: Psychopathology in children with intellectual disability. *Journal of Child Psychology and Psychiatry* 41:407–417.

———. 2003. Anxiety, fears, and phobias in persons with Williams syndrome. *Developmental Neuropsychology* 23:291–316.

Dykens, E. M., and Hodapp, R. M. 1997. Treatment issues in genetic mental retardation syndromes. *Professional Psychology: Research and Practice* 28:263–270.

———. 2001. Research in mental retardation: Toward an etiologic approach. *Journal of Child Psychology and Psychiatry* 42:49–71.

Dykens, E. M., and Rosner, B. A. 1999. Refining behavioral phenotypes: Personality-motivation in Williams and Prader-Willi syndromes. *American Journal on Mental Retardation* 104:158–169.

Dykens, E. M., and Smith, A. C. M. 1998. Distinctiveness and correlates of maladaptive behavior in children and adolescents with Smith-Magenis syndrome. *Journal of Intellectual Disability Research* 42:481–489.

Dykens, E. M., and Volkmar, F. R. 1997. Medical conditions associated with autism. In *Handbook of autism and pervasive developmental disorders*, 2nd ed., ed. D. J. Cohen and F. R. Volkmar, 388–407. New York: John Wiley.

Dykens, E. M., Leckman, J. F., and Cassidy, S. B. 1996. Obsessions and compulsions in Prader-Willi syndrome. *Journal of Child Psychology and Psychiatry and Allied Disciplines* 37:995–1002.

Dykens, E. M., Hodapp, R. M., and Finucane, B. M. 2000. *Genetics and mental retardation: A new look at behavior and interventions.* Baltimore: Brookes.

Dykens, E. M., Rosner, B. A., Ly, T., and Sagun, J. In press. *Music and anxiety in Williams syndrome: A harmonious or discordant relationship?*

Einfeld, S. L., and Tonge, B. J. 1992. *Manual for the Developmental Behaviour Checklist: Primary carer version.* Sydney: School of Psychiatry, University of New South Wales.

———. 1996. Population prevalence of psychopathology in children and adolescents with intellectual disability: II. Epidemiological findings. *Journal of Intellectual Disability Research* 40:99–109.

Einfeld, S. L., Tonge, B. J., and Florio, T. 1997. Behavioral and emotional disturbance in individuals with Williams syndrome. *American Journal on Mental Retardation* 102:45–53.

Einfeld, S. L., Tonge, B. J., and Rees, V. W. 2001. Longitudinal course of behavioral and emotional problems in Williams syndrome. *American Journal on Mental Retardation* 106:73–81.

Elgar, K., and Campbell, R. 2001. Annotation: The cognitive neuroscience of face recognition: Implications for developmental disorders. *Journal of Child Psychology and Psychiatry* 42:705–717.

Gillberg, C., and Rasmussen, P. 1994. Brief report: Four case histories and a literature review of Williams syndrome and autistic behavior. *Journal of Autism and Developmental Disorders* 24:381–393.

Gosch, A., and Pankau, R. 1994. Social-emotional and behavioral adjustment in children with Williams syndrome. *American Journal of Medical Genetics* 53:335–339.

———. 1997. Personality characteristics and behavior problems in individuals of different ages with Williams syndrome. *Developmental Medicine and Child Neurology* 39:527–533.

Gostason, R. 1985. Psychiatric illness among the mentally retarded: A Swedish population study. *Acta Psychiatrica Scandinavica* 71 (suppl. 318): 1–117.

Grice, S. J., Spratling, M. W., Karmiloff-Smith, A., Halit, H., Csibra, G., de Haan, M., and Johnson, M. D. 2001. Disordered visual processing and oscillatory brain activity in autism and Williams syndrome. *NeuroReport* 12:2697–2700.

Grizenko, N., Cvejic, H., Vida, S., and Sayegh, L. 1991. Behaviour problems of the mentally retarded. *Canadian Journal of Psychiatry* 36:712–717.

Gullone, E., King, N. J., and Cummins, R. A. 1996. Self-reported fears: A comparison study of youths with and without intellectual disability. *Journal of Intellectual Disability Research* 40:227–240.

Hodapp, R. M., and Fidler, D. L. 1999. Special education and genetics: Connections for the 21st century. *Journal of Special Education* 33:130–137.

Jacobson, J. W. 1982. Problem behavior and psychiatric impairment within a developmentally delayed population: I. Behavioral frequency. *Applied Research in Mental Retardation* 3:121–139.

Kerr, T., Walsh, J., and Marshall., A. 2001. Emotional change processes in music-assisted reframing. *Journal of Music Therapy* 38:193–211.

King, N. J., Ollendick, T. H., Gullone, E., Cummins, R. A., and Josephs, A. 1990. Fears and phobias in children and adolescents with intellectual disabilities: Assessment and intervention strategies. *Australian and New Zealand Journal of Developmental Disabilities* 16:97–108.

King, N. J., Josephs, A., Gullone, E., Madden, C., and Ollendick, T. H. 1994. Assessing the fears of children with disability using the Revised Fear Survey Schedule for Children: A comparative study. *British Journal of Medical Psychology* 67:377–386.

Korenberg, J. R., Chen, X., Hirota, H., Lai, Z., Bellugi, U., Burian, D., Roe, B., and Matsuoka, R. 2001. *Journey from cognition to brain to gene*, 147–178. Cambridge: MIT Press.

Leckman, J. F., Sholomskas, D., Thompson, D., Belanger, A., and Weissman, M. W. 1982. Best estimate of lifetime psychiatric diagnosis. *Archives of General Psychiatry* 39:879–883.

Lewinsohn, P. M., Gotlib, I. H., Lewinsohn, M., Seeley, J. R., and Allen, N. B. 1998. Gender differences in anxiety disorders and anxiety symptoms in adolescents. *Journal of Abnormal Psychology* 107:109–117.

Lott, I. T., and Head, E. 2001. Down syndrome and Alzheimer's disease: A link between development and aging. *Mental Retardation and Developmental Disabilities Research Reviews* 7:172–178.

Milne, J. M., Garrison, C. Z., Addy, C. L., McKeown, R. E., Jackson, K. L., Cuffe, S. P., and Waller, J. L. 1995. Frequency of phobic disorder in a community sample of adolescents. *American Journal of Child and Adolescent Psychiatry* 34:1202–1211.

Moss, S. C. 1999. Assessment: Conceptual issues. In *Psychiatric and behavioural disorders in developmental disabilities and mental retardation,* ed. N. Bouras, 18–37. Cambridge: Cambridge University Press.

Moss, S., Prosser, H., Ibbotson, B., and Goldberg, D. 1996. Respondent and infor-
mant accounts of psychiatric symptoms in a sample of patients with learning
disability. *Journal of Intellectual Disability Research* 40:457–465.

Moss, S. C., Emerson, E., Bouras, N., and Holland, A. 1997. Mental disorders and
problematic behaviors in people with intellectual disability: Future directions for research. *Journal of Intellectual Disability Research* 41:440–447.

Murphy, K. C., and Owen, M. J. 2001. Velo-cardio-facial syndrome: A model for understanding the genetics and pathogenesis of schizophrenia. *British Journal
of Psychiatry* 179:397–402.

O'Brien, G., and Yule, W., eds. 1995. *Behavioral phenotypes*. London: MacKeith
Press.

Ollendick, T. H., and King, N. J. 1998. Empirically supported treatments for children with phobic and anxiety disorders: Current status. *Journal of Clinical
Child Psychology* 27:156–167.

Ollendick, T. H., King, N. J., and Frary, R. B. 1989. Fears in children and adolescents: Reliability and generalizability across age, gender, and nationality. *Behavior Research and Therapy* 27:19–26.

Philips, I., and Williams, N. 1975. Psychopathology and mental retardation: A study
of 100 mentally retarded children: I. Psychopathology. *American Journal of
Psychiatry* 132:1265–1271.

Pober, B. R., and Dykens, E. M. 1996. Williams syndrome: An overview of medical,
cognitive, and behavioral features. *Child and Adolescent Psychiatric Clinics of
North America* 5:929–943.

Power, T. J., Blum, N. J., Jones, S. M., and Kaplan, P. E. 1997. Brief report: Response
to methylphenidate in two children with Williams syndrome. *Journal of
Autism and Developmental Disorders* 27:79–87.

Reich, W., Shayka, J. J., and Taibelson, C. 1991. *Diagnostic Interview Schedule for
Children and Adolescents, parent version*. St. Louis: Washington University.

Reiss, S. 1988. *Reiss Screen for Maladaptive Behavior*. Chicago: International Diagnostic Systems.

———. 1990. Prevalence of dual diagnosis in community-based day programs in
the Chicago metropolitan area. *American Journal on Mental Retardation*
94:578–585.

———. 1994. *Handbook of challenging behavior: Mental health aspects of mental retardation*. Worthington, OH: IDS Publishing.

Reiss, S., Levitan, G. W., and Szyszko, J. 1982. Emotional disturbance and mental retardation: Diagnostic overshadowing. *American Journal on Mental Retardation* 86:567–574.

Reiss, A. L., Feinstein, C., Rosenbaum, K. N., Borengasser-Caruso, M. A., and Gold-
smith, B. 1985. Autism associated with Williams syndrome. *Journal of Pediatrics* 106:247–249.

Rumsey, J. M. 1996. Neuroimaging studies of autism. In *Neuroimaging: A window to
the neurological foundations of learning and behavior in children*, ed. G. Rein
Lyon and J. M. Rumsey, 119–146. Baltimore: Brookes.

Rutter, M., Tizard, J., Yule, W., Graham, P., and Whitmore, K. 1976. Research report:
Isle of Wight studies, 1964–1974. *Psychological Medicine* 6:313–332.

Sovner, R. 1986. Limiting factors in the use of DSM-III with mentally ill/mentally
retarded persons. *Psychopharmacology Bulletin* 22:1055–1059.

Spence, S. H., and McCathie, H. 1993. The stability of fears in children: A two-year
prospective study: A research note. *Journal of Child Psychology and Psychiatry*
34:579–585.

Szymanski, L. S., King, B. H., Goldberg, B., Reid, A. H., Tonge, B. J., and Cain, N.

1998. Diagnosis of mental disorders in people with mental retardation. In *Psychotropic medications and developmental disabilities: The international consensus handbook,* ed. S. Reiss and M. G. Aman, 3–17. Columbus: Ohio State University Press.

Tomc, S. A., Williamson, N. K., and Pauli, R. M. 1990. Temperament in Williams syndrome. *American Journal of Medical Genetics* 36:345–352.

Udwin, O. 1990. A survey of adults with Williams syndrome and idiopathic infantile hypercalcemia. *Developmental Medicine and Child Neurology* 32:129–141.

Udwin, O., Yule, W., and Martin, N. 1987. Cognitive abilities and behavioral characteristics of children with idiopathic infantile hypercalcemia. *Journal of Child Psychology and Psychiatry* 13:232–244.

Van Borsel, J., Curfs, L. M. G., and Fryns, J. P. 1997. Hyperacusis in Williams syndrome: A sample survey. *Genetic Counseling* 8:121–126.

Wiggs, L., and Stores, G. 1996. Severe sleep disturbances and daytime challenging behaviour in children with severe learning disabilities. *Journal of Intellectual Disability Research* 40:518–528.

Williams, J. C., Barrett-Boyes, B. G., and Lowe, J. B. 1961. Supravalvular aortic stenosis. *Circulation* 24:1311–1318.

Sleep Patterns in Williams-Beuren Syndrome

13

Thornton B. A. Mason II, M.D., Ph.D.,
and Raanan Arens, M.D.

There is an increasing awareness of the importance of normal sleep patterns in pediatric health. For example, obstructive sleep apnea, a decreased or absent airflow during sleep because of obstruction, has been recognized in a large number of children. The American Academy of Pediatrics (2002) has published recommendations for the diagnosis and management of childhood obstructive sleep apnea, as a clinical practice guideline. Concomitantly, researchers have found associations between sleep disturbances, behavioral changes, and memory impairment. The parents of children with Williams-Beuren syndrome (WBS) have reported anecdotally that their children have sleep problems such as difficulty falling asleep and restless and disrupted sleep. Preliminary data collected at the Children's Hospital of Philadelphia suggest that at least a subset of children with WBS have abnormal sleep. By extrapolation from the developing literature on the clinical effects of sleep disorders, we can conclude that children with WBS and disturbed sleep may be at risk for further changes in behavior and cognitive function.

Sleep Findings in Children with Williams-Beuren Syndrome

As reported in an earlier study (Arens et al. 1998), the parents of twenty-eight patients with WBS (mean age, 4.7 ± 2.3 years) participated in a telephone survey to detect possible sleep dysfunction and to differentiate between sleep-disordered breathing (table 13.1, questions 1 and 2) and a possible movement arousal disorder (table 13.1, questions 3–8). From this survey, the profile of sixteen children with WBS (57%) was consistent with a possible motor disorder of sleep. The most commonly reported symptoms were awakenings, restless sleep, and difficulty initiating sleep.

Seven of these children suspected of having a motor disorder of sleep (mean age, 3.9 ± 2.2 years; range, 1.8–7 years) subsequently underwent polysomnography—that is, a multichannel recording of physiologic data

Table 13.1.
Telephone Survey of 28 Families of Children with Williams-Beuren Syndrome

To What Extent Does Your Child Have:	Never	Sometimes (≤1/wk.)	Often (2–5/wk.)	Always (6–7/wk.)	Don't Know
1. Difficulty breathing when asleep?	23	3	2	0	0
2. Snoring or noisy breathing?	17	6	1	4	0
3. Difficulty falling asleep at night (>30 min.)?	10	6	2	10	0
4. Restless tossing and turning in sleep?	9	5	3	10	1
5. Awakenings from sleep?	3	9	4	12	0
6. Discomfort in legs before sleep?	15	1	3	5	4
7. Repetitive leg movement during sleep?	14	2	4	2	6
8. Excessive daytime sleepiness?	15	3	2	3	5

associated with sleep, including the monitoring of brain activity, eye movements, respiratory effort, respiratory gas exchange, muscle activity, and heart rate. Also studied was a control group of ten children without WBS (mean age, 5.3 ± 2.0 years; range, 2–9 years; $P = 0.18$ vs. children with WBS) who had no suggestion of sleep-disordered breathing or a movement disorder of sleep, based on the same survey administered to the WBS group. All control subjects had no history of respiratory, cardiac, or neurologic disease. The WBS and control groups underwent overnight polysomnography under identical conditions. In addition to respiratory monitoring, electroencephalogram (EEG), electro-oculogram, and submental electromyogram (EMG), we monitored leg movements with a bilateral anterior tibialis EMG. Body movements and awakenings were also confirmed by visual inspection with a low-light camera and videotape recording. Respiratory variables, sleep stages, arousals from sleep, and periodic limb movements of sleep were scored using established criteria (Marcus et al. 1992; American Thoracic Society 1996; Rechtschaffen and Kales 1968; American Sleep Disorders Association [ASDA] and Sleep Research Society 1992; Mograss et al. 1994; Coleman 1982). The periodic limb movements in sleep index (PLMI) was defined as the number of periodic limb movements in sleep (PLMS) per hour of sleep. Also scored were the number of PLMS leading to an arousal or awakening per hour of sleep (PLMS-arousal index and PLMS-awake index, respectively).

The polysomnograms indicated that the mean respiratory values were normal overall, the subjects with WBS having results similar to those of the control subjects, except for a mild increase in baseline end-tidal (end-expiratory) pCO_2 (39 ± 3 mm Hg vs. 34 ± 3 mm Hg). Table 13.2 shows the sleep architecture results for the two groups—that is, the division of total sleep time between the sleep stages (including non-REM stages 1–4 and REM sleep, as explained below) and arousals/awakenings. The subjects with WBS had increased wake time, decreased stage 1 to 2, and increased stage 3 to 4 sleep compared with controls. There also seemed to be a trend for these sub-

Table 13.2.
Sleep Architecture in Children with Williams-Beuren Syndrome and Control Subjects (group means ± SD)

	Subjects with WBS (N = 7)	Control Subjects (N = 10)
Total sleep time (min.)	422 ± 54	473 ± 67
Sleep efficiency (%)	83 ± 10	89 ± 7
Sleep latency (min.)	44 ± 38	25 ± 23
Wake (% SPT)	10 ± 7*	4 ± 5
Stage 1–2 (% SPT)	41 ± 8**	59 ± 9
Stage 3–4 (% SPT)	34 ± 7**	20 ± 5
REM (% SPT)	14 ± 9	15 ± 9
Arousal index (no./hr.)	6 ± 3	7.4 ± 3
Awakening index (no./hr.)	1.2 ± 0.7	1.2 ± 0.6

Abbreviation: SPT, sleep period time.
* $P < 0.05$; ** $P < 0.001$.

jects to have less total sleep time and less sleep efficiency than the control children. The children with WBS had a significantly higher number of PLMS jerks and PLMS episodes than controls, with a fivefold greater PLMI (table 13.3). In addition to the higher mean PLMI, the children with WBS had a greater variability in PLMI than control subjects (fig. 13.1).

These preliminary data demonstrate (1) parental awareness of dysfunctional sleep in children with WBS; (2) a PLMI fivefold greater in a selected group of subjects with WBS than in control subjects, with a large amount of variability; and (3) a greater percentage of sleep time spent awake in children with WBS compared with controls.

Overview of Sleep, with Implications for Children with Williams-Beuren Syndrome
Sleep and Learning/Memory

REM and Non-REM Sleep. In general, sleep can be divided into two main categories: rapid eye movement (REM) sleep and non-REM (NREM) sleep. REM sleep is characterized on polysomnography by a low-voltage, mixed-

Table 13.3.
Limb Movements during Sleep in Children with Williams-Beuren Syndrome and Control Subjects (group means ± SD)

	Subjects with WBS (N = 7)	Control Subjects (N = 10)
Total leg jerks	158 ± 58*	65 ± 23
PLMS jerks	108 ± 57**	23 ± 15
PLMS episodes	12.6 ± 4.8*	4.3 ± 2.7
PLMI (no./hr.)	14.9 ± 6.2**	2.8 ± 1.9
PLMI-NREM (no./hr.)	12.2 ± 4.5**	2.2 ± 1.8
PLMI-REM (no./hr.)	2.7 ± 3.1	0.6 ± 1.1
PLMI-arousal index (no./hr.)	4.5 ± 3.1**	1.0 ± 0.9
PLMS-awake index (no./hr.)	1.1 ± 0.7*	0.3 ± 0.2

Abbreviations: PLMS, periodic limb movements in sleep; PLMI, PLMS index; NREM, non-REM sleep.
* $P < 0.05$; ** $P < 0.001$.

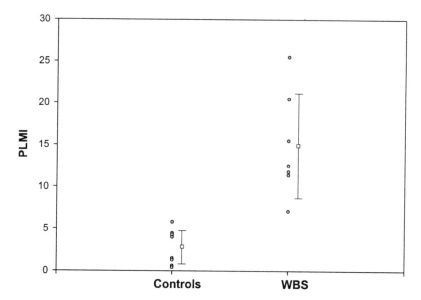

Fig. 13.1. PLMI indices (PMLI), showing means (open squares) and one standard deviation. Note that children with WBS have a higher mean and a wider SD (greater variability).

frequency EEG; a relatively low-amplitude chin EMG (consistent with skeletal muscle hypotonia); and episodes of rapid eye movements. During the night, there are usually three to five episodes of REM sleep, and the episodes tend to increase in duration as sleep progresses. Dreams are more common during REM sleep and usually more complex than in NREM sleep. NREM sleep has four stages. Stages 1 and 2 are light sleep, and stages 3 and 4 are delta or slow-wave sleep (SWS). SWS is considered deeper NREM sleep, marked by high-amplitude broad waves in the EEG.

The polysomnography results described in tables 13.2 and 13.3 support the conclusion that children with WBS can have both NREM sleep stages 1 to 4 and REM sleep. The REM sleep component as a percentage of sleep time seems not to differ from that of control children. The data suggest, however, that SWS may be relatively increased in WBS, whereas lighter sleep (stages 1 and 2) may be relatively decreased. Further studies are needed to determine whether these NREM sleep findings are characteristic of children with WBS.

When one considers the possible clinical implications of sleep disturbances in WBS, many important questions on sleep in normal individuals have yet to be answered. For example, why does sleep in all individuals consist of NREM and REM stages? And, a larger question, why do we need sleep? Multiple hypotheses on the function of sleep have been proposed: brain thermoregulation, energy conservation, brain detoxification (Inoue et al. 1995), replenishment of brain energy stores (Benington and Heller 1995), and the fostering of plastic cerebral changes that underlie learning and memory (Maquet 2001). If there is an important relationship between sleep and learning/ memory, disturbed sleep might be expected to affect performance in many spheres. For children with WBS, the common cognitive profile (relative strengths in auditory rote memory and language ability, with marked weakness in visuospatial constructional ability) may be related to or influenced by disturbed sleep.

Sleep and Memory Consolidation. The conventional view is that sleep processes are involved in the consolidation of memory (Maquet 2001). Memory consolidation can be thought of as a time-dependent process that converts labile memory traces into permanent and/or enriched forms. Accordingly, information acquired while awake is actively restructured, altered, and strengthened during sleep (Peigneux et al. 2001). The mechanisms whereby memory traces are consolidated during sleep are not known, although some researchers suggest that gene transcription and protein synthesis are involved (Ribeiro et al. 1999). With neuronal activity, there might be a local release of many types of molecules such as adenosine, nitric oxide, and various cytokines that may signal an increased need for sleep. Hence, a use-dependent sleep drive may be in place (Maquet et al. 2002).

Declarative and Nondeclarative Memory. Memory has two categories that may be linked to sleep: declarative and nondeclarative memory. *Declarative memory* is involved in acquiring and recalling specific events (episodic memory) and new facts (semantic memory) over periods of days to weeks. The neuroanatomic structures involved in declarative memory include the hippocampus and adjacent parahippocampal, entorhinal, and perirhinal cortices (Plihal and Born 1999). *Nondeclarative memory* refers to a heterogeneous group of memory abilities that are assumed to be independent of the hippocampal region structures. Procedural memory forms part of nondeclarative memory, in which skillful behaviors or habits require repeated practicing of a perceptual, cognitive, or motor skill task (as in acquiring superior athletic performance) (Plihal and Born 1999). In some studies, declarative memory (e.g., as tested through paired association word lists) seems to improve to a greater extent over periods of early (as opposed to late) nocturnal sleep; in other cases, declarative memory tasks have not shown any sleep dependence (Stickgold et al. 2001). In contrast, mirror tracing skills (nondeclarative memory) are apparently facilitated by late nocturnal sleep more than by early sleep (Plihal and Born 1999). These findings suggest that early sleep (dominated by SWS) has consolidating effects that enhance declarative memory, whereas nondeclarative memory may benefit from late sleep with REM predominance.

It is intriguing to note that, given the preliminary data demonstrating a relative increase in SWS among children with WBS, sleep characteristics might contribute to their enhanced declarative memory. Indeed, auditory rote memory abilities seem to provide a firm foundation for both grammatical development and vocabulary acquisition in WBS (Mervis et al. 1999).

Sleep Deprivation. One experimental approach for testing the sleep-memory association has been sleep deprivation. Smith (1996) noted that sleep-deprivation studies (usually the REM type) show mixed results. When the material to be learned included word tests or paired associations, no deprivation effects were reported. With more complex manipulations of symbols or words that required a new behavioral strategy, sleep deprivation has been reported to impair memory processes, interfering with memory consolidation (Smith 1996; Stickgold et al. 2000; Maquet 2001). It seems that procedural/implicit tasks and declarative/explicit tasks are differentially sensitive to sleep loss. Further studies support the suggestion that performance is impaired only if sleep deprivation occurs during specific windows of time during REM (paradoxical) sleep (Smith 1996) and even support a two-step process in memory formation in humans, involving SWS and REM sleep sequentially (Gais et al. 2000). One concern raised in the interpretation of studies employing a sleep-deprivation paradigm is the potential contamination by nonspecific effects of sleep deprivation. These effects, such as a systemic stress response or decreased motivation and arousal, could also be associated with memory impairment or with altered REM sleep in the absence of any particular learning task (Maquet 2000; Seigel 2001).

Visual Texture Discrimination Tasks. Mednick et al. (2002) examined performance in visual texture discrimination tasks. They found that, with repeated testing within a single day, perceptual thresholds progressively increased, with worsening performance over four testing sessions. If the target stimuli were shifted to an untrained region of visual space (i.e., a novel stimulus location) or if the subject took a midday nap, this worsening of performance was prevented. Performance deterioration did not seem to be linked to decreased motivation or the difficulty of the task. Whereas the authors believed that SWS most likely played a central role in reversing the performance decrement, a function for REM sleep could not be excluded. In the near future, the respective roles of NREM and REM sleep in consolidating distinct memory types may be better defined (Peigneux et al. 2001).

For children with WBS, the sleep research performed to date raises other interesting issues. At least some of the research studies support the enhancement of nondeclarative memory with REM-predominant late sleep. Similarly, disturbances in REM sleep could be expected to adversely affect nondeclarative memory (such as skilled motor tasks). As children with WBS have extreme difficulty with tasks involving visuospatial construction (e.g., drawing and block design) (Wang et al. 1995; Bellugi et al. 1994), there could be concomitant REM sleep disturbances. The preliminary polysomnography data for children with WBS did not show differences in REM sleep as a percentage of sleep time compared with controls, but the quality of REM sleep may be decreased in WBS. Subtle disruptions of REM sleep (microarchitectural changes) that do not produce body movement–associated arousals or awakenings could be important here. By extension, improving the quality of REM sleep in children with WBS might lead to enhanced procedural memory and stronger performance in visuospatial construction tasks.

Sleep Disorders

Many disorders can affect sleep, including so-called intrinsic sleep disorders (disorders that either originate or develop within the body or that arise from causes within the body) and extrinsic sleep disorders (disorders that originate or develop from causes outside the body) (ASDA 1997). From a genetics perspective, intrinsic sleep disorders are particularly important. The preliminary data strongly support the higher prevalence of PLMS, an intrinsic sleep disorder, in individuals with WBS than in controls. Other intrinsic sleep disorders that may affect total sleep/REM sleep in WBS are restless legs syndrome and obstructive sleep apnea.

Periodic Limb Movements in Sleep. PLMS was originally termed *nocturnal myoclonus;* it consists of rhythmic and highly stereotyped flexion movements of the lower and sometimes upper extremities (ASDA 1997). In the lower extremities, PLMS occurs as rhythmic extensions of the big toe, with ankle dorsiflexion and knee/hip flexion, and clusters in episodes that may last minutes to hours. Hundreds of these PLMS may occur per night in some individuals. The subset of children with WBS in the study described earlier had a mean number of PLMS of 108 (SD = 57) (Arens et al. 1998).

Leg movements are recorded by overnight polysomnography and analyzed by standard criteria (table 13.3) (Bonnet et al. 1993; ASDA 1997). These movement episodes may predominate in the first half of the night and tend to occur during stages 1 and 2 of sleep. Periodic limb movements can, however, recur during any period of sleep (Nicolas et al. 1999). Intense movements may produce arousals from sleep; if numerous, these arousals/awakenings may result in nonrestorative sleep. Subtle arousals may be underrecognized, as suggested earlier. PLMS may occur in up to 6% of the general population, increasing in prevalence with advancing age (Hening et al. 1999a).

Restless Legs Syndrome. PLMS is commonly associated with restless legs syndrome (RLS) in adults, although the relationship between these two conditions in children has not been defined. RLS is estimated to affect at least 5% of adults. Four clinical features characterize RLS: (1) episodes of periodic, distressing paresthesias ("crawling" sensations) with irresistible urges to move the extremities (usually the legs); (2) temporary relief of sensations by moving the affected extremity; (3) episodes of periodic and repetitive movements of the affected extremity; and (4) symptoms that show diurnal fluctuation, with worsening in the evening (International Restless Legs Syndrome Study Group 1995). Sensory manifestations of RLS are intensely uncomfortable, and dysesthesias include crawling, burning, tingling, aching, and itchy sensations, mostly between the knees and ankles. Associated motor restlessness may include tossing/turning in bed, leg stretching, pacing, leg flexion, body rocking, and foot rubbing. Although most individuals with RLS have associated PLMS (80%–90%) (Montplaisir et al. 1997), RLS may occur as an isolated phenomenon. In adults, PLMS and RLS are associated with a wide range of wake-sleep complaints, including insomnia and daytime sleepiness (Montplaisir et al. 2000).

Given the high prevalence of PLMS in Williams-Beuren syndrome, RLS may also be increased. Because RLS is established by subjective criteria, the diagnosis is difficult to establish in childhood in general, and the task may be more difficult in WBS. Reliable and valid questionnaires need to be developed to explore RLS in pediatric populations.

The Pathogenesis of PLMS and RLS. The pathogenesis of PLMS is unknown. Systemic, vascular, peripheral nervous system, genetic, and central nervous system etiologies have been proposed (Hening et al. 1999a; Tayag-Kier et al. 2000). The leg movements of PLMS occur with remarkable periodicity and suggest the presence of an underlying central nervous system pacemaker or generator (Lugaresi et al. 1972). Studies have reported a twenty- to forty-second periodicity for blood pressure, intraventricular fluid pressure, respiration, and pulse frequency during normal sleep. The periodicity of these phenomena overlaps with PLMS, and all these functions can be synchronous (Montplaisir et al. 2000). These data suggest that, in PLMS, a normal pacemaker (brainstem or spinal cord) becomes disinhibited. Further support for the involvement of spinal mechanisms comes from observations of PLMS in patients with complete spinal cord injury and from the close resemblance of periodic limb movements to spinal cord flexor responses (Yokota et al. 1991; Bara-Jiminez et al. 2000). More recent studies provide evidence that RLS may have an autosomal dominant mode of inheritance in families with early age at onset, although no candidate gene has been established (Winkelmann et al. 2002). A contributing factor to RLS may be a reduction in the relative availability of iron in the brain (Sun et al. 1998; Earley et al. 2000).

Obstructive Sleep Apnea. The sleep disorder known as obstructive sleep apnea (OSA) is common in childhood, affecting approximately 2% of all children (Marcus 2001). Seven to twelve percent of children snore habitually and may have a particularly high risk for sleep-disordered breathing (Chervin et al. 2002a). Increased upper airway resistance and the inability to maintain a patent airway during sleep result in hypopneas (partial obstructive events) and apneas (cessation of airflow). In turn, these respiratory events may lead to hypoxia, hypercarbia, and frequent arousals; neurocognitive and behavioral disruptions may result. Parents may report that their affected children have prominent snoring, gasping, observed apneas, restlessness, and unusual sleeping patterns (e.g., sleeping upright). The peak age of childhood OSA is between two and six years, when tonsils and adenoids are largest in relation to airway size; however, polysomnography is necessary to establish the diagnosis, as the degree of adenotonsillar hypertrophy may not correlate with the presence or severity of sleep apnea. Although tonsillectomy/adenoidectomy remains the best treatment for childhood OSA, other treatment modalities include weight loss and noninvasive ventilatory support (e.g., continuous positive airway pressure [CPAP]) (Marcus 2001; American Academy of Pediatrics 2002).

As yet, OSA has not been shown to be prominent in WBS, but it should be assessed in future studies. Given the prevalence of OSA in the general population, in a larger sample size some children with WBS would be expected to have OSA.

Attention Deficit Hyperactivity Disorder and Sleep. Attention deficit hyperactivity disorder (ADHD) is one of the most common neuropsychiatric disorders of childhood and adolescence, with a prevalence estimated at 3% to 5% in the United States and Europe. ADHD is especially common in WBS, with approximately 70% of individuals affected (Osborne 1999).

Although the etiology of ADHD remains unclear, abnormalities related to sleep and wakefulness mechanisms have been hypothesized, as well as a primary alteration of alertness (hypoarousal with repetitive tasks and hyperarousal with new stimuli or immediate reward). Excessive motor activity may represent a strategy to stay alert and awake (Weinberg and Harper 1993). Excessive movement in sleep was listed in *Diagnostic and Statistical Manual–III* (DSM-III) as one of five possible behavioral markers of hyperactivity used in establishing the diagnosis of ADHD; neither DSM-III-R nor DSM-IV, however, list sleep problems as a marker for ADHD or as an associated feature. Sleep problems are frequently reported by parents of children with ADHD and other neurodevelopmental disorders (Marcotte et al. 1998), but studies using objective measures of sleep have often not provided sufficient evidence to support these subjective reports (Corkum et al. 1998).

Gruber et al. (2000) used actigraphy (motion sensors that record body movement and, by extension, periods of activity/wakefulness vs. inactivity/ sleep) and sleep diaries to study boys meeting DSM-IV criteria for ADHD and a group of controls. No significant differences were found in averaged actigraphic sleep measures (such as sleep onset time, sleep duration, night awakenings, percentage of time asleep) and no differences between the control and ADHD groups in subjective sleep measures (e.g., sleep quality, tiredness during the day). There were statistically significant group differences, however, in night-to-night variability of actigraphic sleep measures (duration of sleep, true sleep time, and sleep onset time). The clinical implications of this apparent instability of the sleep-wake schedule are unclear.

Several studies support an association between ADHD and specific intrinsic sleep disturbances. Periodic limb movements in sleep and restless legs syndrome have been reported to be more prominent in children with ADHD compared with controls (Picchietti and Walters 1999; Picchietti et al. 1999). Walters and colleagues (2000) found that dopaminergic therapy not only was effective for pediatric PLMS and/or RLS but also was associated with improvement in several scales of daytime behavior and performance (supporting an improvement in ADHD). Other studies have indicated an association between ADHD symptoms and sleep-disordered breathing (Guilleminault et al. 1982; Ali et al. 1996; Chervin and Archbold 2001; Chervin et al. 2002a, 2002b). The mechanism by which sleep-disordered breathing might contribute to hyperactive behavior in such children is uncertain, but sleep deprivation, sleep disruption, inadequate oxygen saturation, and perhaps many other variables could be involved (Chervin et al. 2002a).

Treatment Options for ADHD, PLMS, and RLS. Classes of medications that have been used for treatment of RLS/PLMS in the general population include benzodiazepines, dopaminergic agents, anticonvulsants, and opiates (Chesson et al. 1999).

Four of five patients with WBS and PLMS who were given a trial of clonazepam showed immediate and sustained improvement, including a significant decrease in the average PMLI in three of three patients in follow-up studies (Arens et al. 1998). When evaluating the efficacy of clonazepam and other benzodiazepines, however, there may be difficulty in differentiating nonspecific effects on sleep from specific actions on PLMS (Hening et al. 1999b).

PLMS is responsive to dopaminergic therapy, providing general clues to the pathways involved as well as to effective treatment options. Numerous reports demonstrate the effectiveness of dopaminergic agents in the treatment of PLMS and/or RLS (Montplaisir et al. 1996, 1999; Brodeur et al. 1988; Walters et al. 1988). Of these dopaminergic agents, pramipexole, a newly developed D$_3$ receptor agonist, is reported to be the most effective (Montplaisir et al. 1999). To date, no randomized, placebo-controlled trials of therapy for PLMS or RLS have been conducted in children, but pediatric use of L-dopa, carbidopa, and benserazide-levodopa has been reported in many published studies and case reports (Greene et al. 2000; Procianoy et al. 1999; Dionisi-Vici et al. 2000). Overall, L-dopa seems to be fairly well tolerated in the pediatric population, and side effects in children diminish with dose adjustments. Combinations of L-dopa and carbidopa are available in standard and long-acting formulations. Walters and colleagues (2000) suggest that RLS and PLMS should comprise part of the differential diagnosis of the child with ADHD and that patients could potentially benefit from dopaminergic therapy.

Clinical Implications

The data presented here support several important inferences. First, children with WBS may be at risk for sleep disruption, due to periodic limb movements in sleep, restless legs syndrome, or sleep-disordered breathing. Second, the clinical evaluation of children with WBS should include a sleep history to probe the quality and quantity of sleep, as well as for the presence of a specific sleep disorder. Third, overnight polysomnography, the "gold standard" of assessment, may provide critical information necessary for the diagnosis of a sleep disorder. Fourth, drug treatment (for RLS/PLMS) and surgical treatment (tonsillectomy/adenoidectomy for OSA) are available options. Finally, disturbed sleep may adversely affect cognitive functioning, memory consolidation, and behavior; therefore, management/treatment of sleep disorders may result in improved social interactions and academic performance.

Future Directions

Given that the general field of sleep medicine is young, the area of pediatric sleep medicine is still in its infancy. The next several years should afford an opportunity for children with WBS to be evaluated thoroughly for sleep disorders. It may be that sleep disturbances affect a significant number of individuals with WBS and, if so, disturbed sleep could contribute to the overall phenotype of WBS. Indeed, it would be especially informative to develop a large cross-sectional study of sleep in children with WBS that includes a prospective component; a large, matched cohort of normally developing children could also be evaluated as a comparison. Such expanded samples would allow more reliable estimates of the point prevalence and variability of different sleep disorders among children with WBS. Baseline neuropsychometric testing should be compared with testing after various interventions for sleep disorders; improvement would indicate the effects of associated sleep problems and demonstrate the relative effectiveness of different treatment strategies. The rapidly developing field of functional neuroimaging could provide further insight into the relationship between disturbed sleep and cognitive function in WBS. Research on sleep in WBS also has great potential for increasing our understanding of pathways that may be implicated in intrinsic sleep disorders such as PLMS and RLS. Of the many genes identified so far in the WBS critical region of 7q11.23, one or more may play roles in sleep physiology pathways (such as influencing monoaminergic neurotransmitter levels). These findings could, in turn, affect the care of patients with or without WBS.

ACKNOWLEDGMENTS

We thank Dr. Allan Pack and Dr. Paige Kaplan for their helpful suggestions and support in the study of sleep in children with WBS. This work was made possible in part by grant K23 RR16566-01 from the National Institutes of Health to Dr. Mason.

REFERENCES

Ali, N. J., Pitson, D. J., and Stradling, J. R. 1996. Sleep disordered breathing: Effects of adenotonsillectomy on behaviour and psychological functioning. *European Journal of Pediatrics* 155:56–62.

Allen, R. P., Barker, P. B., Wehrl, F., Song, H. K., and Earley, C. J. 2001. MRI measurement of brain iron in patients with restless legs syndrome. *Neurology* 56:263–265.

American Academy of Pediatrics. 2002. Clinical practice guideline: Diagnosis and management of childhood obstructive sleep apnea. *Pediatrics* 109:704–712.

American Sleep Disorders Association. 1997. *The International Classification of Sleep Disorders, revised: Diagnostic and coding manual.* Rochester, MN: The Association.

American Sleep Disorders Association and Sleep Research Society. 1992. EEG arousals: Scoring rules and examples. A preliminary report from the Sleep Disorders Task Force of the American Sleep Disorders Association. *Sleep* 15:173–184.

American Thoracic Society. 1996. Standards and indications for cardiopulmonary sleep studies in children. *American Journal of Respiratory and Critical Care Medicine* 153:866–878.

Arens, R., Wright, B., Elliott, J., Zhao, H., Wang, P. P., Brown, L. W., Namey, T., and Kaplan, P. 1998. Periodic limb movements in sleep in children with Williams syndrome. *Journal of Pediatrics* 133:670–674.

Bara-Jiminez, W., Aksu, M., Graham, B., Sato, S., and Hallet, M. 2000. Periodic limb movements in sleep: State-dependent excitability of the spinal flexor reflex. *Neurology* 54:1609–1615.

Bellugi, U., Wang, P. P., and Jernigan, T. L. 1994. Williams syndrome: An unusual neuropsychological profile. In *Atypical cognitive deficits in developmental disorders: Implications for brain function,* ed. S. H. Broman and J. Grafman, 23–56. Hilldale, NJ: Erlbaum.

Benington, J. H., and Heller, H. C.. 1995. Restoration of brain energy metabolism as the function of sleep. *Progress in Neurobiology* 45:347–360.

Bonnet, M., Carley, D., Carskadon, M., Easton, P., Guilleminault, C., Harper, R., Hayes, B., Hirshkowitz, M., Ktonas, P., Keenan, S., Pressman, M., Roehrs, T., Smith, J., Walsh, J., Weber, S., and Westbrook, P. (ASDA Atlas Task Force). 1993. Recording and scoring leg movements. *Sleep* 16:748–759.

Brodeur, C., Montplaisir, J., Marinier, R., and Godbout, R. 1988. Treatment of RLS and PLMS with l-DOPA: A double-blind controlled study. *Neurology* 35:1845–1848.

Chervin, R. D., and Archbold, K. H. 2001. Hyperactivity and polysomnographic findings in children evaluated for sleep-disordered breathing. *Sleep* 24:313–320.

Chervin, R. D., Archbold, K. H., Dillon, J. E., Panahi, P., Pituch, K. J., Dahl, R. E., and Guilleminault, C. 2002a. Inattention, hyperactivity, and symptoms of sleep-disordered breathing. *Pediatrics* 109:449–456.

Chervin, R. D., Archbold, K. H., Dillon, J. E., Pituch, K. J., Panahi, P., Dahl, R. E., and Guilleminault, C. 2002b. Associations between symptoms of inattention, hyperactivity, restless legs, and periodic leg movements. *Sleep* 25:213–218.

Chesson, A. L., Jr., Wise, M., Davila, D., Johnson, S., Littner, M., Anderson, W. M., Hartse, K., and Rafecas, J. 1999. Practice parameters for the treatment of restless legs syndrome and periodic limb movement disorder: An American Academy of Sleep Medicine Report, Standards of Practice Committee of the American Academy of Sleep Medicine. *Sleep* 22:961–968.

Coleman, R. M. 1982. Periodic movements in sleep (nocturnal myoclonus) and restless leg syndrome. In *Sleeping and waking disorders: Indications and techniques*, ed. C. Guilleminault, 265–295. Menlo Park, CA: Addison-Wesley.

Corkum, P., Tannock, R., and Moldofsky, H. 1998. Sleep disturbances in children with attention-deficit/hyperactivity disorder. *Journal of the American Academy of Child and Adolescent Psychiatry* 37:637–646.

Dionisi-Vici, C., Hoffmann, G. F., Leuzzi, V., Hoffken, H., Brautigam C., Rizzo, C., Steebergen-Spanjers, G. C., Smeitink, J. A., and Wevers, R. A. 2000. Tyrosine hydroxylase deficiency with severe clinical course: Clinical and biochemical investigations and optimization of therapy. *Journal of Pediatrics* 136:560–562.

Earley, C. J., Connor, J. R., Beard, J. L., Malecki, E. A., Epstein, D. K., and Allen, R. P. 2000. Abnormalities in CSF concentrations of ferritin and transferrin in restless legs syndrome. *Neurology* 54:1698–1700.

Gais, S., Plihal, W., Wagner, U., and Born, J. 2000. Early sleep triggers memory for early visual discrimination skills. *Nature Neuroscience* 3:1335–1339.

Greene, P. E., Bressman, S. B., Ford, B., and Hyland, K. 2000. Parkinsonism, dystonia, and hemiatrophy. *Movement Disorders* 15:537–541.

Gruber, R., Sadeh, A., and Raviv. 2000. Instability of sleep patterns in children with attention-deficit/hyperactivity disorder. *Journal of the American Academy of Child and Adolescent Psychiatry* 39:495–501.

Guilleminault, C., Winkle, R., Korobkin, R., and Simmons, B. 1982. Children and nocturnal snoring—evaluation of the effects of sleep related respiratory resistive load and daytime functioning. *European Journal of Pediatrics* 139:165–171.

Hening, W., Allen, R., Earley, C., Kushida, C., Picchietti, D., and Silber, M. 1999a. The treatment of restless legs syndrome and periodic limb movement disorder. *Sleep* 22:970–999.

Hening, W. A., Allen, R., Walters, A. S., and Chokroverty, S. 1999b. Motor functions and dysfunctions of sleep. In *Sleep disorders medicine: Basic science, technical considerations, and clinical aspects,* 2nd ed., ed. S. Chokroverty, 441–507. Boston: Butterworth Heinemann.

Inoue, S., Honda, K., and Komoda, Y. 1995. Sleep as neuronal detoxification and restitution. *Behavioral Brain Research* 69:91–96.

International Restless Legs Syndrome Study Group (Arthur S. Walters MD—Group Organizer and Correspondent). 1995. Towards a better definition of the restless legs syndrome. *Movement Disorders* 10:634–642.

Lugaresi, E., Coccagna, G., Mantovani, M., and Lebrun, R. 1972. Some periodic phenomena arising during drowsiness and sleep in man. *Electroencephalography and Clinical Neurophysiology* 32:701–705.

Maquet, P. 2000. Sleep on it! *Nature Neuroscience* 3:1235–1236.

———. 2001. The role of sleep in learning and memory. *Science* 294:1048–1051.

Maquet, P., Peigneux, P., Laureys, S., and Smith, C. 2002. Be caught napping: You're resting more than your eyes. *Nature Neuroscience* 5:618–619.

Marcotte, A. C., Thacher, P. V., Butters, M., Bortz, J., Acebo, C., and Carscadon, M. A. 1998. Parental report of sleep problems in children with attention and learning disorders. *Journal of Developmental and Behavioral Pediatrics* 19:178–186.

Marcus, C. 2001. Sleep-disordered breathing in children. *American Journal of Respiratory and Critical Care Medicine* 164:16–30.

Marcus, C. L., Omlin, K. J., Basinski, D. J., Bailey, S. L., Rachal, A. B., Von Pechmann, W. S., Keens, T. G., and Ward, S. L. 1992. Normal polysomnogram values for children and adolescents. *American Review of Respiratory Disease* 146:1235–1239.

Mednick, S. C., Nakayama, K., Cantero, J. L., Atienza, M., Levin, A. A., Pathak, N., and Stickgold, R. 2002. The restorative effect of naps on perceptual deterioration. *Nature Neuroscience* 5:677–681.

Mervis, C. B., Morris, C. A., Bertrand, J., and Robinson, B. F. 1999. Williams syndrome: Findings from an integrated program of research. In *Neurodevelopmental disorders,* ed. H. Tager-Flusberg, 65–110. Cambridge: MIT Press.

Mograss, M. A., Ducharme, F. M., and Brouillette, R. T. 1994. Movement/arousals: Description, classification, and relationship to sleep apnea in children. *American Journal of Respiratory and Critical Care Medicine* 150:1960–1966.

Montplaisir, J., Boucher, S., Gosselin, A., Pourier, G., and Lavigne, G. 1996. Persistence of repetitive EEG arousals (K-alpha complexes) in RLS patients treated with l-dopa. *Sleep* 19:196–199.

Montplaisir, J., Boucher, S., Poirier, G., Lavigne, G., Lapierre, O., and Lasperance, P. 1997. Clinical, polysomnographic, and genetic characteristics of restless legs syndrome: A study of 133 patients diagnosed with new standard criteria. *Movement Disorders* 12:61–65.

Montplaisir, J., Nicolas, A., Denesle, R., and Gomez-Mancilla, B. 1999. Restless legs syndrome improved by pramipexole, a double-blind randomized trial. *Neurology* 52:938–943.

Montplaisir, J., Nicolas, A., Godbout, R., and Walters, A. 2000. Restless legs syndrome and periodic limb movement disorder. In *Principles and practice of sleep medicine,* ed. M. H. Kryger, T. Roth, and W. C. Dement, 742–752. Philadelphia: Saunders.

Nicolas, A., Michaud, M., Lavigne, G., and Montplaisir, J. et al. 1999. The influence of sex, age and sleep/wake state on characteristics of periodic leg movements in restless legs syndrome patients. *Clinical Neurophysiology* 110:1168–1174.

Osborne, L. R. 1999. Williams-Beuren syndrome: Unraveling the mysteries of a microdeletion disorder. *Molecular Genetics and Metabolism* 67:1–10.

Peigneux, P., Laureys, S., Delbeuck, X., and Maquet, P. 2001. Sleeping brain, learning brain: The role of sleep for memory systems. *NeuroReport* 12:A111–A124.

Picchietti, D. L., and Walters, A. S. 1999. Moderate to severe periodic limb movement disorder in childhood and adolescence. *Sleep* 22:297–300.

Picchietti, D. L., Underwood, D. J., Farris, W. A., Walters, A. S., Shah, M. M., Dahl, R. E., Trubnick, L. J., Bertocci, M. A., Wagner, M., and Hening, W. A. 1999. Further studies on periodic limb movement disorder and restless legs syndrome in children with attention-deficit hyperactivity disorder. *Movement Disorders* 14:1000–1007.

Plihal, W., and Born, J. 1999. Effects of early and late nocturnal sleep on priming and spatial memory. *Psychophysiology* 36:571–582.

Procianoy, E., Fuchs, F. D., Procianoy, L., and Procianoy, F. 1999. The effect of increasing doses of levodopa on children with strabismic amblyopia. *Journal of the American Association for Pediatric Ophthalmology and Strabismus* 3:337–340.

Rechtschaffen, A., and Kales, A. 1968. *A manual of standardized terminology, techniques and scoring systems for sleep stages of human subjects.* Washington, DC: National Institutes of Health.

Ribeiro, S., Goyal, V., Mello, C. V., and Pavlides, C. 1999. Brain gene expression during REM sleep depends on prior waking experience. *Learning and Memory* 6:500–508.

Seigel, J. M. 2001. The REM sleep-memory consolidation hypothesis. *Science* 294:1058–1063.

Smith, C. 1996. Sleep states, memory processes and synaptic plasticity. *Behavioral Brain Research* 78:49–56.

Stickgold, R., James, L., and Hobson, J. A. 2000. Visual discrimination learning requires sleep after training. *Nature Neuroscience* 3:1237–1238.

Stickgold, R., Hobson, J. A., Fosse, R., and Fosse, M. 2001. Sleep, learning, and dreams: Off-line memory processing. *Science* 294:1052–1057.

Sun, E. R., Chen, C. C., Ho, G., Early, C. J., and Allen, R. P. 1998. Iron and the restless legs syndrome. *Sleep* 21:371–377.

Tayag-Kier, C. E., Keenan, G. F., Scalzi, L. V., Schultz, B., Elliot, J., Zhao, H., and Arens, R. 2000. Sleep and periodic limb movement in sleep in juvenile fibromyalgia. *Pediatrics* 106:e70.

Walters, A. S., Hening, W. A., Chokroverty, S., and Gidro-Frank, S. 1988. A double-blind randomized crossover trial of bromocriptine and placebo in restless legs syndrome. *Annals of Neurology* 24:455–458.

Walters, A. S., Mandelbaum, D. E., Lewin, D. S., Kugler, S., England, S. J., Miller, M., and Dopaminergic Therapy Study Group. 2000. Dopaminergic therapy in children with restless legs/periodic limb movements in sleep and ADHD. *Pediatric Neurology* 22:182–186.

Wang, P. P., Doherty, S., Rourke, S. B., and Bellugi, U. 1995. Unique profile of visuopeceptual skills in a genetic syndrome. *Brain and Cognition* 29:54–65.

Weinberg, W. A., and Harper, C. R. 1993. Vigilance and its disorders. *Neurology Clinics* 11:59–78.

Winkelmann, J., Muller-Myhsok, B., Wittchen, H. U., Hock, B., Prager, M., Pfister, H., Strohle, A., Eisensehr, I., Dichgans, M., Gasser, T., and Trenkwalter, C. 2002. Complex segregation analysis of restless legs syndrome provides evidence for autosomal dominant mode of inheritance in early age at onset families. *Annals of Neurology* 52:297–302.

Yokota, T., Hirose, K., Tanabe, H., and Tsukagoshi, H. 1991. Sleep-related periodic leg movements (nocturnal myoclonus) due to spinal cord lesion. *Journal of the Neurological Sciences* 104:13–18.

The Neurobiology of Williams-Beuren Syndrome

14

Carl Feinstein, M.D., and Allan L. Reiss, M.D.

Traditionally, the study of the brain in disorders of behavior and cognition has served several purposes. Initially, and in general, there has been the search for an increased understanding of these disorders based on knowledge of their associated central nervous system pathophysiology. An increasingly important rationale for the study of brain morphology and function in these conditions has been the need to establish biological validation, or at least biological correlation, for these behaviorally defined syndromes. Ultimately, however, the greatest scientific challenge is to integrate brain morphologic and functional data with genetic, molecular biological, histologic, cognitive, and behavioral data as they mutually interact over the course of development. It is only through this integration that the relationship between genes, neurodevelopment, cognition, and behavior can be fully understood. Furthermore, such a comprehensive understanding is the most likely basis for a new generation of biologically based interventions that can improve the clinical and adaptive outcomes for individuals born with neurodevelopmental disorders.

Neurobiological studies of Williams-Beuren syndrome (WBS), related to the unique clinical characteristics of this disorder, offer an outstanding opportunity for advances in our understanding of the relationship between genetic mechanisms, neurodevelopment, cognition, and behavior. Exciting advances in the study of WBS are beginning to reveal insights, particularly, into the interactions of genes, brain, and behavior with regard to the biological foundations of visuospatial perception, language, social drive, cognition, and emotions. This new information both enhances our clinical understanding of WBS and advances the study of brain-behavior relationships in general.

An Integrated Clinical Neuroscience Approach

Williams-Beuren syndrome is a genetically based disorder, occurring in 1 in 20,000 live births, which is associated with both numerous medical complications and prominent neurodevelopmental, behavioral, and cognitive abnormalities. It is caused by a contiguous hemizygous microdeletion on chromosome 7q11.23 (Bellugi et al. 1990; Morris et al. 1993; Korenberg et al. 2000). In this chapter, we focus on brain structure and morphometry derived from magnetic resonance imaging (MRI) research, functional brain physiologic findings based on functional magnetic resonance imaging (fMRI) and electrophysiologic (evoked response potentials [ERP]) studies, and neurohistologic and cytoarchitectonic findings based on autopsy studies. Most of the recent advances in our neurobiological understanding of WBS have come through carefully targeted research based on the highly distinctive clinical profile for this syndrome, one of profound deficits in certain cognitive abilities and preserved or even heightened abilities in others. Here we summarize briefly the highlights of this distinctive profile to orient the reader to the unified, cross-disciplinary context that has characterized clinical neuroscience research in WBS, focusing on the main implications for current and future neurobiological research.

Individuals with WBS share a unique cognitive profile, frequently referred to as the Williams syndrome cognitive profile. In the context of overall reduced intelligence, most commonly in the range of mild to moderate mental retardation, people with WBS show distinctive strengths in language skills but marked impairments in visuospatial processing (Bellugi et al. 2000; Mervis and Klein-Tasman 2000). This evidence in support of modularity in these dissociated cognitive functions has led to numerous studies of brain structure, physiology, and cytoarchitecture with specific reference to the brain regions known to subserve them.

Even within the domain of visual-perceptual function, individuals with WBS manifest a unique profile of strengths and weaknesses. In relation to their overall intellectual level, affected individuals demonstrate severe impairment in their ability to process visuospatial stimuli yet significant strengths in face-processing abilities (Atkinson et al. 1997, 2001; Nakamura et al. 2002; Paul et al. 2002). These two distinct components of visual processing are mediated by different neuroanatomic and cytoarchitectonic structures and pathways: the "dorsal pathway," including the magnocellular layers of the lateral geniculate nucleus for visuospatial perception, and the "ventral pathway," including the parvocellular layers of the lateral geniculate nucleus. Consequently, studies of brain structure have focused on carefully defining abnormalities in these two distinct pathways and their component structures (Atkinson et al. 1997; Galaburda et al. 2001).

The emotional functioning of individuals with WBS also demonstrates a distinctive and unique profile. It has been repeatedly noted that these children and adults are overfriendly and "hypersocial" (Bellugi et al. 1999; Jones et al. 2000; Einfeld et al. 2001). Individuals with WBS manifest excessive linguistic affect during conversations and when giving narratives (Jones et al. 2000; Losh et al. 2000; Reilly et al. 2004). They also are known to experience heightened emotional reactions to music and certain classes of noise (Gosch et al. 1994; Einfeld et al. 1997; Hopyan et al. 2001). In addition, recent findings suggest that the relative preservation of linguistic function in individuals with WBS may be specific for the emotional aspects of language (Pearlman-Avnion and Eviatar 2002). Observed patterns of psychiatric vulnerability and disorder in individuals with WBS highlight anxiety, overarousal, and inappropriately intense affect (Davies et al. 1998; Einfeld et al. 2001). These findings on emotionality and clinical disorder have led to specific structural and functional imaging of brain regions known to underlie emotional processing and regulation, such as the amygdala, hippocampus, parahippocampal gyrus, cingulate, insula, nucleus accumbens, and orbital frontal cortex.

In discussing the WBS cognitive phenotype, we also need to mention briefly some aspects of the molecular biology of the deletion site. WBS is most commonly the result of a hemizygous 1.6 Mb contiguous deletion of approximately twenty genes at chromosome 7q11.23, surrounding the elastin gene (*ELN*) (Francke 1999; Osborne 1999; Korenberg et al. 2000; Peoples et al. 2000; Hoogenraad et al. 2002; Merla et al. 2002). This region is referred to as the WBS critical region (WSCR). It seems to consist of two nested duplicated regions flanking a largely single-copy region. Cytomolecular techniques (Botta et al. 1999; Galaburda et al. 2002) can be used to study the expression of the genes in the WSCR in normal human tissue specimens, but recent identification of WBS patients with atypical deletions has created unique opportunities for studying the effects of some of the genes in the WSCR on both WS and on normal brain development.

At least two common deletion breakpoints have been reported, including one or more at either end of the deletion site. Recent research in this area has identified a small number of atypical, highly informative variations in size and number of genes included in the chromosomal deletion of some patients with WBS (Botta et al. 1999a, 1999b; Osborne 1999; Tassabehji et al. 1999). In these individual cases, therefore, the individuals retain one or more genes that are normally deleted in WBS and may express a partial phenotype of the disorder. Investigators have been quick to realize the research opportunity to study the general effects of specific genes in the WSCR on neurodevelopment, cognition, and affective function. In particular, structural and functional neuroimaging or neurohistologic studies in autopsy specimens offer the chance to observe direct gene effects on neurodevelopment. In at least one case, that of mouse gene *Cyln2*, a mouse knockout model has been created that implicates this gene specifically in some of the neurodevelopmental abnormalities characteristic of WBS (Hoogenraad et al. 2002). Also, in a few reported cases, there is an inversion of the WSCR rather than a deletion, which results in a subset of the WBS clinical phenotype (Osborne et al. 2001). In summary, these recent and ongoing findings create an almost unparalleled opportunity for dissecting out the genetic effects on normal brain development, structure, and function of at least a few genes that happen to be located in the WBS deletion site.

Brain Tissue Findings in Williams-Beuren Syndrome

In 1994, Gallaburda et al. first reported neurohistologic findings from a WBS autopsy specimen. The focus of this early study was on the primary visual cortex in the occipital lobes. The visual cortex is a high-priority area for study in WBS because of the striking pattern of visuospatial deficits in people with this syndrome. The overall volume of the posterior brain appeared markedly diminished. Cytoarchitectonic analysis in primary visual cortical area 17 revealed prominent anomalies—a horizontal organization of neurons with layers, increased packing cell density, and abnormally clustered and oriented neurons. Although these anomalies were most dramatic in area 17, they also were found in other areas of the posterior brain. This initial finding thus linked brain anatomic and microanatomic findings to a specific deficit observed in WBS.

Gallaburda and colleagues (2002) later reported the results of cytologic studies of the primary visual cortex in autopsy specimens of three adults with WBS, comparing them with three matched, normally developed control brains. This effort sought to refine the study of the visual cortex, tracking the well-established clinical finding that peripheral field visuospatial processing in WBS is highly impaired, while central representation of objects is relatively spared. Specifically, these researchers examined primary visual cortex area 17, halfway between the splenium of the corpus callosum and the occipital pole along the calcarine sulcus. This sample would represent mostly peripheral (dorsal) visual pathways that mediate visuospatial perception. They found that neuronal differences between the WBS and control specimens in the primary visual cortex affect the left hemisphere more than the right, particular layer IV. The left visual cortex of the WBS brains had more small and fewer large neurons than the control brains in layers IV, V, and VI and showed increased cell-packing density in left layer IVC.

Although these findings confirm that there are cytoarchitectonic differences in the visual cortex in WBS when compared with normally developed brains, correlating the specific anomalous histology of these areas of the visual cortex with specific impairments in peripheral versus central visual processing remains a difficult challenge. This is partly because the overall reduced size and altered shape of the occipital cortex (see below) in WBS leaves open the possibility that peripheral and central processing fields in the visual cortex are arranged differently and are organized along anomalous functional pathways, when compared with the visual cortex in normal brains. Future directions for research are likely to expand the brain areas studied with these histologic techniques, comparing WBS and normally developed brains, as well as tracking other known cognitive or emotional abnormalities and exploiting findings from structural and functional brain imaging. The examination of gene expression (of genes from the WSCR) with immunohistochemical and molecular biological techniques to compare gene expression in specific brain areas in WBS with that in matched control brains seems another likely way of correlating gene-brain-behavior relationships.

Brain Structure in Williams-Beuren Syndrome

Neuroimaging studies with MRI in the early 1990s established that the brains of individuals with WBS have smaller total volume than normally developed controls (Jernigan and Bellugi 1990; Jernigan et al. 1993). However, these studies also noted that reduction in brain volume is regionally uneven, with relative preservation of temporal-limbic and cerebellar volumes and superior temporal auditory cortex (Jernigan et al. 1993). Other investigators reported evidence that gray matter might be preferentially preserved in WBS (Harris-Collazo et al. 1997).

In 2000, we systematically replicated and extended these early findings using higher-resolution MRI and compared young adult males with WBS and age- and gender-matched normally developed control subjects (Reiss et al. 2000). We found total brain volume in the WBS subjects to be decreased 13% compared with the matched controls. However, as previous reports had suggested, we found that reduction in brain volume is uneven across different brain regions. Cerebellar volume, for example, was reduced only 7% and was not statistically different from that of controls. In fact, the ratio of cerebellar to cerebral volume was significantly higher in the WBS group than in the controls, indicating relative preservation of cerebellar volume.

Brainstem tissue volumes were 20% reduced in WBS compared with controls. This reduction is proportionately greater than that observed for overall brain tissue volumes. A previous suggestion of a disproportionate decrease in cerebral white matter, with relative sparing of gray matter, was replicated in this study. Reduction of cerebrospinal fluid volume in WBS was found to be proportional to overall cerebral volume reduction. In the cerebellum, however, we found no disproportionate reduction in white matter or sparing of gray matter.

Analysis of right versus left brain asymmetry revealed group differences between WBS subjects and controls only for the occipital lobes. In the occipital lobes of subjects with WBS, there is an overall shift in the ratio of brain tissue from right to left, with a disproportionate reduction in right occipital gray matter, whereas relative symmetry was found in controls. In this study, we found no other evidence of unusual asymmetries, including hemispheric and individual lobe gray and white matter volumes, subcortical gray matter volumes, and ventricular volumes. In contrast to the decrease in volume of the occipital lobes, a brain region that processes visual information (a cognitive function impaired in WBS), the volume of the superior temporal gyrus is preserved. The superior temporal gyrus is involved in the processing of auditory verbal and music stimuli, functions that are cognitive strengths in WBS. In fact, superior temporal gyrus gray matter as a proportion of the total volume of cerebral gray matter is increased in WBS, when compared with controls.

The earlier findings of Galaburda and Bellugi and their colleagues describing distortions in the overall shape of WBS brains observed at autopsy became the basis of an MRI replication study of brain shape in WBS (Galaburda et al. 2001). This study showed abnormal cerebral curtailment in the posterior-parietal and occipital regions. The investigators described a dysmorphism in cortical folding, with a short central sulcus that does not become opercularized in the interhemispheric fissure, suggesting a developmental anomaly in the dorsal half of the cerebral hemispheres. They also found that the normally occurring asymmetry of the planum temporale was absent in WBS.

Following this, we worked with the Galaburda group to further elucidate the distortions in the dorsal forebrain anatomy in WBS, using MRI (Galaburda et al. 2001). Comparing brains of young adults with WBS and age- and gender-matched controls, we found that WBS brains are far less likely to have central sulci that reach the interhemispheric fissure. This difference in the central sulcus involves only the dorsal end; the ventral end of WBS and control brains is identical. The failure of opercularization of the dorsal central sulcus in WBS was interpreted as being due to generalized abnormalities in dorsomedial opercularization of the hemispheres. The finding that only the dorsal area of the central sulcus is curtailed and the ventral extension is normal is consistent with the cognitive profile of WBS, in which visuospatial functions are impaired while visual object and face recognition, speech, and language (all primarily ventral brain mediated) are relatively conserved.

Schmitt et al. (2001a), also using MRI, further defined the brain shape abnormality in WBS, comparing it with age- and gender-matched controls. They specifically measured the difference between the groups in linear length and angle of curvature (the "bending angle") for both right and left hemispheres and for the corpus callosum. Using this information and data collected from additional analyses, these investigators (Galaburda et al. 2001; Schmitt et al. 2001b) determined that the cerebral hemispheres and corpus callosum in WBS had shorter midline lengths than those in the control brains, a finding consistent with previously described decreases in dorsal occipital-parietal brain volume in WBS. Both the cerebral hemispheres and the corpus callosum in WBS were noted to have reduced curvature (bending angle is increased) in comparison to normal controls. The reduction in corpus callosum midline length seemed to be secondary to a decrease in both the splenium and isthmus (posterior body). It is noteworthy that the splenium anatomically connects left and right parieto-occipital lobe regions, areas that are reduced in WBS. This also correlates with the well-documented decrement in visuospatial skills in WBS.

Similar findings of dysgenesis in the posterior portion of the corpus callosum have been reported by Tomaiulo et al. (2002). Although dysgenesis of the corpus callosum has been described in several neurogenetic, psychiatric, and neurologic disorders (Bodensteiner et al. 1994; Gabrielli et al. 1998), reduction in size of these structures is consistent with both the known decrease in size of the occipital lobe in WBS and the impairments in visuospatial processing. Tomaiulo and colleagues (2002) also compared the area of the corpus callosum in WBS with normal controls. They found an overall smaller volume of the corpus callosum in WBS, particularly in the splenium and in the caudal part of the callosal body, as well as the shape anomaly described above. In addition, they used voxel-based morphometry techniques—MRI-based techniques that use statistical methods developed for use in functional neuroimaging (Ashburner and Friston 2000)—to study white matter density; they found increased density in the midsection of the corpus callosum in WBS.

As discussed by Schmitt et al., this highly distinctive brain shape abnormality in WBS (fig. 14.1) is most likely caused by aberrant brain development and is therefore a key link in the understanding of the pathogenesis of this syndrome. For example, it has been shown that both the cerebral hemispheres and the corpus callosum develop in a rostrocaudal direction (Barkovich and Norman 1988; Huttenlocher 1990). Abnormally early termination of brain development on the rostral-caudal axis could produce cortical shapes similar to that found in WBS.

Several genes in the 7q11.23 deletion site, including the syntaxin gene (*STX1A*), *CYLN2*, the LIM kinase 1 gene (*LIMK1*), *WBSCR11*, and *GTF2I*, are differentially expressed in the brain (Hoogenraad et al. 1998; Nakayama et al. 1998; Osborne et al. 1999; P. P. Wang 1999). Hemizygosity for one or more of these genes in WBS may account for the deviant brain development underlying the abnormal shape and morphology of the brain. Another gene in the WSCR, *FZD9*, is expressed strongly in the adult brain and is likely to be involved in global brain development (Cadigan and Nusse 1997; Y. K. Wang et al. 1999). Hemizygosity of this gene also may account, in part, for neurodevelopmental abnormalities observed in WBS.

Most recently, Schmitt et al. (2002) have studied abnormal patterns of

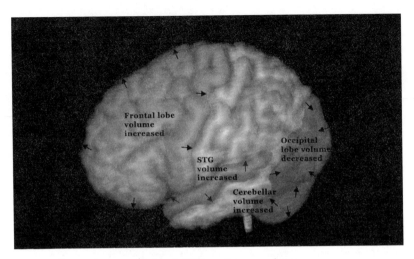

Fig. 14.1. Aberrant brain morphology in Williams-Beuren syndrome.

cortical gyrification in WBS. Evidence for excessive and convoluted patterns of cortical gyrification in this syndrome had been described previously for a small number of postmortem WBS brains (Gallaburda et al. 2001). This finding, if confirmed, might further clarify the type and timing of the deleterious effects of hemizygosity of genes in the WSCR on the brain shape deformity in WBS.

Cortical surface folding resulting in gyrification begins in the fifth month of gestation, when neuronal migration is largely complete, and may be a consequence of the rapid expansion of cortical gray matter and the development of interconnecting circuits (Ono et al. 1990; Magnotta et al. 1999). Schmitt and colleagues (2002) found significantly increased cortical gyrification globally in WBS, with abnormalities especially pronounced in the right parietal, right occipital, and left frontal regions.

As previously described, the volume of the cerebellum in WBS is preserved despite an overall decrease in brain volume. However, additional neuroimaging studies have targeted the neocerebellum (which includes the posterior vermis, cerebellar tonsils, and the neocerebellar cortex). The neocerebellum is evolutionarily and developmentally distinct from the anterior cerebellar regions (Yachnis and Rorke 1999). Neocerebellar activation has been associated in several studies with language ability, verbal fluency, and possibly socioemotional behavior (Ackermann et al. 1998; Saitoh and Courchesne 1998; Schlosser et al. 1998; Levitt et al. 1999). These are all areas of relative strength in WBS.

Earlier studies of the neocerebellum in WBS described increases in the size of the posterior cerebellar vermis lobules VI and VII and of the cerebellar tonsils (Jernigan and Bellugi 1990; P. P. Wang et al. 1992). Schmitt and colleagues (2001c), comparing young adults with WBS and matched controls, found the cerebellar vermis to be proportionately larger in WBS. This was due to the increased volume of posterior vermis lobules VI to X. More recently, Hesselink et al. (2002) were able to perform MRI imaging on very young children (mean age, 21 months) with WBS and matched controls. This study of cerebellar size in young children, although not based on standardized morphometric analysis, is significant in that it found overall cerebellar enlargement already evident at a relatively early stage of development.

Clearly, much progress has been made in describing the abnormal morphology of certain brain regions in WBS, neurodevelopmentally based distortions in brain shape, and the proportion of various regions to the whole brain, but further advances are possible. One research strategy would be to study other brain structures that are likely to be affected as suggested by the WBS cognitive profile. To date, the structure, size, and intactness of several components of both the visual and auditory and the language pathways have been described. The amygdala and hippocampal structures would seem to be promising regions to study, given the heightened emotionality and proneness to anxiety that are common clinical findings in WBS. In the light of the previously reported 30% reduction in volume of the brainstem in WBS and the morphologic differences in the cerebellum, a more fine-grained analysis of brainstem structure might be informative.

New specialized MRI techniques also could be brought to bear to advance our understanding of the brain in WBS. As is clear from the corpus callosum abnormalities in WBS and the disproportionate reduction in brain white matter, a more intensive study of white matter tracts is needed. Diffusion tensor imaging, an MRI technique designed to visualize white matter pathways in the brain (Pierpaoli et al. 1996), could prove a valuable new research tool for studying the abnormalities in brain white matter in WBS. Furthermore, given the findings of Galaburda and colleagues on the cytoarchitectonic abnormalities in occipital gray matter, it is reasonable to hypothesize that, in addition to measuring volume and shape of gray matter brain structures, a study of gray matter density and shape in regions of special interest (when compared with matched, normally developed controls) would be useful. Voxel-based morphometry is also well suited for any search for abnormalities in gray matter density.

As described above, individuals with WBS who have atypical breakpoints in the 7q11.23 deletion that result in retained gene(s) may manifest variations in the WBS cognitive-behavioral phenotype. These individuals are of particular scientific interest. Study of such cases could provide highly specific information about the influence of the nondeleted genes. Structural brain imaging research comparing the brains of these atypical subjects with the brains of full-WBS-deletion individuals, as well as with matched controls, could help unravel the effects of both the retained gene(s) and the other genes in the deletion site on brain development.

Magnetic Resonance Spectroscopy, Functional Magnetic Resonance Imaging, and Electrophysiologic Studies

A single study by Rae et al. (1998) used magnetic resonance spectroscopy (MRS) to compare the brain biochemistry of individuals with WBS, over a wide age range, with age-matched controls. MRS is a brain-imaging technique that offers poor spatial resolution but provides rich information about brain biochemistry, including numerous substances involved in neuronal activity. This study found significant differences between WBS subjects and controls in several neuroactive substances localized in the cerebellum and correlated these findings with neuropsychological test results. Unfortunately, it was not possible with this approach to determine whether the localized differences in brain chemistry factors were specific to the cerebellum or were a reflection of more global differences in brain neurochemistry between the WBS and control groups.

Functional magnetic resonance imaging, as a technique for observing and measuring the topography of brain activation involved in perceptual, cognitive, or emotion-processing tasks, offers great promise for the study of neurocognitive functioning in WBS. Because the WBS cognitive and emotional profile is so distinctive and characterized by peaks and valleys of functioning, there are likely to be associated differences between brain-activation patterns in WBS and in matched controls, reflecting these cognitive-behavioral anomalies. To date, however, only one fMRI study has been reported. Levitin et al. (2003) investigated the neural correlates of auditory perception in WBS, illustrating how important fMRI is likely to become in delineating the highly altered and atypical brain functional structures and pathways of this neurodevelopmental disorder.

Levitin and colleagues examined the neural basis of auditory processing of music and noise in individuals with WBS and age-matched controls. Both hyperacusis and heightened emotional reactions to music and certain classes of noises are well-known traits in WBS. These researchers found that normal controls, as expected, processed music and noise patterns primarily in the superior and middle temporal gyri, the major auditory-processing brain centers. Remarkably, the participants with WBS showed a very different neural organization of noise and music processing. Noise and music processing in WBS involves a widely distributed network of brain activation. There is markedly less activation of the temporal lobes than in normal controls, coupled with significantly greater activation in the right amygdala and activation of the cerebellum, pons, and brainstem. These findings establish an anomalous neurofunctional basis for auditory processing in WBS that seems to be correlated with the intense emotionality with which individuals with this syndrome respond to music.

The findings on noise and music processing in WBS suggest that, in addition to research correlating areas of cognitive deficit with brain abnormalities, the study of "spared" cognitive processes with neurophysiologic techniques may shed equally valuable light on how the 22q11.23 deletion results in a brain that is organized differently from the normal brain, even for areas of intact cognitive functioning. The success of fMRI in delineating the functional organization of the brain in WBS will most likely lead to further efforts to correlate unique patterns of neurofunction associated with other traits, such as processing of faces, increased affectivity in language, poor visuospatial functioning, and strong social drive.

The findings thus far from a small number of electrophysiologic studies of brain function in WBS, using evoked response potentials, have similarly revealed unique and abnormal patterns of brain pathways and structural specialization (these findings are summarized in Mills et al. 2000). ERP studies, while offering only limited topographic resolution, record underlying brain electrophysiologic processing of specific cognitive tasks with extremely high temporal resolution. This methodology allows very fine-grained comparisons of spatiotemporal processing of stimuli between individuals with normal cognitive functioning and those with a variety of disorders and neurodevelopmental syndromes, including WBS.

ERP studies of grammatical language functioning in WBS (a relatively spared area of cognitive functioning) in the 1990s indicated an abnormal brain organization of language systems (Neville et al. 1994). In normally developed adults and school-aged children, ERPs of grammatical function display a left-anterior asymmetry from at least nine years of age. In contrast, children and adults with WBS do not show this pattern of asymmetry. In addition, subjects with WBS also showed an abnormally organized ERP response to the processing of semantic information in auditory sentences. The N400 wave (previously shown to be linked to integration of word meaning) was larger over anterior than posterior regions and was larger from the left hemisphere than from the right. By contrast, in normally developed adults the N400 is larger over posterior regions of the right hemisphere.

More recent electrophysiologic studies of human face processing and face recognition in WBS also indicate an abnormal cerebral organization for this relatively spared visual cognitive function (Mills et al. 2000). Before these studies, it had been established that, in normally developed adults, different brain systems mediate matching of identical versus nonidentical faces when shown upright, as compared with when they are inverted. A task involving recognition of mismatched upright faces elicits a prominent negative wave at 320 msec (N320) that is most prominent over the anterior regions of the right hemisphere, whereas a task involving recognition of mismatched inverted faces elicits a positive wave at 500 msec (P500) with a symmetric bilateral posterior distribution.

This information strongly suggests a different brain functional organization for these two tasks. This, in turn, seems to be related to neuropsychological data indicating that, for adults, the upright face-matching task is accomplished by global configuration pattern recognition, whereas the inverted face-matching involves a local, detail-oriented cognitive approach. Young, normally developing children, however, show the same N320 ERP pattern for both upright and inverted face-matching, a pattern that correlates with their use of local detail visual-processing strategy. Adults with WBS exhibit the N320 ERP pattern for both upright and inverted faces, the pattern seen in normally developing children but not in adults, and also show a unique N100 wave that seems to correlate with the increased attention to faces characteristic of people with WBS.

Future Directions

Williams-Beuren syndrome is a unique neurodevelopmental disorder caused by a hemizygous deletion of chromosome 7q11.23. This deletion of genetic material results in a striking profile of cognitive deficits and strengths, heightened social motivation, and a distinctive infusion of hyperemotionality into language and other aspects of neurobehavioral functioning. Advances in molecular biology, neuroimaging, and neurophysiology, only recently available, have facilitated a rapidly expanding body of research that integrates genetic, neurobiological, cognitive, and behavioral approaches in the elucidation of gene-brain-behavior interactions and pathways. This integrated multidisciplinary research effort has shed light on many aspects of the pathogenesis of WBS.

Perhaps even more exciting for the burgeoning field of clinical neuroscience is the evidence that fundamental insights into the genetic and neurodevelopmental foundations of visual perception, language functioning, the interactions between emotional and cognitive processing, and social drive can be gleaned from the study of WBS. It seems clear that numerous lines of additional research, now on the horizon, will soon add further to our understanding of the neurobiology of these core human traits.

REFERENCES

Ackermann, H., Wildgruber, D., Daum, I., and Grodd, W. 1998. Does the cerebellum contribute to cognitive aspects of speech production? A functional magnetic resonance imaging (fMRI) study in humans. *Neuroscience Letters* 247:187–190.

Ashburner, J., and Friston, K. J. 2000. Voxel-based morphometry—the methods. *NeuroImage* 11 (6, pt. 1): 805–821.

Atkinson, J., King, J., Braddick, O., Nokes, L., Anker, S., and Braddick, F. 1997. A specific deficit of dorsal stream function in Williams' syndrome. *NeuroReport* 8:1919–1922.

Atkinson, J., Anker, S., Braddick, O., Nokes, L., Mason, A., and Braddick, F. 2001. Visual and visuospatial development in young children with WBS. *Developmental Medicine and Child Neurology* 43:330–337.

Barkovich, A. J., and Norman, D. 1988. Anomalies of the corpus callosum: Correlations with further anomalies of the brain. *AJR American Journal of Roentgenology* 151:171–179.

Bellugi, U., Bihrle, A., Jernigan, T., Trauner, D., and Doherty, S. 1990. Neuropsychological, neurological, and neuroanatomical profile of WBS. *American Journal of Medical Genetics Supplement* 6:115–125.

Bellugi, U., Adolphs, R., Cassady C., and Chiles, M. 1999. Towards the neural basis for hypersociability in a genetic syndrome. *NeuroReport* 10:1653–1657.

Bellugi, U., Lichtenberger, L., Jones, W., Lai, Z., and St. George, M. 2000. The neurocognitive profile of WBS: A complex pattern of strengths and weaknesses. *Journal of Cognitive Neuroscience* 12 (suppl. 1): 7–29.

Bodensteiner, J., Schaefer, G. B., Breeding, L., and Cowan, L. 1994. Hypoplasia of the corpus callosum: A study of 445 consecutive MRI scans. *Journal of Child Neurology* 9:47–49.

Botta, A., Novelli, G., Mari, A., Novelli, A., Sabani, M., Korenberg, J., Osborne, L. R., Diglio, M. C., Giannotti, A., and Dallapiccola, B. 1999a. Detection of an atypical 7q11.23 deletion in WBS patients which does not include the STX1A and FZD3 genes. *Journal of Medical Genetics* 36:478–480.

Botta, A., Sangiuolo, F., Calza, L., Giardino, L., Potenza, S., Novelli, G., and Dallapiccola, B. 1999b. Expression analysis and protein localization of the human HPC-1/syntaxin 1A, a gene deleted in WBS. *Genomics* 62:525–528.

Cadigan, K. M., and Nusse, R. 1997. Wnt signaling: A common theme in animal development. *Genes and Development* 11:3286–3305.

Davies, M., Udwin, O., and Howlin, P. 1998. Adults with WBS: Preliminary study of social, emotional and behavioural difficulties. *British Journal of Psychiatry* 172:273–276.

Einfeld, S. L., Tonge, B. J., and Florio, T. 1997. Behavioral and emotional disturbance in individuals with WBS. *American Journal on Mental Retardation* 102:45–53.

Einfeld, S. L., Tonge, B. J., and Rees, V. W. 2001. Longitudinal course of behavioral and emotional problems in WBS. *American Journal on Mental Retardation* 106:73–81.

Francke, U. 1999. Williams-Beuren syndrome: Genes and mechanisms. *Human Molecular Genetics* 8:1947–1954.

Gabrielli, O., Coppa, G. V., Manzoni, M., Carloni, I., Kantar, A., Maricotti., M., and Salvolini, U. 1998. Minor cerebral alterations observed by magnetic resonance imaging in syndromic children with mental retardation. *European Journal of Radiology* 27:139–144.

Galaburda, A. M., Wang, P. P., Bellugi, U., and Rossen, M. 1994. Cytoarchitectonic anomalies in a genetically based disorder: WBS. *NeuroReport* 5:753–757.

Galaburda, A. M., Schmitt, J. E., Atlas, S. W., Eliez, S., Bellugi, U., and Reiss, A. L. 2001. Dorsal forebrain anomaly in WBS. *Archives of Neurology* 58:1865–1869.

Galaburda, A. M., Holinger, D. P., Bellugi, U., and Sherman, G. F. 2002. WBS: Neuronal size and neuronal-packing density in primary visual cortex. *Archives of Neurology* 59:1461–1467.

Gosch, A., Stading, G., and Pankau, R. 1994. Linguistic abilities in children with Williams-Beuren syndrome. *American Journal of Medical Genetics* 52:291–296.

Harris-Collazo, M., Archibald, S., Lai, Z., Bellugi, U., and Jernigan, T. 1997. *Morphological differences on quantitative MRI in WBS.* New Orleans: Society for Neuroscience.

Hoogenraad, C. C., Eussen, B. H., Langeveld, A., van Haperen, R., Winterberg, S., Wouters, C. H., Grosveld, F., De Zeeuw, C. I., and Galjart, N. 1998. The murine CYLN2 gene: Genomic organization, chromosome localization, and comparison to the human gene that is located within the 7q11.23 WBS critical region. *Genomics* 53:348–358.

Hoogenraad, C. C., Koekkoek, B., Akhmanova, A., Krugers, H., Dortland, B., Miedema, M., van Alphen, A., Kistler, W. M., Jaegle, M., Koutsourakis, M., Van Camp, N., Verhoye, M., van der Linden, A., Kaverina, I., Grosveld, F., De Zeeuw, C. I., and Galjart, N. 2002. Targeted mutation of *Cyln2* in the WBS critical region links *CLIP-115* haploinsufficiency to neurodevelopmental abnormalities in mice. *Nature Genetics* 32:116–127.

Hopyan, T., Dennis, M., Weksberg, R., and Cytrynbaum, C. 2001. Music skills and the expressive interpretation of music in children with Williams-Beuren syndrome: Pitch, rhythm, melodic imagery, phrasing, and musical affect. *Neuropsychology, Development, and Cognition. Section C, Child Neuropsychology* 7:42–53.

Huttenlocher, P. R. 1990. Morphometric study of human cerebral cortex development. *Neuropsychologia* 28:517–527.

Jernigan, T. L., and Bellugi, U. 1990. Anomalous brain morphology on magnetic resonance images in WBS and Down syndrome. *Archives of Neurology* 47:529–533.

Jernigan, T., Bellugi, U., Sowell, E., Doherty, S., and Hesselink, J. R. 1993. Cerebral morphologic distinctions between Williams and Down syndromes. *Archives of Neurology* 50:186–191.

Jones, W., Bellugi, U., Lai, Z., Chiles, M., Reilly, J., Lincoln, A., and Adolphs, R. 2000. Hypersociability in WBS. *Journal of Cognitive Neuroscience* 12 (suppl. 1): 30–46.

Jones, W., Hesselink, J., Courchesne, E., Duncan, T., Matsuda, J., and Bellugi, U. 2002. Cerebellar abnormalities in infants and toddlers with WBS. *Developmental Medicine and Child Neurology* 44:688–694.

Korenberg, J. R., Chen, X. N., Hirota, H., Lai, Z., Bellugi, U., Burian, D., Roe, B., and Matsuoka, R. 2000. Genome structure and cognitive map of WBS. *Journal of Cognitive Neuroscience* 12 (suppl. 1): 89–107.

Levitin, D. J., Menon, V., Schmitt, J. E., Eliez, S., White, C. D., Glover, G. H., Kadis, J., Korenberg, J. R., Bellugi, U., and Reiss, A. L. 2003. Neural correlates of auditory perception in WBS: An FMRI study. *NeuroImage* 18:74–82.

Levitt, J. G., Blanton, R., Capetillo-Cunliffe, L., Gutherie, D., Toga, A., and McCracken, J. T. 1999. Cerebellar vermis lobules VIII–X in autism. *Progress in Neuropsychopharmacology and Biological Psychiatry* 23:625–633.

Losh, M., Bellugi, U., Reilly, J., and Anderson, D. 2000. Narrative as a social engagement tool: The excessive use of evaluation in narratives from children with WBS. *Narrative Inquiry* 10(2):1–26.

Magnotta, V. A., Andreasen, N. C., Schultz, S. K., Harris, G., Cizadlo, T., Heckel, D., Nopoulos, P., and Flaum, M. 1999. Quantitative in vivo measurement of gyrification in the human brain: Changes associated with aging. *Cerebral Cortex* 9:151–160.

Merla, G., Ucla, C., Guipponi, M., and Reymond, A. 2002. Identification of additional transcripts in the Williams-Beuren syndrome critical region. *Human Genetics* 110:429–438.

Mervis, C. B., and Klein-Tasman, B. P. 2000. WBS: Cognition, personality, and adaptive behavior. *Mental Retardation and Developmental Disabilities Research Reviews* 6:148–158.

Mills, D. L., Alvarez, T. D., St. George, M., Applebaum, L. G., Bellugi, U., and Neville, H. 2000. Electrophysiological studies of face processing in WBS. *Journal of Cognitive Neuroscience* 12 (suppl. 1): 47–64.

Morris, C. A., Thomas, I. T., and Greenberg, F. 1993. WBS: Autosomal dominant inheritance. *American Journal of Medical Genetics* 47:478–481.

Nakamura, M., Kaneoke, Y., Watanabe, K., and Kakigi, R. 2002. Visual information process in WBS: Intact motion detection accompanied by typical visuospatial dysfunctions. *European Journal of Neuroscience* 16:1810–1818.

Nakayama, T., Matsuoka, R., Kimura M., Hirota, H., Mikoshiba, K., Shimuzu, N., and Akagawa, K. 1998. Hemizygous deletion of the HPC-1/syntaxin 1A gene (STX1A) in patients with WBS. *Cytogenetics and Cell Genetics* 82:49–51.

Neville, H. J., Mills, D. L., and Bellugi, U. 1994. Effects of altered auditory sensitivity and age of language acquisition on the development of language-related neural systems: Preliminary studies of WBS. In *Atypical cognitive deficits in developmental disorders: Implications for brain function*, ed. S. Broman and J. Grafman, 67–83. Hillsdale, NJ: Erlbaum.

Ono, M., S. Kubic, Abernathey, C. D., and Yasargil, M. G. 1990. *Atlas of the cerebral sulci*. New York: Thieme Medical Publishers.

Osborne, L. R. 1999. Williams-Beuren syndrome: Unraveling the mysteries of a microdeletion disorder. *Molecular Genetics and Metabolism* 67:1–10.

Osborne, L. R., Campbell, T., Daradich, A., Scherer, S. W., and Tsui, L. C. 1999. Identification of a putative transcription factor gene (WBSCR11) that is commonly deleted in Williams-Beuren syndrome. *Genomics* 57:279–284.

Osborne, L. R., Li, M., Pober, B., Chitayat, D., Bodurtha, J., Mandel, A., Costa, T., Grebe, T., Cox, S., Tsui, L. C., and Scherer, S. W. 2001. A 1.5 million-base pair inversion polymorphism in families with Williams-Beuren syndrome. *Nature Genetics* 29:321–325.

Paul, B. M., Stiles, J., Passarotti, A., Bavar, N., and Bellugi, U. 2002. Face and place processing in WBS: Evidence for a dorsal-ventral dissociation. *NeuroReport* 13:1115–1119.

Pearlman-Avnion, S., and Eviatar, Z. 2002. Narrative analysis in developmental social and linguistic pathologies: Dissociation between emotional and informational language use. *Brain and Cognition* 48:494–499.

Peoples, R., Franke, Y., Wang, Y. K., Perez-Jurado, L., Paperna, T., Cisco, M., and Francke, U. 2000. A physical map, including a BAC/PAC clone contig, of the Williams-Beuren syndrome–deletion region at 7q11.23. *American Journal of Human Genetics* 66:47–68.

Pierpaoli, C., Jezzard, P., Basser, P. J., Barnett, A., and Di Chiro, G. 1996. Diffusion tensor MR imaging of the human brain. *Radiology* 201:637–648.

Rae, C., Karmiloff-Smith, A., Lee, M. A., Dixon, R. M., Grant, J., Blamire, A. M., Thompson, C. H., Styles, P., and Radda, G. K. 1998. Brain biochemistry in WBS: Evidence for a role of the cerebellum in cognition? *Neurology* 51:33–40.

Reilly, J., Losh, M., Bellugi, U., and Wulfeck, B. 2004. Frog where are you? Narratives in children with specific language impairment, early focal brain injury and WBS. *Brain and Language* 88:229–247.

Reiss, A. L., Eliez, S., Schmitt, J. E., Straus, E., Lai, Z., Jones, W., and Bellugi, U. 2000. Neuroanatomy of WBS: A high-resolution MRI study. *Journal of Cognitive Neuroscience* 12 (suppl. 1): 65–73.

Saitoh, O., and Courchesne, E. 1998. Magnetic resonance imaging study of the brain in autism. *Psychiatry and Clinical Neuroscience* 52 (suppl. 1): 219–222.

Schlosser, R., Hutchinson, M., Joseffer, S., Rusinek, H., Saarimaki, A., Stevenson, J., Dewey, S. L., and Brodie, J. D. 1998. Functional magnetic resonance imaging of human brain activity in a verbal fluency task. *Journal of Neurology, Neurosurgery, and Psychiatry* 64:492–498.

Schmitt, J. E., Eliez, S., Bellugi, U., and Reiss, A. L. 2001a. Analysis of cerebral shape in WBS. *Archives of Neurology* 58:283–287.

Schmitt, J. E., Eliez, S., Warsofsky, I. S., Bellugi, U., and Reiss, A. L. 2001b. Corpus callosum morphology of WBS: Relation to genetics and behavior. *Developmental Medicine and Child Neurology* 43:155–159.

———. 2001c. Enlarged cerebellar vermis in WBS. *Journal of Psychiatric Research* 35:225–229.

Schmitt, J. E., Watts, K., Eliez, S., Bellugi, U., Galaburda, A. M., and Reiss, A. L. 2002. Increased gyrification in WBS: Evidence using 3D MRI methods. *Developmental Medicine and Child Neurology* 44:292–295.

Tassabehji, M., Metcalfe, K., Karmiloff-Smith, A., Carette, M. J., Grant, J., Dennis, N., Reardon, W., Splitt, M., Read, A. P., and Donnai, D. 1999. WBS: Use of chromosomal microdeletions as a tool to dissect cognitive and physical phenotypes. *American Journal of Human Genetics* 64:118–125.

Tomaiuolo, F., Di Paola, M., Caravale, B., Vicari, S., Petrides, M., and Caltagirone, C. 2002. Morphology and morphometry of the corpus callosum in WBS: A T1-weighted MRI study. *NeuroReport* 13:2281–2284.

Wang, P. P. 1999. Cognitive dissection of WBS. *American Journal of Medical Genetics* 88:103–104.

Wang, P. P., Hesselink, J. R., Jernigan, T. L., Doherty, S., and Bellugi, U. 1992. Specific neurobehavioral profile of Williams' syndrome is associated with neocerebellar hemispheric preservation. *Neurology* 42:1999–2002.

Wang, Y. K., Sporle, R., Paperna, T., Schughart, K., and Francke, U. 1999. Characterization and expression pattern of the frizzled gene Fzd9, the mouse homolog of FZD9 which is deleted in Williams-Beuren syndrome. *Genomics* 57:235–248.

Yachnis, A. T., and Rorke, L. B. 1999. Cerebellar and brainstem development: An overview in relation to Joubert syndrome. *Journal of Child Neurology* 14:570–573.

Absolute Pitch and Neuroplasticity in Williams-Beuren Syndrome

15

Howard M. Lenhoff, Ph.D.

> Because psychologists have been able to discover,
> exactly as in a slow-motion picture,
> the way the human creature acquires knowledge and habits,
> the normal child has been vastly helped by what the retarded have taught us.
> —Pearl Buck, *The Child Who Never Grew*

Only in recent years have empirical peer-reviewed reports on the musical abilities of people with Williams-Beuren syndrome (WBS) been published (Don et al. 1999; Levitin and Bellugi 1998; Lenhoff et al. 2001; Levitin et al. 2003). In this chapter, after describing some anecdotal observations (Stambaugh 1996; Lenhoff 1998) that preceded the current research on music in WBS, I focus primarily on the study of absolute pitch in individuals with WBS, with some attention to their abilities in relative pitch and in the retention of melody and lyrics. In chapter 16, Levitin and Bellugi focus on rhythm, timbre, hyperacusis, and brain function (Levitin et al. 2003) in individuals with WBS.

Absolute pitch (AP) is the rare ability, present in 1 in 10,000 normally developed individuals in Western cultures (Bachem 1955; Takeuchi and Hulse 1993), to identify a wide range of specific musical tones (Baggaley 1974; Ward 1999). It is generally believed that, to possess AP as adults, individuals must be trained in music during a "critical period" between the ages of approximately three to six years (Takeuchi and Hulse 1993; Brown et al. 2000).

Our research data quantifying the AP abilities of individuals with WBS demonstrated that they can score higher in tests for AP than do highly trained, normally developed musicians who claim to have AP; as a population, they possess a higher incidence of AP than do populations of normal individuals; and they can acquire AP at an age when people with normal cognition can no longer do so (Lenhoff et al. 2001). This research on absolute pitch in WBS also led us to consider some basic questions. Are humans born with AP? What roles do genes play in AP? Can cognitively impaired individuals possess high levels of musical intelligence? Are there advantages for research scientists in studying AP in individuals with WBS?

Anecdotal Reports of Musical Interests and Abilities
of People with Williams-Beuren Syndrome

Researchers paid no serious attention to the musical interests of individuals with WBS until the late 1990s. Nonetheless, anecdotal reports of musical interests of children with WBS started to appear as early as 1964 (Von Arnim and Engel 1964). In subsequent years, sporadic mentions were made of these special interests in both professional and general publications dealing with WBS. A survey returned in 1997 by more than 200 of 388 parents of children with WBS confirmed reports that these children are more interested in listening to music, singing, and dancing than are their normally developing siblings who are closest in age and that these differences in interest are statistically significant ($P < 0.001$ in all cases) (B. Sandeen, L. Levine, and H. Lenhoff, unpublished results). Possession of strong musical interests and abilities was not considered one of the shared traits of WBS until 1990, however, when a thirty-five-year-old musician (GML), newly diagnosed with WBS, performed before WBS researchers at their biannual professional meeting.

As pointed out in the Preface, I am the father of a daughter who is a WBS musical savant; she is GML, Ms. Gloria M. Lenhoff. Because of my daughter and other WBS musicians I have observed during the past fifteen years, I changed my research direction from biochemistry and invertebrate behavior to the study of music cognition in WBS. Hence, my starting point was a rich anecdotal information base provided by parents and teachers as well as by individuals with WBS themselves.

Most important, in 1994, with a few other parents, we formed a yearly weeklong music camp for individuals with WBS, their ages ranging from ten to forty-eight, in Lenox, Massachusetts, at Belvoir Terrace, a premier music camp for high-functioning young women. Since then, reports on the musicality of individuals with WBS have become more and more common (Lenhoff 1998; Stambaugh 1996). Such accounts have noted, for example, the following points:

- Whereas children with WBS have short attention spans for most subjects, their attention span for listening to music and participating in musical activities is long.
- Although most cannot read musical notation, many are said to have absolute and relative pitch.
- Some have uncanny rhythm, being able to learn complex drum beats, such as 7/4, in a short session.
- They seem to have an excellent sense of timing, as when two experienced vocalists were able to perform a complex classical duet nearly perfectly at their first practice together.
- Many are able to retain complex music (some in a variety of languages), including both the words of many verses of long ballads and the melodies, for periods of years ranging into decades.

- Those who learn to sing in foreign languages have near perfect accents.
- Experienced WBS musicians have a facility with harmony.
- Some can improvise and compose lyrics with great facility.
- As a final plus, virtually all WBS performers lack stage fright.

One child with WBS expressed this interest in music to Audrey Don (Don et al. 1999), the first researcher to carry out a rigorous and systematic study of musical abilities of children with WBS, with the memorable statement, "Music is my favorite way of thinking." My primary research asked how children with WBS "think" about musical pitch.

Studies on Some Musical Abilities: Results and Discussion of Data

Details of the experiments and measurements on the participants in this study are described in Lenhoff et al. 2001.

Absolute Pitch

Quantitative measurements of absolute pitch were possible after we found five people with WBS who were able to name musical notes and associate them with tones. Most musicians with WBS do not name musical notes. The average IQ for the group was 58. Their ages at the time of testing were 13, 17, 19, 21, and 43; none could read music. Three played the piano and/or the keyboard, one the guitar, and one the accordion. The older two were also experienced vocalists. Because my daughter (the only female and the oldest in the group) was one of the participants, all tests were given by a coworker.

Selecting proper comparison or control groups for such studies is relatively complex, as discussed later in the chapter. For this study we used two comparison groups. For one, we compared our findings with a meta-analysis of data obtained in several studies published between 1970 and 1991. Those studies evaluated individuals with normal cognition who claimed to possess AP, most of whom were trained musicians (Takeuchi and Hulse 1993). Second, to make certain that our testing procedures for AP were not slanted toward individuals with WBS, we administered them to six university graduates. Four of them had a range of musical training from none to a moderate amount. The other two participants had graduate training in music and were working for Master of Fine Arts degrees.

On tests for AP, all five in the WBS group performed at or near ceiling, averaging 97.5% correct on a range of tests comprising 1,084 randomized trials. They responded to tones played either on a piano or on a synthesizer programmed for piano tones. One series of tasks tested the participants' ability to identify natural notes, accidental notes, mixed natural and accidental notes in octave 4, and mixed natural and accidental notes in octaves 2 through 6 (fig. 15.1, bar one; Lenhoff et al. 2000). Their average performance on these tasks was 97% correct. In a second series of tasks testing their abil-

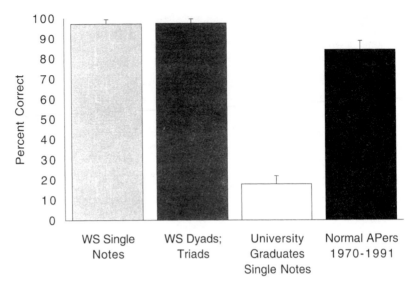

Fig. 15.1. Percentage of correct answers in tests for absolute pitch. Bar 1: Single-note tests of individuals with WBS. Bar 2: Identification of notes in dyads and triads by individuals with WBS. Bar 3: Single-note tests of university graduates. Bar 4: Meta-analysis findings for normally developed musicians with AP. The vertical lines above the bars represent standard error. *Source:* Lenhoff et al. 2000. Preservation of a Normally Transient Critical Period in a Cognitively Impaired Population: Window of Opportunity for Acquiring Absolute Pitch in Williams syndrome. Chapter 19 in Shaw CA and McEachern JC (eds.), *Toward a Theory of Neuroplasticity,* p. 279. Reproduced by permission of Routledge/Taylor & Francis Books, Inc.

ity to identify the individual natural notes presented simultaneously in sets of two (dyads) or three (triads) under a variety of conditions, the WBS group averaged 98% correct (fig. 15.1, bar two). The WBS participants scored much higher than the six non-WBS university graduates we tested (including the two with graduate training in music), who averaged 18% correct (fig. 15.1, bar three). The WBS group also scored well compared with the published performances of trained non-WBS musicians claiming to possess AP, who as a group scored 84.3% correct on tests for AP using piano or synthesized piano tones (fig. 15.1, bar four) (Takeuchi and Hulse 1993).

These results demonstrate that the rare musical ability of AP can be possessed by people with WBS in spite of their severe limitations in other cognitive domains. Whether or not possession of AP accounts for the extraordinary talents of some WBS musicians cannot be concluded from these measurements.

Relative Pitch

Most experienced musicians have high levels of relative pitch (RP), the ability to recognize the relations between pitches (Takeuchi and Hulse 1993). Although not investigated exhaustively in our study focusing primarily on AP, the abilities of individuals with WBS in RP also appeared strong as measured by the tasks we presented. To quantify RP abilities, we devised a production task and an identification task. Preliminary experiments convinced us that the concept of "musical interval" was difficult—that is, too cognitive—for most people with WBS to grasp. Yet these participants performed as follows in recognizing intervals.

The intervals tested were presented in the following order: perfect eighth (P8), perfect fifth (P5), perfect fourth (P4), major third (M3), major second (M2), major sixth (M6), and major seventh (M7). Intervals were presented using the notes ranging from C3 to C5. The tasks were given in blocks of ten trials for each interval. Intervals P8 through M3 and M2 through M7 were presented on two separate days of testing. The WBS participants as a group scored an average of 85% correct in the production tasks and 89% correct in the identification tasks.

Possibly some of their "lower" scores came from the participants' inability to understand the concept of intervals and/or because of the inadequacy of our testing methods. Not scoring uniformly as high in RP tests as in AP tests, however, is not considered unusual for musicians of normal cognition who possess AP (Miyazaki 1995). Miyazaki tested the RP abilities of normal individuals having or lacking AP and concluded that his results "suggest that absolute pitch listeners are weak in relative pitch processing and show a tendency to rely on absolute pitch in relative pitch tasks" (962). Whether Miyazaki's findings on relative pitch in musicians with normal cognition and possessing AP are a generalization also applicable to cognitively impaired musicians who possess AP has yet to be determined.

Retention, Recall, and Transposition

Additional evidence supporting the conclusion that individuals with WBS have skills in RP is found in the results of tests for retention, recall, and transposition. There are abundant anecdotal reports that people with WBS have a remarkable ability to retain and recall melodies. I have three noteworthy examples. First, in the summer of 2002, our daughter, GML, while chatting with a French-speaking visitor, sang for him in correct pitch, timing, and diction the seventy-one-word French chanson "La Charme," by Chausson, which she had learned twenty years ago from a college student—a song that neither my wife, nor Gloria's subsequent voice teachers, nor I recall ever having heard her sing before. We checked the printed music, and she had recited the lyrics without error. Second, in the winter of 2003, we asked her if she would learn Verdi's rendition of "Ave Maria." Her response was, "That is a lovely piece," and she proceeded to sing it faultlessly. She told us she had heard it on one of her compact discs. Third, in preparation for a concert, in the spring of 2003 we asked her to learn Mozart's "Exsultate, Jubilate," a relatively long piece that precedes his famous "Alleluia." Not only did she sing the piece to us in its entirety, but she told us she had listened to it about twenty years ago on a 33⅓ record and had never sung it until we asked her about it that spring. Extraordinary as these examples are, the problem remains for researchers to measure and quantify this ability.

In our studies, to get one type of measurement of retention along with measurements of recall and transposition, we followed the suggestion of a musician who was the mother of one of the WBS participants in our study. We tested the participants' abilities to produce (sing) the melody of a song(s), singing the names of the notes that make up the melody, not the specific words. Specifically, all were asked to sing the names of the musical notes of a number of pieces (vocal or instrumental) of songs they previously had learned to sing or play, usually in the key of C. None of the participants had been told previously the corresponding names of those notes. In addition, some were asked to expand the same task by transposing the melodies into different keys. The tasks varied somewhat for each of the participants. Their responses were recorded. After they had completed these tasks, we compared their responses with the printed musical notation of each piece. The numbers of correct and erroneous responses were scored.

Four of the participants scored 87% correct or better, with two scoring nearly at ceiling. Only one of the five seemed confused by these tasks. Nonetheless, the five averaged 86% as a group for all the recall and transposition tasks, which involved 1,468 notes.

The skill of the WBS participants in producing (i.e., singing) the melodies and correct notes in these recall and transposition tasks also shows clearly that, in the tasks for measuring AP (fig. 15.1), they were not cued to the correct notes by their familiarity with the timbre and characteristics of the piano and keyboard tones (Lockhead and Byrd 1981).

Further Analysis of the Results on Absolute Pitch
Level and Incidence of Absolute Pitch

The results of the AP studies demonstrated that, as a group, the five WBS participants scored at 97.5% correct—that is, near ceiling levels. The results also indicate that the incidence of AP in people with WBS is higher, possibly much higher, than that in the population with normal cognition. As noted above, it is generally accepted that the incidence of AP among normal individuals in Western countries is 1 in 10,000 (Takeuchi and Hulse 1993). In some Asian countries the incidence is thought to be somewhat higher, possibly because, in Japan, for example, children start musical training earlier (Miyazaki 1988) or because some Asian populations speak in tonal languages, such as Vietnamese or Mandarin (Deutsch 2002; Deutsch et al. 2004).

Because all the WBS participants in our study possess AP, the incidence of AP in the WBS population seems to be greater than that in the general population. This conclusion is based on the fact that the five were selected from the known population of about five thousand people with WBS in Canada and the United States, the pool in which we found them. Thus, even if we made the highly conservative assumption that the five individuals in our study were the only people with WBS in the United States and Canada who have AP, the incidence of AP in that population would be about 1 in 1,000, which is more than ten times that presumed to exist in Western populations.

I presume that the incidence of AP in the WBS population is higher, possibly in the neighborhood of 1 in 10. I make that projection because of the increasing number of anecdotal quantitative reports I have received from teachers and parents. As more and more people with WBS begin to study music, learn to name the notes, and are tested, we should get a more accurate estimate of the incidence of AP in Williams-Beuren syndrome.

Critical Period for "Acquiring" Absolute Pitch
May Be Extended in WBS

Individuals with normal cognition who possess AP as adults are said to have had musical training between the ages of three and six (Sergeant 1969; Sergeant and Roche 1973; Cohen and Baird 1990; Takeuchi and Hulse 1993; Baharloo et al. 1998, 2000; Brown et al. 2000). This generalization does not seem to apply to at least four of the five WBS participants in our study, because only one of them started formal training in music before the age of six. The other four participants started music lessons at age nine ($\pm$ 1.8 years), which is after the normal early-childhood "critical period" for acquiring AP.

Thus, the critical period for the development of AP, open to normally developing individuals up to the age of six, seems to be extended in individuals with WBS, possibly into adulthood. Does the possession of AP by individuals with WBS after six years of age require prior training in music? The available evidence (Lenhoff et al. 2001) supports this view, but more data are needed.

Nonetheless, after we published the concept of an extended critical period, it was recognized by three leading researchers who study absolute pitch. Schellenberg and Trehub (2003, 266), when elaborating on the acquisition of pitch labels, allude to "the prolonged critical period" in WBS. Deutsch et al. (2004) apply the concept to non-WBS individuals by proposing that "the acquisition of absolute pitch by rare individuals who speak an intonation language may be associated with a critical period of unusually long duration" (339). We look forward to more reports and supporting evidence for that intriguing concept.

The term *musical training* applied to people with WBS, however, takes on a somewhat different meaning. Unlike most individuals with normal cognition, those with WBS learn primarily through listening. Most do not read music, nor do they understand many of the cognitive aspects of music. Also, their congenital physical and motor problems prevent them from playing a wide range of instruments with dexterity. Thus, their training is quite different from that of most musicians.

As already noted, it becomes more difficult for normal individuals to learn absolute pitch as they pass the age of six (Brady 1970; Sergeant and Roche 1973; Sloboda 1985). Baharloo and colleagues (1998) presented data indicating that early musical training is necessary for the development of AP. They asked 612 classically trained musicians the age at which they first started formal music lessons. Of those starting before age four, 40% reported having absolute pitch, whereas only 3% of those who began after age nine claimed to have absolute pitch. Furthermore, although musicians at most ages can gain abilities in relative pitch, they cannot gain absolute pitch once they are older (Takeuchi and Hulse 1993). Even such eminent composers as Berlioz, Schumann, Wagner, Tchaikovsky, Ravel, and Stravinsky did not possess AP (Langendorf 1992).

Absolute Pitch: Gained or Retained? Its Evolutionary Role

Although it is generally accepted that individuals who possess AP have had musical training before age seven, the question remains of whether they *gained* AP or *retained* it, because there is growing evidence that we are all born with AP. Until that question is resolved, I write "*possess* AP" as adults. If we are born with AP, what evolutionary role has it played?

At least three researchers provide evidence that we are born with abilities in AP. They investigated three unique populations, using their own techniques rather than the standard ones for measuring AP such as identifying and producing specific tones. Levitin (1994), for example, studied the abilities of adults to sing a familiar song in the key in which the song is usually performed in the media. Many could, and his results imply that we are born with a component of AP that he calls pitch memory.

Deutsch, in her classic paper on the "tritone paradox" (1986) and in a later publication (1988), reported that adult speakers of tone languages possess a "partial form of absolute pitch" (see also Deutsch 1992). Saffran, comparing the abilities in absolute and relative pitch in normally developing infants and adults, concludes that infants are born with AP, possibly (referring to the works of Deutsch) to help in learning to speak in tone languages (Saffran and Griepentrog 2001). As they approach age six or seven, children begin to rely more on relative pitch. Deutsch (2002) proposes that "absolute pitch may have evolved as a feature of speech" and that "tone language speakers generally acquire this feature [AP] during the 1st year of life" (200). Accordingly, if people with WBS are also born having AP, we might conclude that they *retain* AP once they have had the requisite musical training. Further investigations with the WBS population, known for their strength in language (see chapter 7), might provide evidence supporting the views of Saffran and Deutsch regarding the evolutionary role of AP in language and speech development.

Possible Role of Genes in Absolute Pitch

Does the high incidence of AP in people with WBS provide any basis for thinking that one or more genes are directly responsible for AP? I do not think so. A more plausible alternative would be that the hemizygous condition of one or more of the genes in the chromosome 7 deletion affects the development of parts of the brain, perhaps those parts dealing with specific auditory phenomena, so that the mechanism that closes the critical period for possessing absolute pitch does not operate normally and, as a result, the critical period does not close. In more general terms we could state that, as the presence of some of those genes in the hemizygous state affects brain development in WBS, causing cognitive impairments, a related anomaly of brain development "jams" the closure of the window of the critical period, allowing for the possession of AP at ages after six.

From our research findings, we do not postulate that the ability to acquire absolute pitch is determined either directly by specific genes or by stimuli from the environment, such as musical training. Instead, we propose that changes in the WBS brain that are associated with the microdeletion may allow the critical period for AP (Cohen and Baird 1990) to remain open. Whether the possession of absolute pitch by adults with WBS is dependent on a certain degree of exposure to music and/or to some kinds of training in music is not known; the five participants in our study (Lenhoff et al. 2001) did have some musical training. Further, humans have about thirty thousand genes, so the thousands of genes other than the twenty or so in the hemizygous state in WBS may also affect abilities in music, just as they might do in any other individuals.

Who Is Considered Musically Intelligent?

In many cultures, psychologists, educators, and the public use the terms *mentally retarded* or *cognitively impaired* to label individuals whose cognitive social skills do not fit the accepted norm and who do not score well in IQ and related tests—that is, in tests designed to show the skills needed for problem solving and recognizing spatial and visual relationships.

Gardner, in his book on multiple intelligences (1983), defines pitch, timbre, and rhythm as major components of musical intelligence. We demonstrated that cognitively impaired musicians with WBS possess such a musical intelligence with regard to pitch (Lenhoff et al. 2001). I believe research will eventually show that people with WBS also possess a high level of musical intelligence with regard to timbre and rhythm. Levitin and Bellugi (1998) have already provided some promising preliminary evidence on their abilities with rhythm.

Geschwind (1984) challenges us to consider how a society in which musical skills were considered the norm would treat individuals of normal or above-normal intelligence who were not musical. His example is a girls' school taught by Antonio Vivaldi in which everyone is expected to be talented and immersed in music. Here, a "dysmusical" individual is considered inept and a failure at the single activity considered most important. Perhaps, Geschwind proposes, like many of the individuals with mental retardation in our society (including the highly talented WBS musicians), this dysmusical individual would be "constantly reminded of . . . [her] incapacity and probably [be] condemned permanently to the kitchens, latrines, baths, and floors." As a footnote, I would add that, today, that individual might be assigned to sorting and packing, custodial chores, or some sort of gardening or yard work.

Advantages of Investigating Music Cognition in People with WBS

There are two major advantages in working with WBS populations in research on music cognition, rather than with other populations with disabilities that may show high incidences of AP, such as those with autism or blindness (Oakes 1955). For one, the WBS population, in contrast to the blind and/or autistic populations, is relatively homogeneous genetically (see chapter 3). Second, people with WBS have an IQ in the range of mild mental retardation, averaging 55, and also share many cognitive and behavioral similarities (see chapter 7). In contrast, autistic and blind individuals with AP have IQs that range over several levels of intelligences. Some of the non-WBS musical savants described in the literature have relatively normal or above-normal cognitive abilities, especially those who are blind. Among the autistic savants studied, some are cognitively impaired but others are rather high-functioning compared with persons with WBS. For example, TR can sight-read music, has a good sense of direction and excellent spatial skills, engages in cryptic crossword puzzles, and has studied chess and mathematics; his IQ is 100 or above, depending on the test administered (Young and Nettelbeck 1995). Even one of these abilities is extremely rare in WBS. Other autistic savants, such as EN (Sloboda et al. 1985) and QC (Mottron et al. 1999), read music. Moreover, the ten individuals with autism who participated in the extensive comparative study by Heaton and colleagues (1998) had IQs ranging from 55 to 127 (mean, 85). Thus far it seems that cognitively impaired individuals with WBS share a common genetic makeup related to their AP abilities. Such is not true for autism or blindness.

Clinical Implications and Future Directions

In chapter 16, Levitin and Bellugi provide an excellent discussion of the clinical implications of the research on music cognition in people with WBS. Here I focus on some implications for future research. From an abundance of anecdotal reports and the few papers published to date, music cognition in Williams-Beuren syndrome seems to be a promising area for research. For those new to working with individuals with WBS, I begin with a few cautionary measures.

Selecting WBS Participants in Research

Selecting appropriate participants for research on music in WBS depends on the questions being asked. For example, if the study aims to determine the degree to which they can perform a specific musical task, it might seem best to test a random cross section of the WBS population. This cross section may give misleading results, however, if the participants vary greatly in the amount of musical training they have received. A more reliable cross section might have as an internal control the condition that all or most of the participants have had relatively equal amounts of musical training. The important point is that, if a study is made up only of WBS participants who have had no or little musical training, we may never know the extent of the musical abilities and potentials of the WBS population.

If the research seeks, instead, to determine the highest levels of musical behavior attainable by individuals with WBS, we may need participants who demonstrate a high level of excellence in music. The rationale and advice of Maslow (1971) and Butler (1992) to that effect are reflected in Maslow's analogy: "If we want to know how fast a human being can run, then it is no use to average out the speed of a 'good sample' of the population; it is far better to collect Olympic gold medal winners and see how well they can do" (Maslow 1971, 7).

Selection of Controls or Comparison Groups

In addition to the various good standard protocols for selecting the proper control or comparison groups, I suggest two other possible approaches when investigating WBS. For our unpublished survey determining parental attitudes and views about the musical interests and abilities of their children with WBS, we compared the parents' attitudes and views about the child's abilities with their views on the same questions asked about the sibling closest in age to the child with WBS (Sandeen, Levine, and Lenhoff, unpublished results). Thus, by including the questioning about a sibling (when possible), we had an internal control for the influence of socioeconomic and cultural background on the individuals being studied.

Another type of control population might be used for other studies, such as those on the critical period for AP. As noted, that critical period usually ends by the age of seven in individuals with normal cognition but may persist in adulthood in WBS. I therefore suggest that, in some studies with WBS participants that involve traits acquired during this critical period, researchers might consider using as controls normally developing children age six and under, rather than individuals of the same chronological age (see, e.g., Bertrand et al. 1997; see also chapter 9).

Problems of Testing Individuals with WBS

Researchers new to working with WBS participants may profit from learning about several difficulties we encountered in our research on pitch. To devise tasks that could be comprehended by the participants, we found it necessary first to get a better understanding of the behavior and thought processes of people with WBS in general and especially of those participating in our research. This was time consuming, sometimes taking days; the time varied with each participant and with the type of pitch studies.

As one example, we needed to modify our testing procedures because of the participants' desire to please, a common characteristic in WBS. Some participants will cooperate more with investigators they like and less so with others. But their desire to please may lead them to twist their answers in a way that they believe (rightly or wrongly) will satisfy an investigator they admire. Frequently, the eyes of the participant are glued on those of the investigator, partly, I believe, because she or he wants to detect how the answers are perceived. Experienced investigators, however, show approval equally for both correct and incorrect answers.

We also noted that our participants had difficulty handling such comparisons as *same* or *different, higher* or *lower,* and *more* or *less.* These problems are similar to those encountered by other researchers trying to assess pitch discrimination by young, normally developing children (Andrews and Madeira 1977).

Uncertainties in Generalizing from the Non-WBS to the WBS Population

Because of the recognized differences in the behavior (see chapter 7) and the brain structure (Jernigan et al. 1993) of the WBS and the normally developed populations, generalizations about music cognition may not be transferable from one group to the other. I have already given a number of examples illustrating this point, such as the differences between the two populations in the incidence of AP and the length of the AP critical period.

Another example concerns the ability to hear a pitch and to give a label to that pitch. It is generally agreed that "Pitch labelling [in people of normal cognition] can be trained more successfully in children than in adults" (Levitin and Rogers 2005, 30). If that is true, then it explains why some of my colleagues were amazed when they learned that my daughter with WBS learned to name and identify the natural notes at age forty-one and the accidental notes at age forty-three (Lenhoff et al. 2001). Those music researchers told me that they did not know of any adult of normal cognition who could accomplish that feat. Knowledge of the names of the notes had not been necessary for her to learn and perform operatic arias; since she already had absolute pitch, she simply learned to attach a name to the notes when I asked her to, after she had reached age forty. Examples such as this one point out why there might be much to learn about music cognition and mechanisms for possessing AP through studying people with WBS.

Societal and Professional Attitudes

Scientists considering initiating research on music cognition in WBS may wish to take into account some societal and professional attitudes before taking the plunge. It is common knowledge that society in general regards cognitively impaired individuals as incapable of significant achievements in processes thought to require high levels of intelligence. Those who do reach certain levels of accomplishment generally are viewed as anomalies.

Unfortunately, similar attitudes appear even among some academics in the field of music cognition. One example illustrates a total misunderstanding of the nature of WBS by a reviewer of a prestigious journal. That reviewer suggested that people with WBS "learned" the rare ability of AP in order to please the researcher. More troublesome are the remarks of two experts whose chapter on AP appeared in the first edition of *The Psychology of Music* (Ward and Burns 1982). The chapter refers to a study of "mentally retarded teenagers [who] apparently have AP" (449). That otherwise outstanding chapter, however, ended with the following statement: "It appears that AP is typical of either musical precociousness or mental retardation. So if you have it, be sure it is for the right reason" (449). As a research scientist and father of a WBS musician, I find such a remark in the academic literature both unscientific and unworthy.

A number of researchers in the music cognition literature refer to music as one of the highest levels of human cognition. Do they perhaps feel that any evidence demonstrating that a cognitively impaired individual can attain a high level of musical ability somehow lessens the significance of their life's work? Just as experimental biologists investigate an atypical system or organism to better understand the normal (genetics, development, physiology, and behavior), we believe cognitive scientists in music likewise will do well when they view cognitively impaired musicians as offering an opportunity to better understand the complexities of the human brain in processing musical information.

Low IQ and Musical Performance

Contrary to what we might expect, could it be that a lower IQ may actually serve to enhance the performance ability of experienced WBS musicians? Perhaps, among individuals with WBS who are well trained in music, those with IQ measurements closer to the mean for WBS (i.e., around 55 [see chapter 7]) are more at ease during performances because their minds are less preoccupied with cognitive distractions occasioned by an ongoing analysis of the music as they perform—distractions that may interfere with performance for those with higher IQs and cognitive abilities. In analogous fashion, premiere athletes of normal intelligence who have a high "bodily kinesthetic" intelligence (Gardner 1983) perform (i.e., compete) better than the next level of athletes whose focus may be distracted by thinking about the many factors required for excellent athletic performance. Using the terminology and analogies of Csikszentmihalyi (1990), we might say that during performances by WBS musicians, the "flow"—that is, "intense concentration" on the music being performed—is less disturbed by the cognitive distractions that often plague normal musicians.

Do Behavioral Mental Asymmetries and Uncovered Intelligences of the "Mentally Retarded" Offer an Approach for Investigating Sequences of Brain Development?

A growing body of evidence, presented in this chapter and in chapter 16, shows that people with WBS have levels of musical intelligence, especially in pitch and probably in timbre and rhythm, that are equal to or greater than those of people considered to be of normal intelligence. Consequently, I propose that we refer to such individuals as *mentally asymmetric* rather than the less accurate and more pejorative *mentally retarded*.

In the past few years I have received a growing number of reports from relatives of individuals representing other cognitively impaired populations who have various levels of enhanced musical abilities. There are some intriguing examples. A fourteen-year-old with the rare chromosome 9 monosomy has AP and studies the cello. A twenty-three-year-old woman with isodicentric 15 is a vocalist reported to have AP as well as "perfect music memory." Parents of children who have a chromosome 22q11.2 microdeletion attest to their children's musicality, one describing an accomplished nineteen-year-old guitarist from South Africa who has AP and has performed widely with major musical groups. More recently there have been reports of individuals with retinopathy of prematurity (ages twelve through twenty-nine), who are blind and have mental retardation, and who are musical savants with prodigious memories. There are also savants among those who are blind because of optic nerve hypoplasia (ages four to twenty-four). I have had the privilege of observing a prodigious musical savant (age twenty-nine) who has retinopathy of prematurity and another (age seven) who has optic nerve hypoplasia. I have been told of a ten-year-old musical savant with Leber's congenital amaurosis. Other individuals I have encountered who show musical abilities similar to those in WBS include some who have been brain damaged while infants by severe accidents or by congenital birth defects.

As more musical individuals having genetic or physically induced brain aberrations are identified, they may offer a unique opportunity to investigate "sequential changes" in development of some parts of the brain. Before leaping to some of the more technological methods available today (e.g., functional magnetic resonance imaging or positron emission tomography scans), researchers may benefit by starting to gather behavioral measurements, such as those used in determining pitch and the timing and lengths of critical periods. This approach might be analogous to that of biochemical geneticists who have investigated an array of bacterial mutants to uncover sequential metabolic pathways. Quantitative investigations of the behaviors of mentally asymmetric genetic populations and some phenocopies may lead to the discovery of sequences in the development of specific regions of the human brain that affect those behaviors. When researchers quantify the extraordinary abilities of individuals from a broad spectrum of such mentally asymmetric populations, rather than focusing on their inabilities, they may find that much of the mystery surrounding the mentally asymmetric disappears and the excitement of a new understanding beckons.

ACKNOWLEDGMENTS

The research on absolute pitch in individuals with WBS was carried out in collaboration with Oligario Perales and Dr. Gregory S. Hickok of the Department of Cognitive Sciences, University of California, Irvine. Most of this chapter was written while I was an adjunct professor in the Department of Psychology, University of Massachusetts, Amherst. I thank coeditor Dr. Paul Wang for his helpful advice and encouragement. For specific sections of this chapter I am grateful for the advice of Dr. Diana Deutsch (University of California, San Diego), Dr. Daniel Levitin (McGill University), and Dr. Daniel Stokols (University of California, Irvine). I thank David Mehnert for introducing me to blind musical savants. The research was supported by grant SBR-9617078 from the National Science Foundation, Division of Human Perception and Cognition, and by the Bernon Family Fund. I thank the Williams Syndrome Foundation, the Williams Syndrome Association, the

Berkshire Hills Music Academy, and the Belvoir Terrace Summer Camp for their cooperation. To my wife, Sylvia, I am once again grateful for her editing and encouragement. I thank the many parents, relatives, and music teachers of individuals with WBS and of individuals having other congenital conditions for sharing their anecdotal observations with me. Most of all, I thank my daughter Gloria and her fellow WBS musicians for developing their talents and changing our views of the abilities of cognitively impaired individuals, thereby helping researchers to delve into some of the mysteries of the human brain.

REFERENCES

Andrews, M. L., and Madeira, S. S. 1977. The measurement of pitch discrimination ability in young children. *Journal of Speech and Hearing Disorders* 42:279–286.
Bachem, A. 1955. Absolute pitch. *Journal of the Acoustical Society of America* 27:1180–1185.
Baggaley, J. 1974. Measurement of absolute pitch. *Psychology of Music* 22:11–17.
Baharloo, S., Johnston, P. A., Service, S. K., Gitschier, J., and Freimer, N. B. 1998. Absolute pitch: An approach for identification of genetic and nongenetic components. *American Journal of Human Genetics* 62:224–231.
Baharloo, S., Service, S. K., Risch, N., Gitschier, J., and Freimer, N. B. 2000. Familial aggregation of absolute pitch. *American Journal of Human Genetics* 67:755–758.
Bertrand, J., Mervis, C., and Eisenberg, J. 1997. Drawing by children with Williams syndrome: A developmental perspective. *Developmental Neuropsychology* 13:41–67.
Brady, P. T. 1970. The genesis of absolute pitch. *Journal of the Acoustical Society of America* 48:883–887.
Brown, S., Merker, B., and Wallin, N. L. 2000. An introduction to evolutionary musicology. In *The origins of music,* ed. N. L. Wallin, B. Merker, and S. Brown, 3–24. Cambridge: MIT Press.
Butler, D. 1992. *The musician's guide to perception and cognition,* 10–12. New York: Schirmer Books.
Csikszentmihalyi, M. 1990. *Flow: The psychology of optimal experience.* New York: Harper and Row.
Cohen, A., and Baird, K. 1990. Acquisition of absolute pitch: The question of critical periods. *Psychomusicology* 9:31–37.
Deutsch, D. 1986. A musical paradox. *Music Perception* 3:275–280.
———. 1988. Pitch class and perceived height: Some paradoxes and their implications. In *Explorations in music, the arts, and ideas: Essays in honor of Leonard B. Meyer,* ed. E. Narmour and R. Solie, 261–294. Hillsdale, NY: Pendragon Press.
———. 1992. Paradoxes of musical pitch. *Scientific American* 267:88–95.
———. 2002. The puzzle of absolute pitch. *Current Directions in Psychological Science* 11:200–204.
Deutsch, D., Henthorn, T., and Dolson, M. 2004. Absolute pitch, speech, and tone language: Some experiments and a proposed framework. *Music Perception* 21:339–356.
Don, A. J., Schellenberg, E. G., and Rourke, B. P. 1999. Music and language skills of children with Williams syndrome. *Child Neuropsychology* 5:154–170.

Gardner, H. 1983. *Frames of mind: The theory of multiple intelligences*, 99–126. New York: Basic Books.

Geschwind, N. 1984. The brain of learning-disabled individuals. *Annals of Dyslexia* 34:319–327.

Heaton, P., Hermelin, B., and Pring, L. 1998. Autism and pitch processing: A precursor for savant musical ability? *Music Perception* 15:291–305.

Jernigan, T. L., Bellugi, U., Sowell, E., Doherty, S., and Hesselink, J. 1993. Cerebral morphologic distinctions between Williams and Down syndromes. *Archives of Neurology* 50:186–191.

Langendorf, F. 1992. Absolute pitch: Review and speculations. *Medical Problems of Performing Arts* 7:6–13.

Lenhoff, H. M. 1998. Insights into the musical potential of cognitively impaired people diagnosed with Williams syndrome. *Music Therapy Perspectives* 16:32–35.

Lenhoff, H. M., Wang, P. P., Greenberg, F., and Bellugi, U. 1997. Williams syndrome and the brain. *Scientific American* 26:42–47.

Lenhoff, H., Perales, O., and Hickok, G. 2000. Preservation of a normally transient critical period in a cognitively impaired population: Window of opportunity for acquiring absolute pitch in Williams Syndrome. In *Toward a theory of neuroplasticity*, ed. C. Shaw and J. McEachin, 275–287. Philadelphia: Psychology Press, Taylor and Francis.

———. 2001. Absolute pitch in Williams syndrome. *Music Perception* 18:491–503.

Levitin, D. J. 1994. Absolute memory for musical pitch: Evidence from the production of learned melodies. *Perception and Psychophysics* 58:927–935.

Levitin, D. J., and Bellugi, U. 1998. Musical abilities in individuals with Williams syndrome. *Music Perception* 15:357–389.

Levitin, D. J., and Rogers, S. E. 2005. Absolute pitch: Perception, coding, and controversies. *Trends in Cognitive Sciences* 9:26–33.

Levitin, D. J., Menon, V., Schmitt, J. E., Eliez, S., White, C., Glover, G., Korenberg, J. R., Bellugi, U., and Reiss, A. L. 2003. Music and noise processing in Williams syndrome: Evidence from fMRI. *NeuroImage* 18:74–82.

Lockhead, G. R., and Byrd, R. 1981. Practically perfect pitch. *Journal of the Acoustical Society of America* 70:387–389.

Maslow, A. H.. 1971. *The farther reaches of human nature*. New York: Viking.

Miyazaki, K. 1988. Musical pitch identification by absolute pitch possessors. *Perception and Psychophysics* 44:501–512.

———. 1995. Perception of relative pitch with different references: Some absolute-pitch listeners can't tell musical interval names. *Perception and Psychophysics* 57:962–970.

Mottron, L., Peretz, I., Belleville, S., and Rouleau, N. 1999. Absolute pitch in autism: A case study. *Neurocase* 5:485–501.

Oakes, W. F. 1955. An experimental study of pitch naming and pitch discrimination reactions. *Journal of General Psychology* 86:237–259.

Saffran, J. R., and Griepentrog, G. J. 2001. Absolute pitch in infant auditory learning: Evidence for developmental reorganization. *Developmental Psychology* 37:74–85.

Schellenberg, E. G., and Trehub, S. E. 2003. Good pitch memory is widespread. *Psychological Science* 14:262–266.

Sergeant, D. 1969. Experimental investigation of absolute pitch. *Journal of Research in Music Education* 17:135–143.

Sergeant, D., and Roche, S. 1973. Perceptual shifts in the auditory information processing of young children. *Psychology of Music* 1:39–48.

Sloboda, J. A. 1985. *The musical mind.* Oxford: Clarendon Press.

Sloboda, J. A., Hermelin, B., and O'Conner, N. 1985. An exceptional musical memory. *Music Perception* 3:155–170.

Stambaugh, L. 1996. Special learners with special abilities. *Music Educators Journal* 83:19–23.

Takeuchi, A. H., and Hulse, S. H. 1993. Absolute pitch. *Psychological Bulletin* 113:345–361.

Von Arnim, G., and Engel, P. 1964. Mental retardation related to hypercalcaemia. *Developmental Medicine and Child Neurology* 6:336–377.

Ward, W. D., and Burns, E. M. 1982. Absolute pitch. In *The psychology of music,* ed. D. Deutsch, 431–451. San Diego: Academic Press.

Young, R. L., and Nettelbeck, T. 1995. The abilities of a musical savant and his family. *Journal of Autism and Developmental Disorders* 25:231–247.

Rhythm, Timbre, and Hyperacusis in Williams-Beuren Syndrome

16

Daniel J. Levitin, Ph.D., and Ursula Bellugi, Ed.D.

Anecdotal reports have long suggested that individuals with Williams-Beuren syndrome (WBS) are especially musical. Recent research has attempted to *quantify* and better understand the nature and extent of these reported musical abilities in an effort to enhance our understanding of the relation among genes, development, brain, and cognitive function. This chapter reports on the extant literature on three of the phenotypic markers of auditory and musical function in WBS: rhythmic ability (both production and perception), timbre perception and memory, and hyperacusis.

Rhythm, along with pitch, is one of the two dissociable attributes of music (Krumhansl 2000; Levitin 2002) and is fundamentally important in distinguishing one musical piece from another. Controlled experiments have been conducted to compare the rhythmic abilities of individuals with WBS with those of typically developing, normal controls, as well as with individuals with Down syndrome and autism. The research on timbre perception has led to both behavioral and neuroimaging research, as reported here. The term *hyperacusis*—an unusual sensitivity to sound—has an unfortunate history of inconsistency of use in both the clinical and research communities; it has been used to describe four vastly different auditory disorders, and we attempt here to clarify and reconcile these reports.

At the outset, the most important observation to stress is that individuals with WBS comprise a heterogeneous group with respect to musical ability and achievement. That is, there is as much individual difference in this population as in a normal population, and it would be inaccurate to claim that all individuals with WBS are "musical." What can be said is that they are more likely to express love for music, to engage in musical activities (either creative or receptive), and to have longer-lasting emotional reactions to music (Don et al. 1999; Levitin et al. 2004).

Rhythm

Rhythm is that aspect of music that encodes the temporal components of a musical piece. In Beethoven's *Fifth Symphony,* for example, the opening phrase consists of four notes played in a rhythm of short-short-short-long (bum-bum-bum-baaaah). If this rhythmic phrase is inverted to long-short-short-short, the piece becomes unrecognizable and has a completely different semantic meaning (Levitin and Menon 2003).

Rhythm Production

We have investigated the rhythmic abilities of individuals with WBS and examined rhythm production and memory (Levitin and Bellugi 1998). Using a series of rhythmic patterns of increasing complexity, we engaged participants in an echo clapping task to assess their mental representations of musical rhythms and their ability to reproduce them. In this task, the experimenter would clap a rhythm and the participant's task was to clap that rhythm back as accurately as possible. The patterns were based on those used in the Gordon Musical Aptitude Profile (Gordon 1965) and by Bruscia (1981) in a similar paradigm, and they provided a wide variety of temporal ratios.

The age of the WBS participants ranged from nine to twenty years (mean, 13.4 years; SD = 3.6 years); there were two female and six male participants. To provide a comparison with mental age–matched, typically developing children, eight participants were recruited from Palo Alto, California, in June 1997: two normally developing girls and six boys, with chronological age ranging from five to seven, two participants for each age category. Given that the WBS participants may have had a greater number of hours of musical exposure because of their greater chronological age, we attempted to balance this by recruiting as controls educationally sophisticated children who had taken at least three years of continuous formal musical instruction, were from one of the highest rated school districts in California, and were currently studying music privately.

Even though not specifically instructed to do so, the WBS participants in this experiment (more so than the control participants) tended to look the experimenter in the eye rather than watching the experimenter's hands during presentation of the examples. This tendency toward eye contact was first documented in the documentary film *Williams Syndrome—A Highly Musical Species* (Wilmowski 1995) by the drum instructor K. B. McConnel. Also, on nearly every trial, the WBS participants clapped back the rhythms immediately in perfect time, without missing a beat, as if their response formed part of the same rhythmic sequence. That is, when the experimenter was finished giving the exemplar, the participants came right in on the next beat without pausing. All of the WBS participants thus seemed to interpret the examples as forming part of a larger musical set; they acted as though they understood there to be an implied time signature and tempo, and they responded to the "first measure" of music played by the experimenter in time for the downbeat (or in some cases pickups) to the "second measure." Moreover, the WBS participants revealed a remarkable ability to track changes in rhythmic pulse, including changes to swing time, straight eighths, triplets, sixteenths, syncopations, and so on. In some cases, the experimenter began the next trial without pausing after the participants' response, giving the experimental session the flavor of a jazz "jam" session of "trading ones," the technical term used to describe musicians who alternate playing measures of a musical phrase.

Surprisingly, we found that the WBS participants performed as well as their mental age–matched controls, and, most interestingly, on the one-third of the trials in which the individuals with WBS made errors, the errors were far more likely to be musically coherent than those of the controls. Put another way, their errors were *musical*, as if completing the rhythmic phrase they were attempting to reproduce. This finding was especially interesting, as it stands in contradiction to Miller's position (1989) that musical savants tend to lack rhythmic ability. In addition, Serafine (1979) argued that metric conservation in normally developing children is correlated with the standard Piagetian conservation tasks; given that most individuals with WBS do not reach this Piagetian stage (Bellugi et al. 1994) but our WBS participants demonstrated conservation of musical time, their performance is especially surprising and challenges important theoretical models of cognitive abilities that couple these two forms of conservation. We concluded our report of this study by suggesting that participants with WBS had evidenced a quality we called rhythmicity or rhythmic musicality.

Rhythm Perception

Four other studies have examined rhythmic perception in WBS. Don et al. (1999), Hopyan et al. (2001), and our research group (D. J. Levitin and U. Bellugi, unpublished data). all administered the Gordon Primary Measures of Musical Audiation (PMMA), a standard rhythm perception test (Gordon 1986). The test is furnished on cassette tape, and participants listen to pairs of examples that consist of short rhythmic phrases that are either identical or slightly different; participants are instructed to respond "same" or "different." Don compared nineteen individuals with WBS (mean age, 10.5 years; SD = 1.83 years; range, 8–13 years) with nineteen typically developing, normal participants (mean age, 7.9 years; SD = 2.3 years; range not given), matched for their levels of general cognitive ability (as indexed by the Peabody Picture Vocabulary Test–Revised [PPVT-R]). The control group performed better than the WBS group on the rhythm subcomponent of the

PMMA, but the statistical analyses employed were subject to question and therefore it is difficult to draw a firm conclusion as to whether the differences are statistically significant. Don and colleagues apparently made multiple post hoc comparisons without appropriate adjustments in significance level, and they failed to report the main effect of group in their analysis of variance statistic.

Hopyan and colleagues (2001) administered the same test to fourteen children with WBS (mean age, 12 years; SD = 3 years) and fourteen chronological age–matched controls (mean age, 12 years; SD = 3 years). This study reported that the control group performed significantly better than the WBS group on the rhythm test. In our own laboratory, in an experiment currently underway, we obtained the same results as Hopyan. But the pattern of errors made by the WBS participants alerted us to a potential confound with the stimulus materials. More often than not, our WBS participants were labeling "different" some pairs of examples that the PMMA had intended to be the same. On closer listening to the examples, we discovered that the cassette tapes contained numerous rhythmic confounds, rendering the rhythmic task more difficult to complete for a careful listener. Specifically, the test as furnished by the manufacturer contains random static and recording artifacts that create unintended spaces and gaps during long tones of the rhythm test. Thus, a reference rhythm and its matched comparison rhythm may in fact seem different to a careful listener when intended to be the same by the test maker. To remove this potential confound from the experiment, we resynthesized and rerecorded all the examples digitally and administered the test to a fresh group of participants.

The participants performed very well on this resynthesized version. To give the comparison group the best possible chance of performing better than our WBS group—in an effort to replicate the findings of Hopyan and colleagues of better rhythm performance among the controls—our control participants were not simply matched on chronological age but were drawn from a pool of true musical experts: students at the Julliard School of Music in New York. In this work we found that WBS and Julliard students performed equivalently on the rhythm tests, evidence that the WBS group was performing significantly above overall cognitive level and, indeed, on a par with chronological age–matched controls (Levitin and Bellugi, unpublished data).

Brochard and colleagues (in press) tested rhythmic sequence discrimination by employing a same/different task in which the "different" examples differed either in meter or gestalt grouping. Although the nine adults with WBS performed more poorly overall than the nine controls (matched for sex and chronological age), the WBS participants showed a relative strength in perceiving the metric rather than the grouping examples. Moreover, the processing of rhythmic pauses was highly disturbed when some musical semantic content was present.

Thus, with the exception of specific impairments on metrical sequences and semantic pauses documented by Brochard et al. (in press), we would argue that *both* rhythm production and rhythm perception are relative strengths in WBS, when bias-free tests are used. Preliminary studies suggest a neuroanatomic basis for this relative sparing of rhythmic ability, as discussed below. The most direct implication of this finding is that caregivers may want to encourage individuals with WBS to play rhythm instruments (percussion, drums, etc.) as a musical outlet. Indeed, a large number of the males at the WBS music camp where we made our observations (Belvoir Terrace) play the drums at a relatively proficient level and play in small bands.

Timbre Perception and Hyperacusis

As has been noted previously, individuals with WBS tend to be unusually sensitive to and interested in sound (Udwin 1990), a characteristic dubbed "soundscape sensitivity" (Levitin and Bellugi 1998) and often referred to by the medical term *hyperacusis*. Because the sensitivity to sound experienced by most individuals with WBS seems to be related to specific tonal colors or timbres of those sounds, we deal with these two topics together.

The medical definition of hyperacusis is "abnormal sensitivity to sound" (Dirckx 2001; Venes et al. 2001) that indicates lowered hearing thresholds (an ability to hear soft sounds that others cannot), but this description does not adequately capture the phenomenology of WBS. Whereas there have been many anecdotal accounts of people with WBS who have lowered hearing thresholds (a claim not yet supported by our own research), three unusual behaviors have additionally been reported in WBS.

The first is aversion to certain types of normal-volume sounds (Morelock and Feldman 2000), such as lawnmowers, leaf blowers, or vacuum cleaners—although the particular sounds seem to be idiosyncratic—and there are many others. The distress extends even to the anticipation of such noises (Hagerman 1999), and typical reactions are for children to put their hands over their ears and cry or attempt to avoid the source of the sound (Udwin 1990). The aversion does not result from the *loudness* of the sounds but from some quality of the sounds that has yet to be completely characterized. Because this shares a conceptual similarity with allodynia, a pathologic state (typically following tissue or nerve damage) in which patients feel pain from stimuli that are not normally perceived as painful, we propose renaming this condition *auditory allodynia,* as first suggested by Levitin et al. (2003). These symptoms have sometimes been referred to in the literature as *phonophobia,* but that term, like *hyperacusis,* also has a history of misuse, and consequently we opted for a new term without prior ambiguous associations.

Second, sounds that are not too loud for others are perceived as painfully loud by individuals with WBS. This is essentially a lowered uncomfortable loudness threshold (LULL); it is not necessarily related to a lowered hearing threshold and should be referred to by the term *odynacusis* (Venes et al. 2001; Dirckx 2001). This is distinct from auditory allodynia because individuals with LULLs react negatively to any sound beyond a certain level, not only to particular sounds that they find idiosyncratically aversive. Third is an intense fascination for certain classes of sounds, often the same sounds that frightened the individual at a younger age (Levitin et al. 2005).

The literature has tended to lump these behaviors together, using the single term *hyperacusis* somewhat indiscriminately to describe these phenomena (Katznell and Segal 2001; Klein et al. 1990; Marriage 1995; Phillips and Carr 1998). Because these symptoms stem from different underlying physiologic correlates and etiologies, it is important to be precise with terms so as not to lead to confusion. Klein and colleagues (1990), for example, used the term *hyperacusis* to describe cases of individuals with WBS who experienced "consistently exaggerated or inappropriate responses or complaints of uncomfortable loudness to sounds that are neither intrinsically threatening nor uncomfortably loud to a typical person . . . these responses would occur on nearly every occasion that the sounds are presented and do not habituate with repeated exposures" (339)—what we have categorized as odynacusis. Hopyan et al. (2001) used *hyperacusis* to mean simply "an abnormally strong affective response to certain categories of sounds" (42).

Aversion: Auditory Allodynia

Recently we have had the opportunity to refine our understanding of auditory sensitivities in WBS through a questionnaire administered to 118 individuals with WBS, 40 individuals with Down syndrome, 30 with autism, and 118 typically developing, normal controls (Levitin et al. 2005). As we have noted, individuals with WBS experience strong aversion to certain types of sounds, independent of their loudness. The sounds tend to be spectrally broad-band sounds, such as those emanating from motors, fans, fireworks, and thunder. Compared with typically developing, normal children and children with Down syndrome or autism, individuals with WBS are more than three times as likely to have suffered from auditory aversions, with 91% of respondents reporting this (compared with 27% of individuals with autism and fewer than 7% of individuals with Down syndrome or normal controls).

Attraction and Auditory Fascinations

Individuals with WBS were also nearly ten times as likely to report auditory fascinations, that is, an unusual attraction to certain sounds, sometimes manifesting as auditory fetishes. Interestingly, this attraction is often toward sounds that the individuals initially found aversive. We also noted that 80% of individuals with WBS (compared with 33% or less in the comparison groups) were reported by their caregivers to have LULLs (sounds that are not too loud for others are perceived as painfully loud) and 5% were reported to experience hyperacusis (here meaning the ability to hear soft sounds that are imperceptible to others), whereas no other group reported this. Previous research (discussed below) has established that peripheral auditory mechanisms in WBS function normally (Neville et al. 1994) and therefore it seems reasonable to infer that the LULLs and hyperacusis are probably mediated by hyperexcitability of cortical neurons in the auditory pathway (Neville et al. 1994; Bellugi et al. 1992).

Timbral Identification

We recently completed a behavioral experiment to quantify the timbral/soundscape-processing abilities of individuals with WBS. Numerous observations have told us that not only are many individuals with WBS attracted to the sounds of motors, but many have learned to classify and label the sounds with great accuracy and precision. We have encountered individuals with WBS who can accurately identify different lawnmowers or vacuum cleaners, based solely on the sound of their motors. To turn this observation into an experiment, we digitally recorded twelve different vacuum cleaners and administered a same/different discrimination task to individuals with WBS (Levitin and Bellugi, unpublished data). For a control group, we used the chronological age–matched Julliard students mentioned above. We found that the performance of the WBS participants was as good as that of these highly selected controls, making timbral identification one of only a small set of tasks at which individuals with WBS perform on a par with typically developing, chronological age–matched equivalents.

Neurobiological Studies

The types of neurobiological studies that have been conducted with individuals with WBS fall into three categories: electrophysiologic (primarily using event-related potentials, taken from scalp recording electrodes), neuroimaging (primarily using magnetic resonance imaging [MRI]), and cytoarchitectonic (study of the arrangement of cells in neural tissue in postmortem brains).

Event-Related Brain Potentials

A series of studies using event-related potentials (ERPs) investigated the timing and organization of neural systems connected with auditory function in WBS (Neville et al. 1994). ERPs are well suited to this type of study because they have very high temporal resolution and thus can track changes in auditory processing of the presented stimuli in nearly real time. Of additional importance is that they are relatively noninvasive, although some individuals report slight discomfort or irritation at having the scalp prepared for the electrode attachment or from the electrodes being taped to the scalp.

One hypothesis tested was that hyperexcitability of neuronal responses at some point along the auditory pathway could account for the clinical symptoms of hyperacusis and LULLs. Tests of the auditory recovery cycle revealed that auditory brainstem-evoked potentials were normal in WBS participants, ruling out auditory hyperexcitability at the level of the brainstem. However, data from an auditory recovery paradigm pointed to a possible cortical mechanism subserving the sensitivity to sounds. This is evident only over temporal cortex and occurs only with auditory input, not visual; WBS participants are indistinguishable from normal controls on a visual recovery paradigm. Taken together, these studies suggest that some of the distinctive auditory symptoms observed in WBS may be mediated by hyperexcitability, specifically within cortical regions associated with auditory processing.

Neuroimaging

Findings from functional MRI (fMRI) studies have pointed to a possible neural substrate subserving musical, timbral, and affective processing in WBS (Levitin et al. 2003). Like ERPs, fMRI is a noninvasive technique, but some participants (both normal and WBS) find the procedure stressful because it requires being confined in a small space and being subjected to the loud operating noise of the scanner. Five participants with WBS were scanned with fMRI (1.5T) and compared with chronological age–matched, typically developing controls. The participants were also matched for musical training, though none had had extensive formal training. Chronological age–matched controls were necessary, as opposed to mental age–matched controls, because the young developing brain has functional neuroanatomic differences from the adolescent or adult brain, so this served as the most rigorous comparison of neural organization. The participants in the study listened to orchestral music and environmental sounds of the type eliciting a positive response in individuals with WBS (fans, motors, running water, etc.). We compared the blood oxygenation–level dependent (BOLD) brain response in the two conditions for the two participant groups.

Our most intriguing finding was that the overall pattern of activation in the whole brain was markedly different between the two groups. An analysis of whole-brain activation patterns revealed that all five control participants showed consistent and overlapping patterns of activation bilaterally in extended areas of the superior temporal gyrus, middle temporal gyrus, and superior temporal sulcus for the processing of music compared with noise, with no other brain regions showing consistent activation among the control participants (fig. 16.1 shows the locations of these brain structures). In contrast, the WBS participants showed substantially decreased activation in these regions, accompanied by more variable patterns of activation throughout the cortex and neocortex and higher activation levels than controls in the paleocortical amygdaloid complex. The WBS group showed significantly higher activation levels in the right amygdala compared with the controls. The WBS participants—but not the controls—all showed consistent cerebellar activation as well as activation in the pons and brainstem.

Thus, we can conclude that the normally developed participants demonstrated a relatively well-defined activation pattern in the neocortex, whereas the WBS participants showed a relatively dispersed pattern of activation involving *both* neocortical and paleocortical regions.

That the amygdala was activated in the WBS group is interesting in the context of findings by Adolphs et al. (1998) that the human amygdala triggers socially and emotionally relevant information in the visual domain. In their study, patients with bilateral amygdala damage showed abnormal responses to unfamiliar faces with a threatening appearance; the patients tended to rate all faces as friendly and, in particular, showed a disproportionate impairment in judging threatening faces. Individuals with WBS also display this behavior; they are socially outgoing and tend to be utterly unable to judge whether a stranger is trustworthy or untrustworthy (see chapter 7), acting in these ways like amygdala-damaged patients. The abnormal emotional responses to sound observed phenotypically in WBS seem to correlate with abnormal amygdala activation in our earlier study (Levitin et al. 2003).

The vermal, pons, and brainstem activation may also be related to affective processing in WBS. Previous research (Griffiths et al. 1999; Levitin et al. 2003) has implicated the posterior vermis in music listening, which may be associated with the emotional component of listening to meaningful sounds (Schmahmann 1997; Blood et al. 1999). These activations are presumably mediated by major connections linking the prefrontal cortex with the basal ganglia and the cerebellar vermis and are consistent with the notion that a region in the right cerebellum may be functionally related to those in the left inferior frontal cortex for semantic processing (Roskies et al. 2001; Levitin and Menon 2003), thus serving to link the cognitive and emotional aspects of music.

Findings from structural scans of the brains of individuals with WBS have revealed additional neuroanatomic differences. Volumetric analyses revealed selective decreases in the posterior cerebrum, with relative sparing of volume in the cerebellum and temporal lobes (Reiss et al. 2000; see also chapter 14). Differences in gray and white matter density were also discovered. Cerebral white matter was disproportionately reduced, and reductions in the posterior portions of the corpus callosum were also observed. Gray matter den-

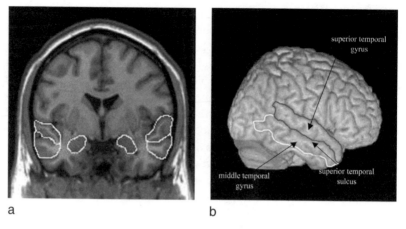

Fig. 16.1. Locations of key neural regions in the text in a typical brain. (*a*) Middle temporal gyrus, superior temporal gyrus, and the amygdala, coronal view. (*b*) Middle temporal gyrus,

sity was reduced in some regions (caudate nucleus and intraparietal sulcus) and increased in others (insular cortex, cingulate gyrus, and cerebellum).

Cytoarchitectonics

Auditory cell-packing density and neuronal size (in area 41) also showed abnormalities in cytoarchitectonic studies of WBS (Holinger et al. 2005). Autopsy specimens from individuals with WBS had an excess of midsize and large cells in layers II in both the left and right hemispheres and in layer VI in the left hemisphere. There was a hemisphere by diagnosis interaction between WBS and control brains in cell-packing density in layer IV, and a hemisphere by diagnosis interaction between WBS and control brains in neuronal size in layer III. In other words, the different participant populations showed complementary hemispheric asymmetries. Larger pyramidal neurons were found bilaterally in layer II and in left layers III and VI and were interpreted as being consistent with a hypothesis of increased connectivity in the WBS auditory cortex. This hyperconnectivity may be related to the relative sparing of language, music, and other auditory functions.

Clinical Implications

Clinicians who are aware of the various auditory phenomena in Williams-Beuren syndrome are in a better position to counsel and advise individuals with WBS and their families. First, rhythmic ability is an area of relative strength in many individuals with WBS, and music in general is something that many find to be especially engaging, comforting, and attractive. Although great individual differences do exist within the WBS phenotype,

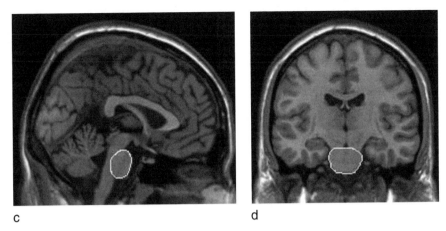

c   d

superior temporal gyrus, and superior temporal sulcus, lateral view. (*c*) Pons, sagittal view.
(*d*) Pons, coronal view. *Source:* Figures prepared by and courtesy of Dr. Vinod Menon.

many people with WBS have become quite proficient at music, and consequently musical activities—particularly those involving rhythm instruments—can be reasonably encouraged. Music can also be used as a reward
in a variety of behavioral situations, whether the reward is the opportunity
to listen to music or to perform it. Music may also be an avenue for learning
certain motor skills. Although many people with WBS have difficulty with
motor action plans and eye-hand coordination in day-to-day activities, such
as buttoning a shirt or tying shoes, these same individuals can execute ar-
guably more difficult motor action sequence plans when they are musical.
There have been anecdotal reports of limited success with teaching motor action sequences, such as tying shoes, if those sequences are set to music and
taught slowly and gradually. Knowing the great comfort to be derived from
music will encourage parents and caregivers to allow music to become a regular routine in the life of individuals with WBS who are in their care. In the
past ten years, several music camps have been developed in Massachusetts,
Michigan, Connecticut, Texas, Canada, Hungary, Spain, and Ireland.

Music may have a psychotherapeutic role for individuals with WBS. The
Berkshire Hills Music Academy (Massachusetts) is now using music to facilitate learning in other domains by building on the musical strengths of individuals with WBS and other cognitively impaired people. The range of uses
of music in a therapeutic setting can include activities as diverse as social
bonding through group singing, motivation for certain tasks, and mental dis-
cipline. Several individuals with WBS perform music in rest homes and hos-
pitals. Such activities, while mentally and logistically challenging, allow the
WBS performers to develop certain skills they might not otherwise develop,

including planning a repertoire, developing stage presence and stage skills, and increasing their consciousness of time and appointment scheduling.

Clinicians and caregivers should understand that certain sounds may cause serious distress in people with WBS and should allow appropriate measures to be taken, which will often include avoidance and coping strategies and, in some cases, simply waiting until the individual grows out of it.

The greatest promise comes from the hope that the type of research reported here will someday be integrated into a deeper understanding of the brain and the relation between brain and behavior. Although this is no doubt in the distant future, such an increased understanding could potentially allow clinicians to propose certain pharmacologic or behavioral interventions that would dramatically improve the lives of individuals with WBS and their families.

Future Directions

Neuroscientific studies in the next few years may find identifiable neural correlates for the processing of music, but we think these neural structures are unlikely to constitute a circumscribed anatomic music "center," any more than language constitutes a "center." That is, there may well be specific componential correlates for things such as musical semantics, musical expectation, tonality, and so forth, but it is unlikely that we will find a "music module." We already know that there are specific brain structures devoted to the processing of pitch, musical timbre, and tempo (Zatorre and Peretz 2001), but these structures are distributed as neural networks spanning several functional areas of the brain—they are not locally isolable blocks of neural tissue. Future work may uncover the affective link between certain sounds and the fear/aversion reaction, and this reaction may be treatable pharmaceutically, perhaps with selective neurotransmitter blocking agents or reuptake inhibitors. Finally, the intense pleasure that WBS people report in response to musical activity may have either a neurochemical or neuroanatomic basis, undoubtedly one that is linked to the microdeletion on chromosome 7. Huron (2001) has speculated that individuals with WBS have fewer inhibitions than most people, perhaps resulting from an underdeveloped "inhibition module." This could explain both the increased sociability of individuals with WBS and their increased musicality—music and sociability have been speculated to share an evolutionary basis.

One question that is often asked is whether there are musical geniuses in the WBS community. A *savant* is defined as a person with a serious mental handicap who exhibits spectacular islands of ability or brilliance that are in stark, incongruous contrast to the handicap (Down 1887; Grossman 1983; Morelock and Feldman 2000; Treffert 1989). Savantism is typically characterized by several common features, including impaired capacity for abstraction, lack of metacognition (Scheerer et al. 1945; Morelock and Feldman 2000), and extraordinary memory (Treffert 1988, 1989). As Tager-Flusberg and Sullivan (2000) note, individuals with neurodevelopmental disorders and mental retardation rarely exhibit absolutely spared cognitive function; rather, the sparing is relative.

To date, we have not been able to verify reports of any individual with WBS who is considered a world-class musician or "musical genius." But we know of dozens who are musical savants—people whose achievements are extraordinary given the deficits they hold in other domains. One individual sings hundreds of songs from memory in twenty-five languages that she doesn't even speak (Lenhoff et al. 1997). Another is a prolific composer and has written several songs for our research team on the spot, songs that conform to structural rules of harmony and form and the lyrical conventions of the popular song (Levitin and Bellugi 1998). Many dozens of Williams-Beuren musicians, as noted above, have relatively preserved musical skills that stand in stark contrast to their lack of skills in other domains, and this is, according to the formal definition, sufficient evidence of savantism.

Conclusions

Music is among a small set of cognitive domains (including language and face processing) that seem to be relatively preserved in individuals with WBS. Apart from this relatively spared ability, individuals with WBS seem to be genuinely *drawn* to music, and this may be because it offers them an opportunity to control structure, sound, and time in ways they cannot do in the rest of their lives.

Our qualitative observations of hundreds of individuals with WBS have confirmed anecdotal reports that they love music and have a more intense relationship with it than most typically developing people. Their relatively preserved rhythmic abilities challenge conventional notions about Piagetian stages and conservation of number and time, and they seem to be equivalent to the abilities of even highly trained, chronological age–matched controls.

Individuals with WBS may suffer from four different auditory abnormalities: lowered uncomfortable loudness levels, hyperacusis, auditory fascinations, and auditory aversions. We argue that the neural basis for some of these behaviors may be in hyperexcitability of cortical neurons. Functional and structural neuroimaging experiments have revealed certain irregularities in the function and structure of specific brain regions in WBS. Compared with normally developed subjects, those with WBS tend to use different regions of their brain for processing music and noise, with a particular emphasis on amygdala activation. Differences in gray and white matter density, as well as cell-packing density and neuronal size, have also been observed in WBS brains. The study of WBS, a neurodevelopmental disorder with a genetic basis, can inform important issues about the evolutionary basis of music.

ACKNOWLEDGMENTS

We are grateful to Howard Lenhoff and Paul Wang for providing valuable comments on several drafts of this manuscript, and to Albert Galaburda, Julie Korenberg, Vinod Menon, and Allan Reiss for conversations that influenced the formulation of our ideas. Some of the research reported herein was supported by grants 410-2003-1255 from the Social Sciences and Humanities Research Council, 228175-00 from the Natural Sciences and Engineering Research Council of Canada, and CFI #2719 from the Canadian Foundation for Innovation to Dr. Levitin; by a grant from the McDonnell Foundation and by a Program Project grant P01 HD33133 to Drs. Bellugi, Julie Korenberg, Debra Mills, Allan Reiss, and Albert Galaburda; and by a grant from the Packard Foundation to Dr. Reiss. We are especially grateful to the families of individuals with WBS who generously gave of their time to assist us in these studies.

REFERENCES

Adolphs, R., Tranel, D., and Damasio, A. 1998. The human amygdala in social judgement. *Nature* 393:470–474.
Bellugi, U., Bihrle, A., Neville, H., Jernigan, T. L., and Doherty, S. 1992. Language, cognition and brain organization in a neurodevelopmental disorder. In *Developmental behavioral neuroscience*, ed. M. Gunnar and C. Nelson, 201–232. Hillsdale, NJ: Erlbaum.
Bellugi, U., Wang, P. P., and Jernigan, T. L. 1994. Williams syndrome: An unusual neuropsychological profile. In *Atypical cognitive deficits in developmental disorders: Implications for brain function*, ed. S. Broman and J. Grafman, 23–56. Hillsdale, NJ: Erlbaum.
Blood, A. J., Zatorre, R. J., Bermudez, P., and Evans, A. C. 1999. Emotional responses to pleasant and unpleasant music correlated with activity in paralimbic brain regions. *Nature Neuroscience* 2:382–387.
Brochard, R., Drake, C., and Robichon, F. In press. Pitch and rhythmic abilities in adults with Williams-Beuren syndrome. *Psychological Research*.
Bruscia, K. E. 1981. Auditory short-term memory and attentional control of mentally retarded persons. *American Journal on Mental Deficiency* 85:435–437.
Dirckx, J. H., ed. 2001. *Stedman's concise medical dictionary for the health professions*. Philadelphia: Lippincott, Williams and Wilkins.
Don, A., Schellenberg, E. G., and Rourke, B. P. 1999. Music and language skills of children with Williams syndrome. *Child Neuropsychology* 5:154–170.
Down, J. L. 1887. *On some of the mental afflictions of childhood and youth*. London: Churchill.
Gordon, E. E. 1965. *Musical Aptitude Profile*. Boston: Houghton Mifflin (audio recording and book).

————. 1986. *Primary Measures of Music Audiation.* Chicago: GIA Publications (audio recording and book).

Griffiths, T. D., Johnsrude, I., Dean, J. L., and Green, G. G. R. 1999. A common neural substrate for the analysis of pitch and duration pattern in segmented sound? *NeuroReport* 10(18):1–6.

Grossman, H. 1983. *Classification in mental retardation.* Washington, DC: American Association on Mental Deficiency.

Hagerman, R. J. 1999. *Neurodevelopmental disorders: Diagnosis and treatment.* New York: Oxford University Press.

Holinger, D. P., Bellugi, U., Mills, D. L., Korenberg, J. R., Reiss, A. L., Sherman, G. F., and Galaburda, A. M. 2005. Relative sparing of primary auditory cortex in Williams syndrome. *Journal of Child Psychology and Psychiatry* 46:514–523.

Hopyan, T., Dennis, M., Weksberg, R., and Cytrynbaum, C. 2001. Music skills and the expressive interpretation of music in children with Williams-Beuren syndrome: Pitch, rhythm, melodic imagery, phrasing, and musical affect. *Child Neuropsychology* 7:42–53.

Huron, D. 2001. Is music an evolutionary adaptation? *Annals of the New York Academy of Sciences* 930:43–61.

Katznell, U., and Segal, S. 2001. Hyperacusis: Review and clinical guidelines. *Otology and Neurotology* 23:321–327.

Klein, A. J., Armstrong, B. L., Greer, M. K., and Brown, F. R. 1990. Hyperacusis and otitis media in individuals with Williams syndrome. *Journal of Speech and Hearing Disorders* 55:339–344.

Krumhansl, C. L. 2000. Rhythm and pitch in music cognition. *Psychological Bulletin* 126:159–179.

Lenhoff, H. M., Wang, P. P., Greenberg, F., and Bellugi, U. 1997. Williams syndrome and the brain. *Scientific American* 277(6): 68–73.

Levitin, D. J. 2002. Memory for musical attributes. In *Foundations of cognitive psychology: Core readings,* ed. D. J. Levitin, 295–310. Cambridge: MIT Press.

Levitin, D. J., and Bellugi, U. 1998. Musical abilities in individuals with Williams syndrome. *Music Perception* 15:357–389.

Levitin, D. J., and Menon, V. 2003. Musical structure is processed in "language" areas of the brain: A possible role for Brodmann area 47 in temporal coherence. *NeuroImage* 20:2142–2152.

Levitin, D. J., Menon, V., Schmitt, J. E., Eliez, S., White, C. D., Glover, G. H., Kadis, J., Korenberg, J. R., Bellugi, U., and Reiss, A. L. 2003. Neural correlates of auditory perception in Williams syndrome: An fMRI study. *NeuroImage* 18:74–82.

Levitin, D. J., Cole, K., Chiles, M., Lai, Z., Lincoln, A., and Bellugi, U. 2004. Characterizing the musical phenotype in individuals with Williams syndrome. *Child Neuropsychology* 10:223–247.

Levitin, D. J., Cole, K., Lincoln, A., and Bellugi, U. 2005. Aversion, awareness and attraction: Investigating claims of hyperacusis in Williams syndrome phenotype. *Journal of Child Psychology and Psychiatry* 46:514–523.

Marriage, J. 1995. Central hyperacusis in Williams syndrome. *Genetic Counseling* 6:152–153.

Miller, L. K. 1989. *Musical savants: Exceptional skill in the mentally retarded.* Hillsdale, NJ: Erlbaum.

Morelock, M. J., and Feldman, D. H. 2000. Prodigies, savants and Williams syndrome: Windows into talent and cognition. In *International handbook of giftedness and talent,* 2nd ed., ed. K. A. Heller, F. J. Mönks, R. J. Sternberg and R. F. Subotnik, 227–241. Amsterdam: Elsevier.

Neville, H. J., Mills, D. L., and Bellugi, U. 1994. Effects of altered auditory sensitivity and age of language acquisition on the development of language-relevant neural systems: Preliminary studies of Williams syndrome. In *Atypical cognitive deficits in developmental disorders: Implications for brain function*, ed. S. H. Broman and J. Grafman, 67–83. Hillsdale, NJ: Erlbaum.

Phillips, D. P., and Carr, M. M. 1998. Disturbances of loudness perception. *Journal of the American Academy of Audiology* 9:371–379.

Reiss, A. L., Eliez, S., Schmitt, J. E., Straus, E., Lai, Z., Jones, W., and Bellugi, U. 2000. Neuroanatomy of Williams syndrome: A high-resolution MRI study. *Journal of Cognitive Neuroscience* 12 (suppl. 1): 65–73.

Roskies, A. L., Fiez, J. A., Balota, D. A., Raichle, M. E., and Petersen, S. E. 2001. Task-dependent modulation of regions in the left inferior frontal cortex during semantic processing. *Journal of Cognitive Neuroscience* 13:829–843.

Scheerer, M., Rothmann, E., and Goldstein, K. 1945. A case of "idiot savant": An experimental study of personality organization. *Psychology Monographs* 58:1–62.

Schmahmann, J. D., ed. 1997. *The cerebellum and cognition.* San Diego: Academic Press.

Serafine, M. L. 1979. A measure of meter conservation in music, based on Piaget's theory. *Genetic Psychology Monographs* 99:185–229.

Tager-Flusberg, H., and Sullivan, K. 2000. A componential view of theory of mind: Evidence from Williams syndrome. *Cognition* 76:59–89.

Treffert, D. A. 1988. The idiot savant: A review of the syndrome. *American Journal of Psychiatry* 145:563–572.

———. 1989. *Extraordinary people: Understanding "idiot savants."* New York: Harper and Row.

Udwin, O. 1990. A survey of adults with Williams syndrome and idiopathic infantile hypercalcaemia. *Developmental Medicine and Child Neurology* 32:129–141.

Venes, D., Thomas, C. L., and Taber, C. W., eds. 2001. *Taber's cyclopedic medical dictionary,* 19th ed. Philadelphia: F. A. Davis.

Wilmowski, W. 1995. *Williams syndrome: A highly musical species.* Germantown, MD: Wayfarer Entertainment (video).

Zatorre, R. J., and Peretz, I., eds. 2001. *The biological foundations of music: Proceedings of the May 20–22, 2000, New York Academy of Sciences Conference.* New York: New York Academy of Sciences.

Index

abdominal aortic obstruction, 116
abdominal pain, 129, 130
Aberrant Behavior Checklist, 274
absolute pitch (AP): critical period for acquiring, 331–332; evolutionary role of, 332–333; explanation of, 325; genes and, 333; level and incidence of, 330–331; Williams-Beuren syndrome and, 327–328
adjectives, comparative, 183–184
adolescents with Williams-Beuren syndrome: academic or vocational training for, 88–89; contractures in, 87; face and visuospatial processing in, 258–259; hypercalcemia in, 130; hypertension in, 92, 118; language ability in, 256–258; number processing in, 259–260; profile of, 255–256; puberty and, 95–97; semantic organization of, 178; social cognition in, 258; theory of mind abilities in, 239, 245–249. See also Williams-Beuren syndrome (WBS)
aging, premature, 136
Alzheimer's disease, 276
amblyopia, 91
American Academy of Pediatrics: sleep apnea recommendations, 294; Williams-Beuren syndrome recommendations, 83
anesthesia, 98–99
Angelman syndrome, 25
anxiety disorders, 284–286
aorta, coarctation of, 115–116
apes, 24
arterial narrowing, 91–92

attention deficit hyperactivity disorder (ADHD): diagnosis of, 282; management of, 89, 154, 286; sleep and, 302–303; treatment options for, 303, 304
auditory allodynia, 348
auditory fascinations, 348–349
autism: explanation of, 283–284; musical ability and, 334, 335

babbling, canonical, 170–171
basic-level categories, 173–174
BAZ1B gene, 36–38, 76
BCL7B gene, 28
behavior: in adults, 136–137; in children, 89, 136; studies of social, 152–153; types of issues related to, 7, 13–14
behavioral neuroscience of Williams-Beuren syndrome: clinical psychology and behavioral medicine and, 154; early observations and, 148; future directions for, 155–156; general cognitive abilities and, 148–149; genetics and, 155; language ability and, 149–151; memory and music and, 153–154; overview of, 147; social cognition and social behavior and, 152–153; visuospatial cognition and, 151–152, 258–259
Berkshire Hills Music Academy, 353
biological motion perception, 215–218
block construction tasks: experimental findings on, 227–231; model for thinking about, 225–227; performance in, 224–225; spatial cognition and, 208–210
bone density studies, 130–131